VOLUME **3**

Diagnosis, Management, and Treatment of Discogenic Pain

VOLUME

3 Diagnosis, Management, and Treatment of Discogenic Pain

Volume Editors

Leonardo Kapural, MD, PhD

Professor of Anesthesiology
Wake Forest University, School of Medicine
Director, Pain Medicine Center
Wake Forest Baptist Health
Winston-Salem, North Carolina

Philip Kim, MD

Medical Director
Center for Interventional Pain & Spine, LLC
Bryn Mawr, Pennsylvania
Newark, Delaware

Series Editor

Timothy R. Deer, MD, DABPM, FIPP

President and CEO
The Center for Pain Relief
Clinical Professor of Anesthesiology
West Virginia University School of Medicine
Charleston, West Virginia

ELSEVIER
SAUNDERS

ELSEVIER
SAUNDERS

1600 John F. Kennedy Blvd.
Ste 1800
Philadelphia, PA 19103-2899

Notices

Knowledge and best practice in this field are constantly changing. As new research and experience broaden our understanding, changes in research methods, professional practices, or medical treatment may become necessary.

Practitioners and researchers must always rely on their own experience and knowledge in evaluating and using any information, methods, compounds, or experiments described herein. In using such information or methods they should be mindful of their own safety and the safety of others, including parties for whom they have a professional responsibility.

With respect to any drug or pharmaceutical products identified, readers are advised to check the most current information provided (i) on procedures featured or (ii) by the manufacturer of each product to be administered, to verify the recommended dose or formula, the method and duration of administration, and contraindications. It is the responsibility of practitioners, relying on their own experience and knowledge of their patients, to make diagnoses, to determine dosages and the best treatment for each individual patient, and to take all appropriate safety precautions.

To the fullest extent of the law, neither the Publisher nor the authors, contributors, or editors, assume any liability for any injury and/or damage to persons or property as a matter of products liability, negligence or otherwise, or from any use or operation of any methods, products, instructions, or ideas contained in the material herein.

Library of Congress Cataloging-in-Publication Data
Interventional and neuromodulatory techniques for pain management.
    p. ; cm.
    Includes bibliographical references and indexes.
    ISBN 978-1-4377-3791-2 (series package : alk. paper)—ISBN 978-1-4377-2216-1 (hardcover, v. 1 : alk. paper)—ISBN 978-1-4377-2217-8 (hardcover, v. 2 : alk. paper)—ISBN 978-1-4377-2218-5 (hardcover, v. 3 : alk. paper)—ISBN 978-1-4377-2219-2 (hardcover, v. 4 : alk. paper)—ISBN 978-1-4377-2220-8 (hardcover, v. 5 : alk. paper)
    1. Pain–Treatment.   2. Nerve block.   3. Spinal anesthesia.   4. Neural stimulation.   5. Analgesia.
I. Deer, Timothy R.
    [DNLM: 1. Pain—drug therapy.   2. Pain—surgery.   WL 704]
    RB127.I587 2012
    616′.0472—dc23
                                                                    2011018904

Acquisitions Editor: Pamela Hetherington
Developmental Editor: Lora Sickora
Publishing Services Manager: Jeff Patterson
Project Manager: Megan Isenberg
Design Direction: Lou Forgione

Printed in China

Last digit is the print number: 9 8 7 6 5 4 3 2 1

For Missy for all your love and support.

For Morgan, Taylor, Reed, and Bailie for your inspiration.

To those who have taught me a great deal:
John Rowlingson, Richard North, Giancarlo Barolat, Sam Hassenbusch,
Elliot Krames, K. Dean Willis, Peter Staats, Nagy Mekhail, Robert Levy, David Caraway,
Kris Kumar, Joshua Prager, and Jim Rathmell.

To my team:
Christopher Kim, Richard Bowman, Matthew Ranson, Doug Stewart,
Wilfredo Tolentino, Jeff Peterson, and Michelle Miller.

Timothy R. Deer

I am eternally grateful to my wife Miranda and to my children Daniella and Luka for their
patience, support, encouragement, and inspiration.

Leo Kapural

To my loving wife, Claire, and my kids who supported me with patience and understanding.

Philip Kim

Contributors

Farshad M. Ahadian, MD
Clinical Professor of Anesthesiology; Medical Director, Center for Pain Medicine, Division of Pain Medicine, Department of Anesthesiology, University of California, San Diego, San Diego, California
Chapter 2, Establishing the Diagnosis of Discogenic Back Pain: An Evidence-Based Algorithmic Approach

Ray M. Baker, MD
Washington Interventional Spine Associates, Bellevue, Washington
Chapter 5, Analgesic Discography

Jeff Buchalter, MD, DABAPM
Chairman, Gulf Coast Pain Specialists; Associate Clinical Professor, Florida State University College of Medicine, Department of Surgery, Pensacola, Florida
Chapter 1, Epidemiology and Etiology of Discogenic Pain: How Big Is the Problem?

Kevin D. Cairns, MD
Attending Physician, Florida Spine Specialists; Medical Director, Pain Medicine, Broward General Medical Center, Fort Lauderdale, Florida
Chapter 12, Current Surgical Options for Intervertebral Disc Herniation in the Cervical and Lumbar Spine

Aaron Calodney, MD, FIPP, ABIPP
Texas Spine and Joint Hospital, Tyler, Texas
Chapter 1, Epidemiology and Etiology of Discogenic Pain: How Big Is the Problem?

Steven P. Cohen, MD
Associate Professor, Department of Anesthesiology, Johns Hopkins School of Medicine, Baltimore, Maryland; Professor, Walter Reed National Military Medical Center, Bethesda, Maryland
Chapter 11, Disc Herniations: Injections and Minimally Invasive Techniques

José De Andrés, MD, PhD, FIPP, EDRA
Anesthesiologist and Chairman of the Anesthesia Critical Care and Multidisciplinary Pain Management Department, General University Hospital; Associate Professor of Anesthesia, Valencia Faculty of Medicine, Valencia, Spain
Chapter 13, Neuromodulation and Intrathecal Therapies for the Treatment of Chronic Radiculopathy Related to Intractable Discogenic Pain

Timothy R. Deer, MD, DABPM, FIPP
President and CEO, The Center for Pain Relief; Clinical Professor of Anesthesiology, West Virginia University School of Medicine, Charleston, West Virginia
Chapter 7, Radiofrequency and Other Heat Applications for the Treatment of Discogenic Pain

Michael DeMarco, DO
Parkway Neuroscience and Spine Center, Hagerstown, Maryland
Chapter 11, Disc Herniations: Injections and Minimally Invasive Techniques

Vincenzo Denaro, MD
Full Professor and Chair, Department of Orthopaedics and Trauma Surgery; Dean of the Faculty of Medicine, University Campus Bio-Medico of Rome, Rome, Italy
Chapter 9, Nucleus Pulposus Replacement and Motion Sparing Technologies

Richard Derby, MD
Medical Director, Spinal Diagnostics and Treatment Center, Daly City, California
Chapter 4, Provocation Discography;
Chapter 5, Analgesic Discography

Alberto Di Martino, MD, PhD
Orthopaedic Surgeon, Department of Orthopaedics and Trauma Surgery, University Campus Bio-Medico of Rome, Rome, Italy
Chapter 9, Nucleus Pulposus Replacement and Motion-Sparing Technologies

Daniel J. Hoh, MD
Department of Neurosurgery, Center for Spine Health, Cleveland Clinic, Cleveland, Ohio
Chapter 8, Arthrodesis and Fusion for the Treatment of Discogenic Neck and Back Pain: Evidence-Based Effectiveness and Controversies

Leonardo Kapural, MD, PhD
Professor of Anesthesiology, Wake Forest University, School of Medicine; Director, Pain Medicine Center, Wake Forest Baptist Health, Winston-Salem, North Carolina
Chapter 7, Radiofrequency and Other Heat Applications for the Treatment of Discogenic Pain

Philip Kim, MD
Medical Director, Center for Interventional Pain & Spine, LLC, Bryn Mawr, Pennsylvania; Newark, Delaware
Chapter 4, Provocation Discography

Milton H. Landers, DO, PhD
Clinical Assistant Professor, Department of Anesthesiology, University of Kansas School of Medicine, Wichita, Kansas
Chapter 4, Provocation Discography

Angela Lanotte, MD
Resident in Orthopaedics and Trauma Surgery, Department of Orthopaedics and Trauma Surgery, University Campus Bio-Medico of Rome, Rome, Italy
Chapter 9, Nucleus Pulposus Replacement and Motion-Sparing Technologies

Thomas M. Larkin, MD
Assistant Professor of Anesthesiology, Walter Reed National Military Medical Center, Bethesda, Maryland; Chief, Pain Service, Parkway Neuroscience and Spine Institute, Hagerstown, Maryland
Chapter 11, Disc Herniations: Injections and Minimally Invasive Techniques

Andrea Luca, MD
Orthopaedic Surgeon, Spine Unit, Schulthess Klinik, Lengghalde, Zurich, Switzerland
Chapter 9, Nucleus Pulposus Replacement and Motion-Sparing Technologies

David P. Martin, MD, PhD
Associate Professor of Anesthesiology, Mayo Clinic College of Medicine, Rochester, Minnesota
Chapter 3, Imaging for Discogenic Pain

Timothy P. Maus, MD
Assistant Professor of Radiology, Mayo Clinic College of Medicine, Rochester, Minnesota
Chapter 3, Imaging for Discogenic Pain

W. Porter McRoberts, MD
Director of Interventional Spine and Pain Medicine, Holy Cross Hospital, Fort Lauderdale, Florida
Chapter 12, Current Surgical Options for Intervertebral Disc Herniation in the Cervical and Lumbar Spine

James L. North, MD
Clinical Assistant Professor, Department of Anesthesiology and Pain Medicine, Wake Forest University Health Sciences; Chief of Pain Medicine, Department of Pain Medicine, Forsyth Medical Center; Attending Physician, Carolinas Pain Institute, Winston-Salem, North Carolina
Chapter 10, Cervical and Thoracic Discogenic Pain: Therapeutic Nonsurgical Options

Stefano Palmisani, MD
Fellow in Pain Medicine, Anesthesia, Critical Care and Multidisciplinary Pain Management Department, General University Hospital, Valencia, Spain; Clinical Research Fellow in Pain Medicine, Pain Management & Neuromodulation Centre, Guy's & St Thomas' Hospital, NHS Foundation Trust, London, United Kingdom
Chapter 13, Neuromodulation and Intrathecal Therapies for the Treatment of Chronic Radiculopathy Related to Intractable Discogenic Pain

Jeffrey D. Petersohn, MD
President and Founder, Pain Care, PC, Linwood, New Jersey; Adjunct Associate Professor, Department of Anesthesiology, Drexel University School of Medicine, Philadelphia, Pennsylvania
Chapter 6, Discogenic Pain: Intradiscal Therapeutic Injections and Use of Intradiscal Biologic Agents

John H. Shin, MD
Department of Neurosurgery, Center for Spine Health, Cleveland Clinic, Cleveland, Ohio
Chapter 8, Arthrodesis and Fusion for the Treatment of Discogenic Neck and Back Pain: Evidence-Based Effectiveness and Controversies

Michael P. Steinmetz, MD
Associate Professor of Surgery, Center for Spine Health, Department of Neurosurgery, Lerner College of Medicine, Cleveland Clinic, Cleveland, Ohio
Chapter 8, Arthrodesis and Fusion for the Treatment of Discogenic Neck and Back Pain: Evidence-Based Effectiveness and Controversies

José Suros, MD
Pain Management Institute, Bethesda, Maryland
Chapter 11, Disc Herniations: Injections and Minimally Invasive Techniques

Mark S. Wallace, MD
Professor of Clinical Anesthesiology; Chair, Division of Pain Medicine, Department of Anesthesiology, University of California, San Diego, San Diego, California
Chapter 2, Establishing the Diagnosis of Discogenic Back Pain: An Evidence-Based Algorithmic Approach

Lee R. Wolfer, MD, MS
Spinal Diagnostics and Treatment Center, Daly City, California
Chapter 4, Provocation Discography;
Chapter 5, Analgesic Discography

Preface

Degeneration of the intervertebral disc, the flexible fibrocartilaginous connection between adjacent vertebrae at the heart of the vertebral motion segment, is universal and occurs in all primates as an inevitable part of the aging process. This degeneration starts with loss of hydration of the central nucleus pulposus in the first few decades of life and progresses through cracking and tearing of the outer annulus fibrosus, ending with complete loss of disc hydration, height, and flexibility in many elderly individuals. The anatomic changes that occur during this degenerative process and the correlates that can be seen on modern imaging studies have been clearly elucidated and are now a part of all spine practitioners' everyday working knowledge. However, correlation between anatomic changes and the occurrence of pain is less than clear. Despite the rapid advances in diagnostic imaging, it is still impossible to determine with certainty that the intervertebral disc itself is the cause for back pain in any given individual. Degenerative anatomic abnormalities are common even in those who are asymptomatic. To compound the problem, treatment for "discogenic pain" is in its infancy. The mainstay of treatment has been surgical vertebral interbody fusion, the theory being that arresting motion in a painful functional spinal unit should eliminate pain arising from anatomic derangement in the disc. However, selecting appropriate patients for fusion and predicting their outcomes has been problematic, and overuse of this aggressive and invasive form of surgical treatment has come under great scrutiny in recent years. Diagnostic provocative discography has been developed as a means to more precisely identify individuals with pain arising from their intervertebral discs, but without a gold standard the validity of this subjective test has been questioned by many experts. New evidence that discography may accelerate disc degeneration has emerged, adding fuel to the raging debate about the safety and usefulness of this test. Despite all of the controversy and remaining questions, there is wide agreement among experts that degenerative disc disease can be the primary source of pain in some individuals and the search for an effective, minimally invasive means to treat discogenic pain goes on.

In this volume, some of the pioneers who have established the scientific basis for diagnosis of discogenic pain and investigated the effectiveness of new treatments for this disorder have written authoritative chapters detailing the evolution of our understanding in this controversial area. Analyses in this text range from the anatomic basis of degenerative disc disease and the epidemiology of low back pain through diagnostic evaluation and treatment. It is clear that the intervertebral disc can be safely accessed percutaneously and we are very likely to find an effective, minimally invasive means to treat discogenic pain that will all but do away with the need for open surgical fusion. Newer techniques, including variants of radiofrequency technology and use of injected biologics, are now in early stages of clinical development; the scientific basis and clinical use of these emerging techniques are described with detail and clarity herein. This volume also includes procedural videos, which can be viewed on the companion website at www. expertconsult.com. This text will serve as a snapshot in time during the early development of treatment for discogenic pain. We will look back on the descriptions found here and understand how these treatments evolved. Some will be found ineffective and disappear, while others will emerge and be refined and adopted as standard care for those suffering with discogenic pain. I commend Dr. Deer and his colleagues for preparing a detailed and authoritative view of this young field and recommend the text to students, practitioners, scientists, and entrepreneurs alike.

James P. Rathmell, MD
Chief, Division of Pain Medicine, Massachusetts General Hospital
Professor of Anaesthesia, Harvard Medical School
Boston, Massachusetts, USA
July 2011

Acknowledgments

I would like to acknowledge Jeff Peterson for his hard work on making this project a reality, and Michelle Miller for her diligence to detail on this and all projects that cross her desk.

I would like to acknowledge Lora Sickora, Pamela Hetherington, and Megan Isenberg for determination, attention to detail, and desire for excellence in bringing this project to fruition.

Finally, I would like to acknowledge Samer Narouze for his diligent work filming and reviewing the procedural videos associated with all of the volumes in the series.

Timothy R. Deer

Contents

1 Epidemiology and Etiology of Discogenic Pain: How Big Is the Problem?

Aaron Calodney and Jeff Buchalter

CHAPTER OVERVIEW

Chapter Synopsis: Although once considered controversial, evidence now clearly shows that intervertebral discs contain their own nerve supply and can be pain generators in their own right. This chapter surveys our current understanding of the epidemiology and etiology of discogenic pain. Back pain in general affects an overwhelming majority of us at some time in our lives—over three quarters of the population. Roughly a quarter of these cases are attributed to discogenic pain. The etiology of discogenic pain contains many elements of chronic pain originating from other areas, including somatosensory and autonomic innervation, sensitization of these fibers through release of inflammatory mediators like substance P, and central sensitization. The discs are comprised of a mix of cell types and connective tissues that provide support and cushioning between the vertebral bodies. With age, discs normally degenerate to some degree, becoming dehydrated and less supple with loss of the supportive proteoglycan molecule. Pathological degeneration can be described in three stages, and can be initiated by multiple microtraumas or by loss of the already limited vascularity. Several risk factors have been proposed for degeneration, ranging from genetics to smoking, obesity, and occupation. Finally, metabolic biomarkers for discogenic pain have been recently identified, which may allow for less invasive diagnostic methods. Discogenic pain is a complex and still incompletely understood condition with contributions from genetic, environmental, and lifestyle factors.

Important Points:
- The intervertebral disc is an independent pain generator of the spine.
- Discogenic pain is the most common cause of recurrent back pain.
- Provocative discography performed with controlled pressure manometry is currently the only definitive diagnostic test available.
- Due to the complex nature of this disease process, no current treatment has been highly successful.
- Genetics is the single most important etiologic factor in determining future risk of developing discogenic pain.

Introduction

Discogenic pain is defined as pain originating from the intervertebral disc itself.[1] It is nonradicular and may occur in the absence of spinal deformity, instability, and signs of neural tension.[2] Although the external outline of the disc may remain intact, multiple processes (e.g., annular tears, degeneration, endplate injury, inflammation) can stimulate multiplication and possibly sensitization of pain nociceptors within the disc independent of nerve root symptoms. The concept of discogenic pain was introduced by Inman and Saunders in 1947,[3] and the term was first used by Fernstrom in 1969 to establish the association between annulus stimulation and back pain perception identified during in vivo studies.[4] Internal disc disorders were originally documented by Crock,[5] who in 1970 was the first to study the mechanism of discogenic pain. He subsequently defined the term *internal disc disruption (IDD)* to describe unremitting lumbar spinal pain that lasted longer than 4 months, was unresponsive to conservative care, and could be reproduced with discography.[6] Epidemiological studies suggest that cervical and lumbar discogenic pain reflect complex diseases (with "disease" defined as any impairment of normal physiological function of an organ or body part)[7] that are accompanied by pathophysiological, biomechanical, psychological, and social implications. Such research offers insight regarding the magnitude of these diseases, their natural history, and the individual and external risk factors associated with each disease process. Even though 15% of the general population is reported to experience thoracic pain, the role of the thoracic disc as a source of chronic pain has not been well researched.[8]

The existence of a nerve supply to the disc and the concept of the intervertebral disc as an independent cause of spinal pain were controversial initially. Both are now well documented in the scientific literature and form the basis of current practice.[9-24] Research by Nachemson, Bogduk, Aprill, Derby, and others has helped define the importance of this complex pain generator over four decades, as illustrated by the following quotes from their respective publications:

"Although practically all anatomic structures in the region of the motion segment have their proponents in the etiology of back pain, the lower intervertebral disc most likely causes the pain."[25] (Nachemson, 1976)

"These anatomical findings (i.e., cervical sinuvertebral nerves that supply the disc) provide the hitherto missing substrate for primary disc pain and the pain of provocation discography."[26] (Bogduk, Windsor, and Inglis, 1988)

"The outer third of the annulus fibrosis is richly innervated, and nerves may extend as deeply as the middle third of the

annulus. This innervation constitutes the anatomic substrate for discogenic pain."[27] *(Schwarzer and associates, 1995)*

"*Different, and independent, techniques point to the same conclusion. IDD has a distinctive morphology that correlates strongly with pain, and IDD has biophysical properties that correlate strongly with pain. For no other cause of low back pain have such multiple and strong correlations been demonstrated.*"[28] *(Bogduk, 2005)*

This chapter provides an overview of the epidemiology and etiology of discogenic pain.

Epidemiology

Epidemiology, as it applies to discogenic pain, studies the distribution of disease in a population. Because very little has been published about the specific epidemiology of discogenic pain, this section first considers the broader epidemiology of chronic back pain, with a focus on the cervical and lumbar spine. It also includes available published epidemiological data specific to discogenic pain.

The epidemiology of cervical and lumbar spinal pain is quite impressive.[29] At some time in their lives, an estimated 60% to 70% of the population will suffer from neck pain, and 65% to 80% of the population will suffer from low back pain.[29-31] The annual prevalence of frequent or persistent neck and low back pain is 2% to 11% and 5% to 20%, respectively.[32,33] In a 2008 survey of U.S. adults, 14% reported neck pain, and 26% reported low back pain within the previous 3 months.[34] Cervical discogenic pain is estimated to be the cause of persistent neck pain in 16% to 41% of patients.[35,36] Discogenic low back pain is cited as the most common cause of chronic low back pain, accounting for approximately 26% to 39% of its incidence.[37,38]

Low back pain is one of the most common health problems in the industrialized world.[39,40] It is estimated that 28% of U.S. industrial workers will experience disabling low back pain at some time in their career and 8% of the entire working population will be disabled by low back pain in any given year, contributing to 40% of all lost work days. After adjustment for inflation, the total estimated medical costs associated with the treatment of neck and back pain is about $86 billion per year.[41]

Etiology

Introduction

Discogenic pain is a complex disease of the spine with profound health care implications. This section (1) reviews normal disc physiology, (2) provides some background information about normal disc aging and degeneration, and (3) discusses each of the potential risk factors for discogenic pain.

The etiology of discogenic pain is as complex as the network of nerves surrounding it. When observing an anatomical dissection of the intervertebral disc, it is clear that its sensory innervation involves branches from the sinuvertebral nerve, anterior primary ramus, gray ramus, and sympathetic chain (**Fig. 1-1**). In addition, the work of Takahashi, Aoki, and Ohtori[42] and Nakamura and associates[43] has demonstrated that there may also be ascending pathways within the sympathetic chain to upper lumbar dorsal root ganglion neurons.

In a diseased disc, pain may be generated from deep within its own tissue. For years it was assumed that the nucleus, inner annulus, and mid annulus were completely avascular and aneural and that only the very outer layers of the posterior and anterolateral

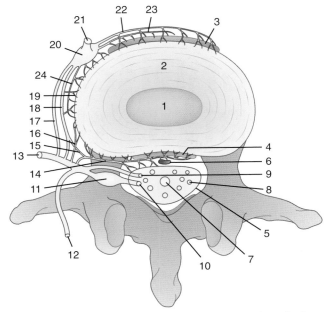

Fig. 1-1 Schematic diagram of innervation of anterior spinal canal and structures of anterior aspect of spinal column. *1*, Nucleus pulposus; *2*, annulus fibrosus; *3*, anterior longitudinal ligament/periosteum; *4*, posterior longitudinal ligament/periosteum; *5*, leptomeninges; *6*, epidural vasculature; *7*, filum terminale; *8*, intrathecal lumbosacral nerve root; *9*, ventral root; *10*, dorsal root; *11*, dorsal root ganglion; *12*, dorsal ramus of spinal nerve; *13*, ventral ramus of spinal nerve; *14*, recurrent meningeal nerve (sinuvertebral nerve of Luschka); *15*, autonomic (sympathetic) branch to recurrent meningeal nerve; *16*, direct somatic branch from ventral ramus of spinal nerve to lateral disc; *17*, white ramus communicans; *18*, gray ramus communicans (multilevel irregular lumbosacral distribution); *19*, lateral sympathetic efferent branches projecting from gray ramus communicans; *20*, paraspinal sympathetic ganglion (PSG); *21*, paraspinal sympathetic chain; *22*, anterior paraspinal afferent sympathetic ramus projecting to PSG; *23*, anterior sympathetic efferent branches projecting from PSG *24*, lateral paraspinal afferent sympathetic ramus projecting to PSG. From Jackson JC 2nd, Winkelman RK, Bickel WH: Nerve endings in the human lumbar spinal column and related structures. *J Bone Joint Surg Am* 48(7):1272-1281, 1966.

annulus contained nerve fibers. It is now clear that these pain-carrying nerve fibers can extend inward, deep into the middle annulus, and even into the nucleus in some cases. Not only has this been observed in degenerative discs, but it has also been linked to discogenic back pain (**Figs. 1-2 and 1-3**).[44]

As early as 1997 Freemont and colleagues[45] observed that 77% of discs that were surgically removed from patients with discography-positive discogenic pain had nerve fiber ingrowth into the middle one third of the annulus. Among the normal control discs, only 6% exhibited this pattern of ingrowth. These pain fibers were also associated with substance P, an active neural transmitter in pain transmission. Brisby[46] identified peripheral sensitization, and thus amplification of the pain response in the sensitized disc, through the secretion of proinflammatory mediators. Increased numbers of mechanoreceptors and pain-producing neurons have also been confirmed both clinically and experimentally in the discs of patients with chronic discogenic pain.[47-49] Given the somatosensory and autonomic neural innervation and the peripheral sensitization and amplification mechanisms impacting the pain response, it is understandable why the etiology and ultimate

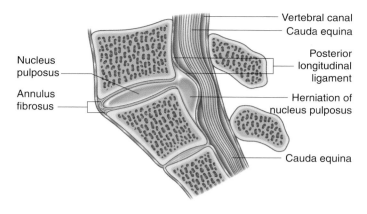

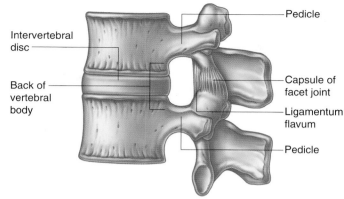

Fig. 1-4   Boundaries of an intervertebral foramen. From Standring et al, editors: *Gray's anatomy: the anatomical basis of clinical practice*, ed 39, 2005, Elsevier Churchill Livingstone, p 742.

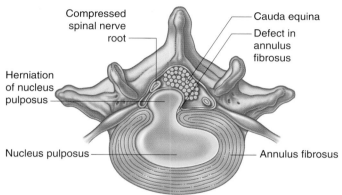

Fig. 1-2   Posterolateral disc prolapsed. From Moore K, Agur AMR: *Essential clinical anatomy*, ed 2, Philadelphia, 2002, Lippincott Williams & Wilkins.

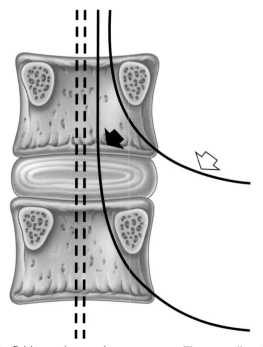

Fig. 1-3   Exiting and traversing nerve roots. The upper line *(open arrow)* is the exiting root at this level: the lower *(arrow)* is the traversing root here, which becomes the exiting root at the level below. The dotted lines are traversing roots of the lower segment. From Standring et al, editors: *Gray's anatomy: the anatomical basis of clinical practice*, ed 39, 2005, Elsevier Churchill Livingstone, p 758.

presentation of discogenic pain is so complex. In fact, as Mooney hypothesized in 1987,[50] "there is something unique about the nerves related to the spine and the spinal canal, which makes the source of pain different from the rest of the musculoskeletal parts of the body." He suggested that the disc is uniquely innervated with a predominantly visceral-type nerve supply.

Normal Disc Physiology

To understand the etiology of discogenic pain, it is helpful to first understand the basic physiology of the normal intervertebral disc. Discs lie between each of the vertebral bodies and link them together (**Fig. 1-4**). In total the discs comprise 25% of the height of the spinal column.[51] In the lumbar region discs are approximately 7 to 10 mm thick and 4 cm in diameter.[52,53] The discs function to resist spinal compression and evenly spread the load on the vertebral bodies while allowing limited movements. The intervertebral disc is comprised of three distinct regions: the nucleus pulposus, the annulus fibrosus, and the endplate (**Figs. 1-5 and 1-6**).[54] The vertebral endplate is considered a component of the intervertebral disc rather than a part of the vertebral body. The endplates are not attached to the subchondral bone of the vertebrae; they are instead strongly interwoven into the annulus of the disc and are therefore considered part of this anatomic structure.[55] The attachment of endplate to vertebral body is less robust and is susceptible to injury.[56] The nucleus pulposus is the gelatinous core of the disc and is normally aneural and avascular.[57] Its matrix is maintained by chondrocyte-like cells, which are stimulated by growth factors to produce constituents, including elastin, type 2 collagen, and proteoglycans.[58] Proteoglycans consist of a core central protein from which chains of glycosaminoglycans (GAGs) project. Multiple proteoglycans are joined by a hyaluronic acid chain to form aggrecan, which is highly hydrophilic. The resulting hydroscopic and hydrostatic properties of the nucleus pulposus are the factors that allow it to accommodate compression.[59,60] Nucleus pulposus cells also inhibit the enzymes responsible for matrix breakdown (e.g., matrix metalloproteinases).[61] Matrix constituents are not static; they continually degrade the matrix and provide it with newly synthesized components.

The nucleus pulposus is encircled by the annulus fibrosus, which is composed of a series of 15 to 25 concentric rings of type 1 collagen that resist pressure from the gelatinous core of the disc.[62] The cells in the outer annulus fibrosus are fibroblast-like, elongated, and thin; and they lie parallel to the collagen fibers. The cells

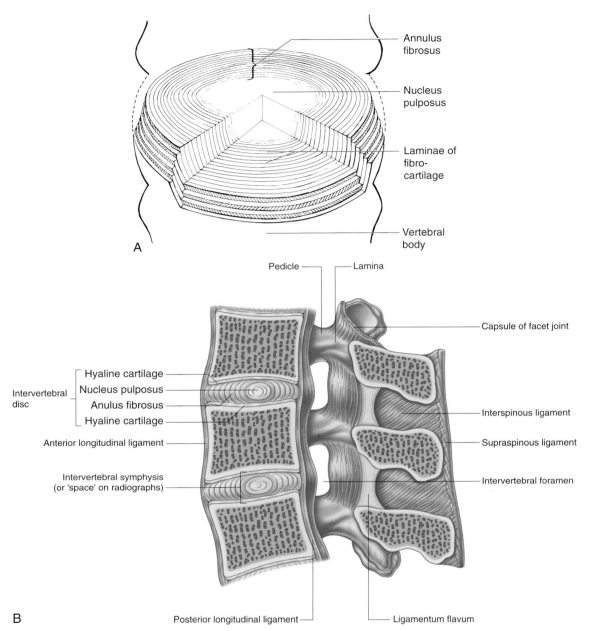

Fig. 1-5 A, Schematic representation of the main structural features of an intervertebral disc. For clarity the number of fibrocartilaginous laminae has been greatly reduced. Note alternating obliquity of collagen fascicles in adjacent laminae (after Inoue). **B,** Median sagittal section through upper lumbar vertebral column showing discs and ligaments. **A** from Inoue H: Three-dimensional observation of collagen framework of the intervertebral discs in rats, dogs and humans, *Arch Histol Jpn* 36:39-56, 1973. **B** from Standring et al, editors: *Gray's anatomy: the anatomical basis of clinical practice*, ed 39, 2005, Elsevier Churchill Livingstone, p 756.

in the inner annulus tend to be more ovular.[63] Innervation of the healthy annulus fibrosus is primarily restricted to the outer lamellae.[64] The posterior annulus and the adhering longitudinal ligament are supplied by the sinuvertebral nerve, which is a mixed autonomic and somatic nerve. The anterior and lateral annuli are supplied by autonomic nerves.[65]

The nucleus pulposus and annulus fibrosus are confined from above and below by the endplates, which lie on the superior and inferior aspect of the discs, adjacent to the vertebral bodies. The endplates are thin, horizontal layers of cartilage that are usually less than 1 mm thick. They are composed of type 2 collagen, proteoglycans, and noncollagenous proteins synthesized by chondrocyte-like cells. The endplates aid in the diffusion of nutrients into the disc and are normally avascular and aneural.

Normal Disc Aging and Degeneration

The most common and striking feature of disc aging and degeneration is the loss of the proteoglycan molecule from the nucleus of the disc. Other signs of aging include progressive dehydration, progressive collagen thickening caused by cross linking and glycation, formation of brown pigmentation, and increased "brittleness" of the disc tissue.[66] These changes are all amplified by the naturally poor vascular supply of the disc via the capillary beds just above the vertebral endplates (**Fig. 1-7**).[67]

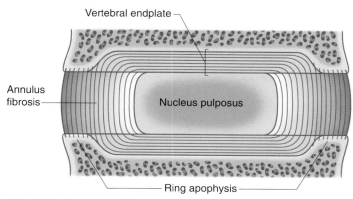

Fig. 1-6 Structure of the vertebral endplate: the collagen fibers of the inner two-thirds of the annulus fibrosus sweep around into the vertebral endplate and form its fibrocartilaginous component. The peripheral fibers of the annulus are anchored into the bone of the ring apophysis. From Bogduk N: *Clinical anatomy of the lumbar spine and sacrum*, ed 3, Edinburgh, 1997, Churchill Livingstone.

The degenerative cascade, described by Kirkaldy-Willis and associates,[68] is a widely accepted pathophysiological model for describing the degenerative process as it affects the lumbar spine and individual motion segments. The process occurs in three phases that comprise a continuum with gradual transition rather than three clearly defined stages. Phase 1 (dysfunctional) is characterized histologically by circumferential tears or fissures in the outer annulus. Tears can be accompanied by endplate separation or failure, blood supply interruption to the disc, and impaired nutritional supply and waste removal. Such changes may be the result of repetitive microtrauma. Since the outer one third of the annular wall is innervated, tears or fissures in the area may lead to discogenic pain. As the disc progresses through phase 2 (unstable) and phase 3 (stabilization), biochemical changes occur that can lead to chronic IDD and disc herniations.

In 2002 Boos and colleagues[69] won the Volvo Award in Basic Science for their observations regarding an idiopathic "obliteration" of parts of the nutrient-providing capillary beds lying just above the vertebral endplates. This auto-destruction begins within the first 2 years of life and increases over the next 8 years. These findings suggest that the initial cause of disc aging and degeneration is "nutritional compromise," which is secondary to the loss of the discal blood supply above the vertebral endplates.

It is not clear why the nucleus of the disc loses much of its vital blood supply during the first decade of life.[70] Without sufficient nutrients (which are transported in the blood) the cells of the disc begin to die, and the disc becomes depleted of water.[71] This correlates with the initial appearance of radial tears seen during the second decade of life, which is also the age when the first signs of discogenic low back pain may occur.[70]

These observations were substantiated by Horner and Urban's Volvo Award–winning study of the viability of living human disc cells under varying conditions.[72] They concluded that, if the cells of the disc failed to get proper nutrients (e.g., oxygen or glucose) or if the pH level of the disc changed (i.e., as a result of increased lactic acid or waste not being diffused out of the disc), its cellular metabolism would be directly affected. More specifically, the disc would stop producing the vital proteoglycan molecules. Proteoglycans are made of a protein core attached to at least one GAG chain. The predominant GAGs in the intervertebral disc are chondroitin-6-sulfate and keratin sulfate. These proteoglycans combine within the disc to produce large-aggregate molecules.[73] Without proteoglycans the disc dehydrates and loses its hydrostatic and osmotic pressure. Several experimental studies have concluded that intervertebral disc cells are very sensitive to the amount of hydrostatic pressure under which they can function.[74,75] Discs perform optimally at approximately 3 atm (44 psi), which is the normal pressure observed in a healthy disc. Any pressure variation either above normal or especially below 1 atm (14.6 psi) impairs disc function. The loss of the proteoglycan content is the most striking feature of disc aging, degeneration, death, and the development of annular tears.[76] Trout, Buckwalter, and Moore[77] confirmed that by adulthood more than 50% of the cells of the disc were dead.

Collagen is the other major structural component of the extracellular matrix of the intervertebral disc (**Fig. 1-8**). It provides tensile strength, allows for stability between vertebrae, and resists excessive disc bulging in response to loads. In younger discs, collagen comprises 67% of the dry weight of the annulus fibrosus and 25% of the nucleus pulposus. There are many types of collagen within the disc; however, types 1 and 2 comprise 80% of the total collagen content of the disc. Type 1 collagen is most abundant within the annulus, and type 2 comprises 80% of the collagen within the nucleus.[73] The loss of optimal intradiscal vascular supply and thus nutrition results in glycation, which is a biochemical reaction during which sugars come in contact with proteins (such as disc collagen) in an avascular and low-oxygen environment. This reaction converts the collagen strands, which are highly stable and have high tensile strength, into bulky, brittle, fibrous-type tissue that is more susceptible to degeneration and annular tears.[73,78] When stained, this tissue is a distinct shade of brown, as noted previously regarding the development of brown pigmentation in the aging disc. These physiological changes result in an intervertebral disc that is more susceptible to injury and possibly the development of discogenic pain.

Over the last decade significant research in the field of nuclear magnetic resonance spectroscopy has enhanced our understanding about the relationship between metabolic biochemical markers and discogenic low back pain.[79-81] In vitro studies have identified multiple potential biochemical and inflammatory markers within the intervertebral discs of patients undergoing back surgery for pain.[82] These markers have included tumor necrosis factor-α, interleukin 1-β, interleukin 6, interleukin 8, and interferon-γ, all of which may play an important role in discogenic pain.[83] Burke and associates[84] detected increased levels of interleukin 6 in disc extracts from patients undergoing fusion for discogenic pain. The identification and quantification of these markers may eventually lead to more definitive biochemical markers and noninvasive diagnostic criteria for discogenic low back pain.[85]

Risk Factors for Discogenic Pain

Why some discs prematurely degenerate and cause chronic pain and others do not is still somewhat controversial; however, it is becoming clear that genetics, a previous history of moderate-to-severe spinal trauma, physically strenuous work, and exposure to whole body vibration are a few of the potential risk factors.[86] Other environmental risk factors such as obesity, smoking, and leisure physical loading have been identified as additional potential independent risk factors for disc degeneration (**Fig. 1-9**).

Genetics

Research by Videman and associates,[87] Battie and colleagues,[88] Matsui and associates,[89] and Postacchini and associates[90] has

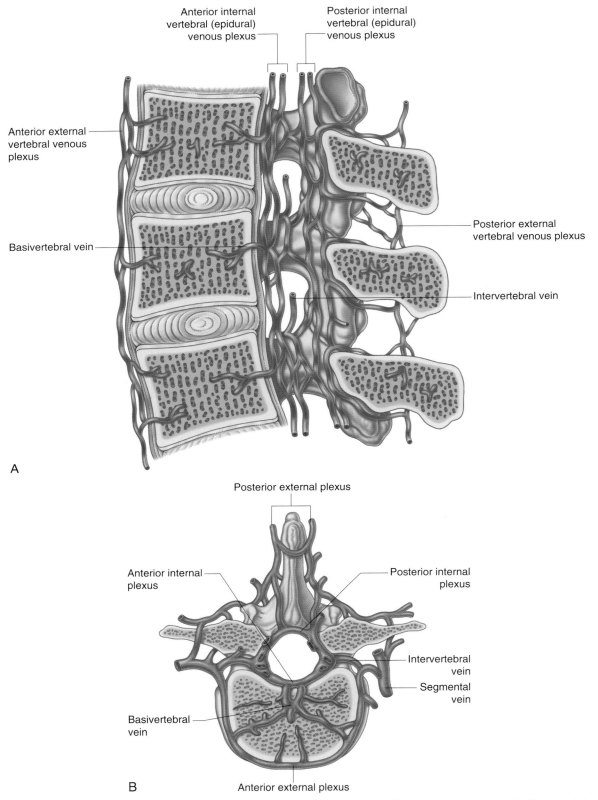

Fig. 1-7 **A** and **B,** Venous drainage of the vertebral column. From Standring et al, editors: *Gray's anatomy: the anatomical basis of clinical practice,* ed 39, 2005, Elsevier Churchill Livingstone, p 739.

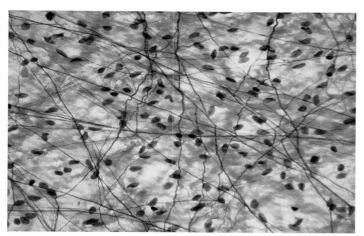

Fig. 1-8 Elastic fibers, seen as fine, dark, relatively straight fibers in a whole-mount preparation of mesentery, stained for elastin. The wavy pink bands are collagen bundles, and oval grey nuclei are mainly of fibroblasts. Photograph by Sarah-Jane Smith.

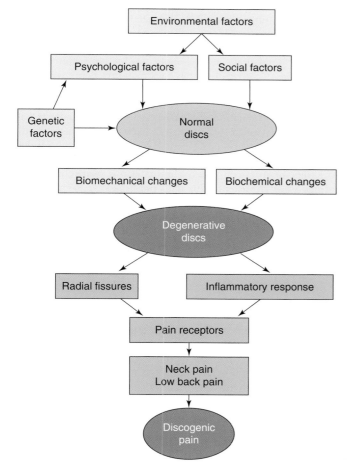

Fig. 1-9 Etiology of discogenic pain.

member will undergo disc surgery. These studies and those of Fejer, Hartvigsen, and Kyvik[91] and MacGregor and associates[92] illustrate the strong familial predisposition to discogenic neck and low back pain and suggest that the etiology of degenerative disc disease and discogenic pain is related to both genetic and environmental factors.

Recent research suggests that there may be "genetic weaknesses" in the collagen framework of the disc and/or genetic influences on blood supply and disc metabolism. Gene mutations occurring within the structural makeup of the disc have been identified. For example, two mutations, COL9A2 and COL9A3, have been identified within the genes that produce discal collagen type 9. Although this type of gene mutation is rare, when it does occur, the association with disc degeneration and sciatica is extremely strong.[93]

Another gene mutation has been associated with the discal proteoglycan aggrecan molecule. Aggrecan is the main proteoglycan responsible for maintaining intradiscal hydrostatic pressure and ultimately intradiscal hydration. This gene mutation produces aggrecan that cannot absorb water, which results in the development of severe disc dehydration and greatly increases the chance of annular tears and disc herniations.[94,95]

Recently a mutation in the vitamin D receptor gene has been associated with disc degeneration; and other gene mutations have been strongly associated with disc bulging, annular tearing, and osteophytosis.[96,97]

Structural Damage

The second major risk factor for developing accelerated disc degeneration and discogenic pain is traumatically induced structural damage to either the annulus fibrosus or the vertebral endplate.[98-100] There is increasing evidence that mechanical load has a profound fundamental influence on disc cell biology. Several investigators have described how any sudden loss of nuclear hydrostatic pressure (as a result of an endplate fracture and/or annular tear) can result in a sudden and devastating axial load shift from the deflated nucleus onto the posterior annulus, ring apophysis, and zygapophyseal joints.[101-103] Axial load shifts can result in visible changes within the annulus that are consistent with early degenerative and biochemical changes such as MMP-3 secretion, which induces the breakdown and weakening of the annulus and can ultimately lead to the development of a painful annular tear (discogenic pain) and/or disc herniation.[104]

The vertebral endplate is susceptible to axial load injuries and repetitive lifting (i.e., fatigue-based injuries). When the motion segment (i.e., two vertebrae and the disc between them) is compressed to the point of failure, the endplates almost always fractures first.[105-108]

Occupation

It is difficult to assess the effect of occupation on the development of discogenic pain since individuals with the same occupation may perform different jobs and therefore may have varying exposure within any given time frame. However, Luoma and associates[109] and Manchikanti[110] conducted an excellent study of the relationship between degenerative disc disease, low back pain, and occupation. They found that occupation was strongly related to lower back pain and/or sciatica but that degenerative disc disease was only somewhat associated with these pain patterns. Heavy physical work was strongly associated with the occurrence of low back pain, with the highest prevalence of low back pain observed in males with physically strenuous occupations.[111-116] No such relationships have been identified between employment status and neck pain, except for a higher rate of incident neck pain among those not working

concluded that the single greatest risk factor for the development of degenerative disc disease is inheritance (i.e., poor genetics). For example, a family history of spine surgery triples the chance that another immediate family member will also suffer low back pain. Even more striking is the fact that a family history of spine surgery increases the chance by tenfold that another immediate family because of ill health or disability at baseline.[117,118] In 1973 Chaffin and Park[119] reported that, when compared to sedentary workers, workers involved in heavy manual lifting were eight times more likely to experience low back injuries. The mechanical loads that accompany heavy manual lifting may lead to disc degeneration and IDD.[120] This in turn can initiate a cycle of persistent inflammation, matrix damage, and sensitization of annular receptors.[121-123] Disc matrix synthesis rates decrease abruptly if the tissue either swells excessively or loses fluid.[124,125] Static loads on the disc result in fluid extrusion, which in turn depends on the size and duration of the load. Prolonged mechanical loading causes a higher rate of intra-discal cell death.[126] These effects of increased mechanical loads on matrix synthesis and cell survival could help explain the increased rate of disc degeneration and annular tears in people who are exposed to increased physical loads such as those with heavy-duty occupations.

Static work postures; whole body vibration; and jobs requiring bending, twisting, and lifting have all been associated with an increased risk of low back pain. For example, it has been reported that males spending more than half their work day in a car experience a threefold increase in the risk of disc herniation. This may be due to the result of the combined effects of sitting and vibration.[127-132] A number of studies have also looked at the association between low back pain and bending, twisting, and lifting.[133] These studies reported that the frequency of low back pain after lifting ranges from 15% to 64%.[134-143] Sudden, unexpected maximum efforts and lifting combined with lateral bending and twisting were found to be particularly harmful.[144,145] When the spine is flexed, this complex motion can lead to annular tears.[146]

The association between whole body vibration and low back pain has been studied for over 30 years, and the results vary. In vitro animal studies suggest that vibration can adversely affect the nutrition and metabolism of the disc, especially if the vibration matches the resonant frequency of the lumbar spine (i.e., 4 Hz to 6 Hz).[147-152] People exposed to whole-body vibration in the resonant range such as helicopter pilots and drivers of trucks, buses, and tractors have a high rate of back pain.[153] A survey among male crane operators suggested that workers in a sedentary position with exposure to whole-body vibration were at a special risk for low back pain.[153] Lings and Leboeuf-Yde[154] conducted a meta-analysis of whole-body vibration and low back pain that included 53 articles. They concluded that, although experimental data supported the hypothesis that whole-body vibration can have a negative effect on the spine, the studies failed to quantify the association between exposure and effect. They also concluded that, based on epidemiological studies, drivers have an increased prevalence of low back pain that is probably dose related, suggesting that long-term exposure to whole-body vibration can contribute to back disorders. Other studies, including a meta-analysis of 45 articles published by Bovenzi and Hulshof,[155] concluded that the epidemiological evidence was not sufficient to support a clear relationship between vibration and low back pain.

Obesity

Although there are several hypotheses linking obesity to the development of neck and low back pain, researchers differ in their conclusions regarding the existence of a direct causal relationship between the two. For example, Deyo and Bass[156] studied the association between back pain and lifestyle factors (i.e., smoking and obesity) using national survey data. They concluded that, even after controlling for other variables, both smoking and obesity were independent risk factors for low back pain. In contrast, Leboeuf-Yde, Kyvid, and Bruun[157] concluded that weight is a potentially weak risk factor and that the data were insufficient to determine if it is a true cause of low back pain. In 2010 Heuch and associates[158] conducted a study using a cross-sectional, population-based design and found that a high body mass index (BMI) was associated with an increased prevalence of low back pain. This association was significant for both genders and was stronger in females than in males. Additional adjustments for age, education, employment status, work type, leisure time, physical activity, and smoking status did not impact the results. The preponderance of evidence suggests no relationship between BMI and the prevalence of neck pain.[159-165]

Tobacco Smoking

Tobacco smoking is considered to be the single most preventable cause of death and disease in the United States.[166] A suspected correlation between smoking and disc degeneration, with its potential to increase the risk of discogenic neck and low back pain, dates back to an epidemiological study conducted by Gyntelberg in 1974.[167] Gyntelberg postulated that chronic bronchitis may induce low back pain resulting from repeated increases in intraspinal pressure from coughing. He also hypothesized that smoking-associated aortic atherosclerosis may cause low back pain. In 1988 Holm and Nachemson's animal research[168] suggested that cigarette smoking not only reduces the solute-exchange capacity of the circulatory system outside the intervertebral disc but also significantly decreases the cellular uptake rate and metabolic production within the disc. Deyo and Bass[169] determined that back pain prevalence was associated with smoking. They found that prevalence increased from 9.6% to 14.1% among those with more than 50 pack years of smoking. This association was strongest in persons under the age of 45. They concluded that the risk of back pain increases steadily with both cumulative exposure and the degree of maximum daily exposure. The study also determined that smoking cessation for more than 10 years completely eliminates this relative risk. These findings were consistent with data published by Frymoyer and associates,[170] who also found that smoking was significantly associated with medically reported episodes of low back pain. In 1991 Battie and colleagues[114] won the Volvo Award for their research showing that smoking increased spinal disc degeneration across all discs by nearly 20%. In 1984 and again in 2001 subsequent studies also consistently identified smoking as an independent risk factor for neck pain.[171,172]

Extensive research has examined the physiological basis for the detrimental effects of smoking on the intervertebral discs and the subsequent development of back pain. Studies by Urban and associates[173] have shown that dogs injected with nicotine in an amount equivalent to that contained in one cigarette may experience a reduction in vertebral body blood flow. Because the disc depends on diffusion through the vertebral endplates for nutrition, smoking may adversely affect discal metabolism.[174,175] For example, nicotine directly inhibited bovine nucleus pulposus disc cell proliferation and the synthesis of extracellular matrix.[176] Similarly, passive smoking in rats resulted in downregulation of collagen genes, which preceded the histological changes of degeneration.[177]

Psychological Pathology

Psychological pathology is an interesting and controversial risk factor that has been implicated as a potential cause for neck and low back pain. Two cohort studies provide consistent evidence that psychological pathology can be a risk factor for neck pain. One phase II cohort study identified poor psychological status as an independent risk factor for neck pain.[178,179] During the past 50 to 60 years, prevailing hypotheses regarding the etiology of back

Table 1-1: Risk Factors for Neck and Back Pain

Type of Pain	Causal Risk Factors	Probable Risk Factors	Possible Risk Factors	Nonrelated Risk Factors
Neck pain	◄———— Genetics		Age (DDD) ◄————	Physical activity
	Smoking		Gender	Work type
			Sleep disturbance	Obesity
		◄———— Prior neck trauma	
		◄———— Psychosocial factors	
Low back pain	◄———— Genetics	◄———— Lifting	Physical activity ◄————
	◄———— Smoking	Vibration	Scoliosis
	◄———— Obesity	Job satisfaction	Kyphosis
	Age (DDD)	Gender	Leg-length discrepancy
		◄———— Heavy physical work	
		◄———— Psychosocial factors	

DDD, Degenerative disc disease.

pain have alternated between mechanical/postural models and behavioral/psychological models.[180-186] In 1983 Roland and Morris published a study of the natural history of low back pain in which they unequivocally concluded that, "Psychological factors are not of great importance in the majority of new presentations of back pain in the general practice. The increased incidence of psychological abnormalities is the result of long-standing pain."[187] Subsequent investigations, including those by Klenerman and associates,[188] Burton and associates,[189] and Gatchel, Polatin, and Mayer[190] provided important information regarding the interdependent role of psychological and physical disorders. For example, Klenerman and associates evaluated the prediction of chronicity in patients with acute low back pain in a general practice setting and found that those who had not recovered within 2 months went on to become chronic low back pain patients. Burton and associates concurrently determined that the identification of psychological problems is an important factor in understanding and preventing the progression to chronicity in patients with low back pain. Finally during the same year, Gatchel, Polatin, and Mayer concluded that preinjury or concomitant psychopathology does not appear to predispose patients to chronic pain disability, although high rates of psychopathology accompanied chronic low back pain. A more recent literature review by Bair and colleagues[191] summarized these findings and concluded that the prevalence of pain in depressed cohorts and depression in pain cohorts is higher than when each of these conditions is examined individually. In addition, when pain is moderate to severe, impairs function, and/ or is refractory to treatment, it is associated with more symptoms of depression and worse depression outcomes. Similarly, depression in patients with pain is associated with more pain complaints and greater impairment. These findings all support the final conclusion that depression and pain share biological pathways and neurotransmitters, which has implications for the concurrent treatment of both. A model that incorporates assessment and treatment of depression and pain simultaneously is necessary for improved outcomes.[191]

By evaluating the full body of literature that focuses on the causes of discogenic pain, one can estimate the relative importance of individual risk factors. No single study can determine if a specific risk factor is causal; however, the arrows in **Table 1-1** indicate an accumulation of literature and the direction of certain specific risk factors identified.

Conclusion

In conclusion, chronic low back pain is among the most important diagnoses in modern industrial societies.[192] IDD is the most common diagnosis leading to chronic low back pain and one of the major causes of chronic neck pain.[193] Discogenic pain is a significant medical challenge in terms of its clinical, social, economic, and public health implications. An extensive body of literature suggests that, rather than being the result of a single process, it is likely to have a number of possible causes. Based on available evidence, the most significant risk factor appears to be genetic inheritance, which is likely accelerated by environmental influences and lifestyle choices. Although the scientific literature conclusively supports the fact that the intervertebral disc is an independent pain generator, research related to the epidemiology of discogenic pain is still in its formative stage, especially when compared to studies of other chronic conditions such as heart disease and cancer. Further investigation is needed to more fully understand the incidence and prevalence of this debilitating condition and the relative contributions of genetic and environmental risk factors.

References

1. Mooney V: Where is the pain coming from? *Spine* 12:754-759, 1987.
2. Rhyne AL et al: Outcome of unoperated discogram-positive low back pain. *Spine* 20:1997-2000, 1995.
3. Inman VT, Saunders JB: Anatomical and physiological aspects of injuries to the intervertebral disc. *J Bone Joint Surg* 29:461, 1947.
4. Fernstrom U: A discographical study of ruptured lumbar intervertebral disc an investigation based on anatomical, pathological, surgical and clinical studies and on experiments in provocation of pain with special reference to simple ruptured lumbar discs and to discogenic pain. *Acta Chirurg Scand* 258(suppl):1-60, 1969.
5. Crock HV: A reappraisal of intervertebral disc lesions. *Med J* 1:983-989, 1970.
6. Daniel K et al, editors: *Surgical management of low back pain*, ed 2, New York, Stuttgart, 2008, Thieme Verlag, p 230.
7. The American Heritage dictionary of the English language, ed 4, Boston, 2000, Houghton Mifflin, updated 2009.
8. Singh V et al: Systematic review of thoracic discography as a diagnostic test for chronic spinal pain. *Pain Physician* 11(5):631-642, 2008.
9. Bogduk N, Tynan W, Wilson AS: The nerve supply to the human lumbar intervertebral discs. *J Anat* 132:39-56, 1981.

10. Bogduk N, Windsor M, Inglis A: The innervations of the cervical intervertebral discs. *Spine* 13:2-8, 1988.

11. Falconer MA, McGeorge M, Begg CA: Observations on the cause and mechanism of symptom production in sciatica and low back pain. *J Neurol Neurosurg Psychiatry* 11:13-23, 1948.

12. Hirsch C, Ingelmark BE, Miller M: The anatomic basis for low back pain. *Acta Orthop Scand* 33:1-17, 1963.

13. Lindblom K: Diagnostic puncture of intervertebral discs in sciatica. *Acta Orthop Scand* 17:231-239, 1948.

14. Nachemson A: A critical look at conservative treatment for low back pain. In Jayson MIV, editor: *The lumbar spine and back pain*, ed 2, Tunbridge Wells, UK, 1980, Pitman Medical Ltd, pp 355-365.

15. Steindler A: *Lectures on the interpretation of pain in orthopaedic practice*, Toronto, 1959, The Ryerson Press (Charles C Thomas).

16. Stolker RJ, Vervest ACM, Groen GJ: The management of chronic spinal pain blockades: a review. *Pain* 58:1-20, 1994.

17. Weinstein JN, Claverie W, Gibson S: The pain of discography. *Spine* 13:1344-1348, 1988.

18. Wilberg G: Back pain in relation to the nerve supply of the intervertebral disc. *Acta Orthop Scand* 19:211-212, 1949.

19. Stillwell DI, Jr: The nerve supply of the vertebral column and its associated structures in the monkey. *Anat Rec* 125:139-169, 1956.

20. Pederson HE, Blunck CFJ, Gardner E: The anatomy of lumbosacral posterior rami and meningeal branches of spinal nerves (sinu-vertebral nerves): with an experimental study of their functions. *J Bone Joint Surg [Am]* 38-A:377-391, 1956.

21. Malinsky J: The ontogenic development of nerve terminations in the intervertebral disc of man. *Acta Anat* ;38:96-113, 1959.

22. Hirsch C, Ingelmark B-E, Miller M: The anatomical basis for low back pain: studies on the presence of sensory nerve endings in ligamentous, capsular and intervertebral disc structures in the human lumbar spine. *Acta Orthop Scand* 33:1-17, 1963.

23. Edgar MA, Nundy S: Innervation of the spinal dura mater. *J Neurol Neurosurg Psychiatry* 29:530-534, 1966.

24. Jackson HC, 2nd, Winkelmann RK, Bickel WH: Nerve endings in the human lumbar spinal column and related structures. *J Bone Joint Surg [Am]* 48-A:1272-1281, 1966.

25. Nachemson ALF L: The lumbar spine: an orthopaedic challenge. *Spine* 1(1):59-71, 1976.

26. Bogduk N, Windsor M, Inglis A: The innervations of the cervical intervertebral discs. *Spine* 13(1):2-8, 1988.

27. Schwarzer AC et al: The prevalence and clinical features of internal disc disruption in patients with chronic low back pain. *Spine* 20(17): 1878-1883, 1995.

28. Bogduk N: *Clinical Anatomy of the Lumbar Spine and Sacrum*, 4th ed. Elsevier Health Sciences, 2005.

29. Manchikanti L: Epidemiology of low back pain. *Pain Physician* 3(2):167-192, 2000.

30. Keshari KR et al: Lactic acid and proteoglycans as metabolic markers for discogenic back pain. *Spine* 33(3):312-317, 2008.

31. Coté P, Cassidy JD, Carroll L: The Saskatchewan health and back pain survey: the prevalence of neck pain and related disability in Saskatchewan adults. *Spine* 1(23)16789-16798, 1998.

32. Zhang Y et al: Clinical diagnosis for discogenic low back pain. *Int J Biol Sci* 5:647-648, 2009.

33. Manchikanti L: Epidemiology of low back pain. *Pain Physician* 3(2)167-192, 2000.

34. Martin BI et al: Expenditures and health status among adults with back and neck problems. *JAMA* 299(6)656-664, 2008.

35. Bogduk N, Aprill C: On the nature of neck pain, discography and cervical zygapophysial joint blocks. *Pain* 54(2):213-217, 1993.

36. Yin W, Bogduk N: The nature of neck pain in a private pain clinic in the United States. *Pain Med* 9:196-203, 2008.

37. Manchikanti L et al: Evaluation of the relative contribution of various structures in chronic low back pain. *Pain Physician* 4(4):308-316, 2001.

38. Schwarzer AC et al: The prevalence and clinical features of internal disc disruption in patients with chronic low back pain. *Spine* 20(17):1878-1883, 1995.

39. Kopec JA, Sayre EC, Esdaile JM: Predictors of back pain in a general population cohort. *Spine* 29(1):70-78, 2003.

40. Manchikanti L: Epidemiology of low back pain. *Pain Physician* 3(2):167-192, 2000.

41. Martin BI et al: Expenditures and health status among adults with back and neck problems. *JAMA* 299:656, 2008.

42. Takahashi K, Aoki Y, Ohtori S: Resolving discogenic pain. *Eur Spine J* 17(suppl) 4:428-431, 2008.

43. Nakamura S-I et al: The afferent pathways of discogenic low-back pain. *J Bone Joint Surg [Br]* 78-B:606-612, 1996.

44. Weishaupt D et al: MR imaging of the lumbar spine: prevalence of intervertebral disk extrusion and sequestration, nerve root compression, end plate abnormalities, and osteoarthritis of the facet joints in asymptomatic volunteers. *Radiology* 209:661-666, 1998.

45. Freemont AJ et al: Nerve ingrowth into diseased intervertebral disc in chronic back pain. *Lancet* 350(9072):178-181, 1997.

46. Brisby H: Pathology and possible mechanisms of nervous system response to disc degeneration. *J Bone Joint Surg [Am]* 88(suppl 2):68-71, 2006.

47. Roberts S et al: Mechanoreceptors in intervertebral discs: morphology, distribution and neuropeptides. *Spine* 20:2645-2651, 1995.

48. Morinaga T et al: Sensory innervations to the anterior portion of lumbar intervertebral disc. *Spine* 21:1848-1851, 1996.

49. Brown MF et al: Sensory and sympathetic innervations of the vertebral endplate in patients with degenerative disc disease. *J Bone Joint Surg [Br]* 79-B:147-153, 1997.

50. Mooney V: Where is the pain coming from? *Spine* 12:754-759, 1987.

51. Williams P, Warwick R: Arthrology. In Williams P, Warwick R, editors: *Gray's anatomy*, Edinburgh, 1980, Churchill Livingstone, pp 444-445.

52. Twomey LT, Taylor JR: Age changes in lumbar vertebrae and intervertebral discs. *Clin Orthop* 224:97-104, 1987.

53. Roberts S, Menage J, Urban JPG: Biochemical and structural properties of the cartilage end-plate and its relation to the intervertebral disc. *Spine* 14:166-174, 1989.

54. Raj PP: Intervertebral disc: anatomy-physiology-pathophysiology-treatment. *Pain Pract* 8(1):18-44, 2008.

55. Yoshizawa H, O'Brien JP, Smith WT, Trumper M: The neuropathy of intervertebral disc removed for low back pain. *Lancet* 350:178-181, 1997.

56. Bogduk N, editor: *Clinical anatomy of the lumbar spine and sacrum*, ed 4, Edinburgh, 2005, Churchill Livingstone, pp 11-18.

57. Freemont AJ: The cellular pathobiology of the degenerate intervertebral disc and discogenic back pain. *Rheumatology (Oxford)* 48(1):5-10, 2009.

58. Freemont AJ: The cellular pathobiology of the degenerate intervertebral disc and discogenic back pain. *Rheumatology (Oxford)* 48(1):5-10, 2009.

59. Eyre DR, Matsui Y, Wu JJ: Collagen polymorphisms of the intervertebral disc. *Biochem Soc Trans* 30:844-848, 2002.

60. Urban JP, Maroudas A: Swelling of the intervertebral disc in vitro. *Connect Tissue Res* 9:1-10, 1981.

61. Matrisian LM: Metalloproteinases and their inhibitors in matrix remodeling. *Trends Genet* 6:121-125, 1990.

62. Marchand F, Ahmed AM: Investigation of the laminate structure of lumbar disc anulus fibrosus. *Spine* 15:402-410, 1990.

63. Bruehlmann SB et al: Regional variations in the cellular matrix of the annulus fibrosus of the intervertebral disc. *J Anat* 201:159-171, 2002.

64. Roberts S et al: Mechanoreceptors in intervertebral discs: morphology, distribution, and neuropeptides. *Spine* 20:2645-2651, 1995.

65. Bogduk N: The innervation of the intervertebral discs. In Boyling JD, Palastanga N, editors: *Grieve's modern manual therapy—the vertebral column*, Edinburgh, UK, 1994, Churchill Livingstone.

66. Banks RA, Bayliss MT, Lafeber FP: Ageing and zonal variation in post-translational modification of collagen in normal human articular cartilage: the age-related increase in non-enzymatic glycation affects biomechanical properties of cartilage. *Biochem J* 330 (Pt 1):345-351, 1998.

67. Hurri H, Karppinen J: Discogenic pain. *Pain* 112(3):225-228, 2004.
68. Kirkaldy-Willis W et al: Pathology and pathogenesis of lumbar spondylosis and stenosis. *Spine* 3(4)318-328, 1978.
69. Boos N et al: Classification of age-related changes in lumbar intervertebral discs: 2002 Volvo Award in Basic Science. *Spine* 27(3):2631-2644, 2002.
70. Hurri H, Karppinen J: Discogenic pain. *Pain* 112(3):225-228, 2004.
71. Coventry M: The intervertebral disc: Part 2. Changes in the intervertebral disc concomitant with age. *J Bone Joint Surg* 27:233-247, 1945.
72. Horner HA, Urban JP: 2001 Volvo Award Winner in Basic Science Studies: effect of nutrient supply on the viability of cells from the nucleus pulposus of the intervertebral disc. *Spine* 26(23):2543-2549, 2001.
73. Cassinelli EH, Hall RA, Kang JD: Biochemistry of intervertebral disc degeneration and the potential for gene therapy applications. *Spine J* 1(3):205-214, 2001.
74. Handa T et al: Effects of hydrostatic pressure on matrix synthesis and matrix metalloproteinase production in the human lumbar intervertebral disc. *Spine* 22:1085-1091, 1997.
75. Ishihara H et al: Effects of hydrostatic pressure on matrix synthesis in different regions of the intervertebral disk. *J Appl Physiol* 80:839-846, 1996.
76. Lyons G et al: Biochemical changes in intervertebral disc degeneration. *Biochim Biophys Acta* 673:443-453, 1981.
77. Trout JJ, Buckwalter JA, Moore KC: Ultrastructure of the human intervertebral disc. II. Cells of the nucleus pulposus. *Anat Rec* 204:307-314, 1982.
78. Bank RA et al: Ageing and zonal variation in post-translational modification of collagen in normal human articular cartilage. *Biochem J* 330:345-351, 1998.
79. Keshari KR et al: Lactic acid and proteoglycans as metabolic markers for discogenic back pain. *Spine* 33(3):312-317, 2008.
80. Majumdar S: Magnetic resonance imaging and spectroscopy of the intervertebral disc. *NMR Biomed* 19:894-903, 2006.
81. Wang C, McArdle E, Fenty M: Validation of sodium magnetic resonance imaging of intervertebral disc. *Spine* 35(5):505-510, 2010.
82. Cuellar JM, Golish SR, Reuter MW, et al: Cytokine evaluation in individuals with low back pain using discographic lavage. *Spine J* 10:212-218, 2010.
83. Hurri H, Karppinen J: Discogenic pain. *Pain* 112(3):225-228, 2004.
84. Burke JG et al: Intervertebral discs which cause low back pain secrete high levels of proinflammatory mediator. *J Bone Joint Surg [Br]* 84(2):196-201, 2002.
85. Cuellar JM et al: Cytokine evaluation in individuals with low back pain using discographic lavage. *Spine J* 10:212-218, 2010.
86. Cassinelli EH, Hall RA, Kang JD: Biochemistry of intervertebral disc degeneration and the potential for gene therapy applications. *Spine J* 1(3):205-214, 2001.
87. Videman T et al: 1998 Volvo Award winner: intragenic polymorphisms of the vitamin D receptor gene associated with intervertebral disc degeneration. *Spine* 23:2477-2485, 1998.
88. Battie MC et al: Similarities in degenerative findings on magnetic resonance images of the lumbar spines of identical twins. *J Bone Joint Surg Am* 77:1662-1670, 1995.
89. Matsui H et al: Familial predisposition for lumbar degenerative disc disease: a case-control study. *Spine* 23:1029-1034, 1998.
90. Postacchini F et al: Familial predisposition to discogenic low-back pain: an epidemiologic and immunogenetic study. *Spine* 13(12):1403-1406, 1988.
91. Fejer R, Hartvigsen J, Kyvik KO: Heritability of neck pain: a population based study of 33,794 Danish twins. *Rheumatology* 45:589-594, 2006.
92. MacGregor AI et al: Structural, psychological, and genetic influences of low back and neck pain: a study of adult female twins. *Arth Rheumatol* 51;160-167, 2004.
93. Cassinelli EH, Hall RA, Kang JD: Biochemistry of intervertebral disc degeneration and the potential for gene therapy applications. *Spine J* 1(3):205-214, 2001.
94. Cooper RG, Freemont AJ: TNF-alpha blockade for herniated intervertebral disc–induced sciatica: a way forward at last? *Rheumatology* 43:119-121, 2004.
95. Kawaguuchi Y et al: Association between an aggrecan gene polymorphism and lumbar disc degeneration. *Spine* 24;2456-2460, 1999.
96. Olmarker K et al: Inflammatogenic properties of nucleus pulposus. *Spine* 20(6):665-669, 1995.
97. Manchikanti L: Epidemiology of low back pain. *Pain Physician* 3(2)167-192, 2000.
98. Adams MA et al: "Stress" distributions inside intervertebral discs: the effects of age and degeneration. *J Bone Joint Surg [Br]* 78:965-972, 1996.
99. Adams MA et al: Mechanical initiation of intervertebral disc degeneration. *Spine* 25(13):1625-1636, 2000.
100. Adams MA et al: *The Biomechanics of back pain*, Edinburgh, UK, 2002, Churchill Livingstone.
101. Adams MA et al: "Stress" distributions inside intervertebral discs: the effects of age and degeneration. *J Bone Joint Surg [Br]* 78:965-972, 1996.
102. Adams MA et al: Mechanical initiation of intervertebral disc degeneration. *Spine* 25(13):1625-1636, 2000.
103. Adams MA et al: *The biomechanics of back pain*, Edinburgh, UK, 2002, Churchill Livingstone.
104. Adams MA et al: Abnormal stress concentrations in lumbar intervertebral discs following damage to the vertebral body: a cause of disc failure? *Eur Spine J* 1:214-221, 1993.
105. Brinckmann P et al: Fatigue fracture of human lumbar vertebrae. *Clin Biomech* 2(2):94-96, 1987.
106. Brinckmann P et al: Prediction of the compressive strength of human lumbar vertebrae. *Spine* 14(6):606-610, 1989.
107. Brinckmann P, Porter RW: A laboratory model of lumbar disc protrusion. *Spine* 19:228-235, 1994.
108. Perry O: Fracture of the vertebral end-plate: a biomechanical investigation. *Acta Orthop Scand* 25:157-165, 1957.
109. Luoma K et al: Low back pain in relation to lumbar disc degeneration. *Spine* 25(4):487-492, 2000.
110. Manchikanti L: Epidemiology of low back pain. *Pain Physician* 3(2)167-192, 2000.
111. Svensson HO, Andersson GBJ: Low back pain in forty to forty-seven year old men: work history and work environment factors. *Spine* 8:272-276, 1983.
112. Behrens V et al: The prevalence of back pain, hand discomfort, and dermatitis in the U.S. working population. *Am J Public Health* 84:1780-1785, 1994.
113. Lloyd MH, Gauld Soutar CA: Epidemiologic study of low back pain in miners and office workers. *Spine* 11:136-140, 1986.
114. Battie MC et al: 1991 Volvo Award in Clinical Sciences: Smoking and lumbar intervertebral disc degeneration: an MRI study of identical twins. *Spine* 16:1015-1021, 1991.
115. Battie MC et al: 1995 Volvo Award in Clinical Sciences: Determinants of lumbar disc degeneration: a study relating lifetime exposures and magnetic resonance imaging findings in identical twins. *Spine* 16:2601-2612, 1995.
116. Pope MN, Magnusson M, Wilder DG: Kappa Delta Award:: Low back pain and whole body vibration. *Clin Orthopaed Rel Res* 354:241-248, 1998.
117. Hogg-Johnson S et al: The burden and determinants of neck pain in the general population. *Eur Spine J* 17, S39-S51, 2008.
118. Croft PR et al: Risk factors for neck pain: a longitudinal study of the general population. *Pain* 93:317-325, 2001.
119. Chaffin DB, Park LS: A longitudinal study of low-back pain associated with occupational weight lifting factors. *Am Ind Hyg Assoc J* 34:513-525, 1973.
120. Cassinelli EH, Hall RA, Kang JD: Biochemistry of intervertebral disc degeneration and the potential for gene therapy applications. *Spine J* 1(3):205-214, 2001.
121. Osti OL, Vernon-Roberts B, Fraser RD: 1990 Volvo Award in experimental studies: Anulus tears and intervertebral disc degeneration: an experimental study using an animal model. *Spine* 15:762-767, 1990.

122. Osti OL et al: Annular tears and disc degeneration in the lumbar spine: a postmortem study of 135 discs. *J Bone Joint Surg Br* 74:678-682, 1992.

123. Ulrich JA et al: Repeated disc injury causes persistent inflammation. *Spine* 32:2812-2819, 2007.

124. Bayliss MT et al: In vitro method for measuring synthesis rates in the intervertebral disc. *J Orthopaed Res* 4:10-17, 1986.

125. Ohshima H, Urban JP, Bergel DH: Effect of static load on matrix synthesis rates in the intervertebral disc measured in vitro by a new perfusion technique. *J Orthopaed Res* 13:22-29, 1995.

126. Rand N et al: *Static hydrostatic loading induces apoptosis In human intervertebral disc cells.* Orlando, Fla, 2000, Orthopaedic Research Society.

127. Kroemer KH, Robinette JC: Ergonomics in the design of office furniture. *Ind Med Surg* 38:115-125, 1969.

128. Bergquist-Ullman M, Larsson U: Acute low back pain in industry: a controlled prospective study with special reference to therapy and confounding factors. *Acta Orthop Scand* 170:1-117, 1977.

129. Svensson HO, Andersson GBJ: The relationship of low-back pain, work history, work environment, and stress: a retrospective cross-sectional study of 38 to 64 year old women. *Spine* 14:517-522, 1989.

130. Westrin CG: Low back pain sick-listing: nosological and medical insurance investigation. *Scand J Soc Med* 7:1-116, 1973.

131. Kelsey JL: An epidemiological study of the relationship between occupations and acute herniated lumbar intervertebral discs. *Int J Epidemiol* 4:197-205, 1975.

132. Hadjipavlou AG et al: The pathophysiology of disc degeneration: a critical review. *J Bone Joint Surg [Br]* 90(10):1261-1270, 2008.

133. Manchikanti L: Epidemiology of low back pain. *Pain Physician* 3(2)167-192, 2000.

134. Chaffin DB, Park LS: A longitudinal study of low-back pain associated with occupational weight lifting factors. *Am Ind Hyg Assoc J* 34:513-525, 1973.

135. Frymoyer JW et al: Epidemiologic studies of low-back pain. *Spine* 5:419-423, 1980.

136. Lloyd MH, Gauld Soutar CA: Epidemiologic study of low back pain in miners and office workers. *Spine* 11:136-140, 1986.

137. Hult L: Cervical, dorsal, and lumbar spine syndromes. *Acta Orthop Scand* 17:1-102, 1954.

138. Bergquist-Ullman M, Larsson U: Acute low back pain in industry: a controlled prospective study with special reference to therapy and confounding factors. *Acta Orthop Scand* 170:1-117, 1977.

139. Kelsey JL: An epidemiological study of the relationship between occupations and acute herniated lumbar intervertebral discs. *Int J Epidemiol* 4:197-205, 1975.

140. Brown JR: Factors contributing to the development of low back pain in industrial workers. *Am Industr Hyg Assoc J* 36:26-31, 1975.

141. Bigos SJ et al: Back injuries in industry: a retrospective study. III. Employee-related factors. *Spine* 11:252-256, 1986.

142. Troup JD, Martin JW, Lloyd DC: Back pain in industry: a prospective study. *Spine* 6:61-69, 1981.

143. Walsh K et al: Occupational causes of low-back pain. *Scand J Environ Health* 15:1-26, 1989.

144. Brown JR: Factors contributing to the development of low back pain in industrial workers. *Am Industr Hyg Assoc J* 36:26-31, 1975.

145. Magora A: Investigation of the relation between low back pain and occupation. 3. Physical requirements: sitting, standing, and weight lifting. *Ind Med Surg* 41:5-9, 1972.

146. Adams MA, Hutton WG: The mechanical function of the lumbar apophysial joints. *Spine* 8:327-330, 1983.

147. Hirano N et al: Analysis of rabbit intervertebral disc physiology based on water metabolism. II: changes in normal intervertebral discs under axial vibratory load. *Spine* 13:1297-1302, 1988.

148. Holm S, Nachemson A: Nutrition of the intervertebral disc: effects induced by vibration. *Orthop Trans* 9:525, 1985.

149. Frymoyer JW et al: Epidemiologic studies of low-back pain. *Spine* 5:419-423, 1980.

150. Kelsey J: An epidemiological study of the relationship between occupations and acute herniated lumbar intervertebral discs. *Int J Epidemiol* 4:197-205, 1975.

151. Kelsey JL: An epidemiological study of the relationship between occupations and acute herniated lumbar intervertebral discs. *Int J Epiemiol* 4:197-205, 1975.

152. Bovenzi M, Zadini A: Self-reported low back symptoms in urban bus drivers exposed to whole-body vibration. *Spine* 17:1048-1059, 1992.

153. Bongers PM et al: Back pain and exposure to whole body vibration in helicopter pilots. *Ergonomics* 33:1007-1026, 1990.

154. Lings S, Leboeuf-Yde C: Whole-body vibration and low back pain: a systematic, critical review of the epidemiological literature 1992-1999. *Int Arch Occup Environ Health* 73(5):290-297, 2000.

155. Bovenzi M, Hulshof CT: An updated review of epidemiologic studies on the relationship between exposure to whole-body vibration and low back pain (1986-1997). *Int Arch Occup Environ Health* 72(6):35-65, 1999.

156. Deyo RA, Bass JE: Lifestyle and low-back pain: the influence of smoking and obesity. *Spine* 14(5):501-506, 1989.

157. Leboeuf-Yde C, Kyvik KO, Bruun NH: Low back pain and lifestyle. Part II. Obesity: information from a population-based sample of 29,424 twin subjects. *Spine* 24:779-783, 1999.

158. Heuch I et al: The impact of body mass index on the prevalence of low back pain: the HUNT study. *Spine* 35(7):764-768, 2010.

159. Andersson H, Ejlertsson G, Leden I: Chronic pain in a geographically defined general population: studies of differences in age, gender, social class, and pain localization. *Clin J Pain* 9:174-182, 1993.

160. Cote P, Cassidy JD, Carroll L: The Saskatchewan Health and Back Pain Survey: the prevalence of neck pain and related disability in Saskatchewan adults. *Spine* 23:1689-1698, 1998.

161. Hartvigsen J, Christensen K, Frederiksen H: Back and neck pain exhibit many common features in old age: a population-based study of 4,486 Danish twins 70-102 years of age. *Spine* 29:576-580, 2004.

162. Makela M et al: Prevalence, determinants, and consequences of chronic neck pain in Finland. *Am J Epidemiol* 134:1356-1367, 1991.

163. Webb R et al: Prevalence and predictors of intense, chronic, and disabling neck and back pain in the UK general population. *Spine* 28:1195-1202, 2003.

164. Niemi S et al: Neck and shoulder symptoms and leisure time activities in high school students. *J Orthop Sports Phys Ther* 24:25-29, 1996.

165. Vikar A et al: Neck or shoulder pain and low back pain in Finnish adolescents. *Scand J Public Health* 28:164-173, 2000.

166. Klesges RC et al: The relationship between smoking and body weight in a population of young military personnel. *Health Psycol* 17:454-458, 1998.

167. Gyntelberg F: One year incidence of low back pain among residents of Copenhagen aged 40-59. *Dan Med Bull* 21:30-36, 1974.

168. Holm A, Nachemson AL: Nutrition of the intervertebral disc: acute effects of cigarette smoking. An experimental animal study. *Ups J Med Sci* 93:91-99, 1988.

169. Deyo RA, Bass JE: Lifestyle and low-back pain: the influence of smoking and obesity. *Spine* 14(5):501-506, 1989.

170. Frymoyer JW et al: Epidemiologic studies of low-back pain. *Spine* 5:419-423, 1980.

171. Croft PR et al: Risk factors for neck pain: a longitudinal study in the general population. *Pain* 93:317-325, 2001.

172. Kelsey JL et al: An epidemiological study of acute prolapsed cervical intervertebral disc. *J Bone Joint Surg [Am]* 66:907-914, 1984.

173. Urban JP et al: Nutrition of the intervertebral disc: an in vivo study of solute transport. *Clin Orthop* 129:101-114, 1977.

174. Frymoyer JW et al: Risk factors in low-back pain. *J Bone Joint Surg* 65A:213-218, 1983.

175. Holm S, Nachemson A: Nutrition of the intervertebral disc: effects induced by vibration. *Orthop Trans* 9:525, 1985.

176. Akmal M et al: Effect of nicotine on spinal disc cells: a cellular mechanism for disc degeneration. *Spine* 29:568-575, 2004.

177. Uei H et al: Gene expression changes in an early stage of intervertebral disc degeneration induced by passive cigarette smoking. *Spine* 31: 510-514, 2006.

178. Croft PR et al: Risk factors for neck pain: a longitudinal study in the general population. *Pain* 93:317-325, 2001.

179. Siivola SM et al: Predictive factors for neck and shoulder pain: a longitudinal study in young adults. *Spine* 19:1662-1669, 2004.

180. Jayson MIV: Why does acute back pain become chronic? *Spine* 10:1053-1056, 1997.

181. Klenerman L et al: The prediction of chronicity in patient with an acute attack of low back pain in a general practice setting. *Spine* 20:278-282, 1994.

182. Hanvik LJ: MMPI profiles in patients with low back pain. *J Consult Clin Psychol* 15:350-353, 1951.

183. Polatin PB et al: Psychiatric illness and chronic low back pain: the mind and the spine—which goes first? *Spine* 18:66-71, 1993.

184. Wiltse LL, Rocchio PD: Preoperative psychological tests as predictors of success of chemonucleolysis in the treatment of low back pain. *J Bone Joint Surg [Am]* 57:478-483, 1975.

185. Wolkind SN, Forrest AJ: Low back pain: a psychiatric investigation. *Postgrad Med J* 48:76-79, 1972.

186. Troup JDG: Causes, prediction and prevention of back pain at work. *Scand J Work Environ Health* 10:419-428, 1984.

187. Roland M, Morris R: A study of the natural history of low-back pain. *Spine* 8:145-150, 1983.

188. Klenerman L et al: The prediction of chronicity in patient with an acute attack of low back pain in a general practice setting. *Spine* 20:278-282, 1995.

189. Burton AK et al: Psychosocial predictors of outcome in acute and subchronic low back trouble. *Spine* 20:722-728, 1995.

190. Gatchel RJ, Polatin PB, Mayer TG: The dominant role of psychosocial risk factors in the development of chronic low back pain disability. *Spine* 20:2702-2709, 1995.

191. Bair MJ et al: Depression and pain comorbidity: a literature review. *Arch Intern Med* 163:2433-2445, 2003.

192. Singh V et al: Percutaneous disc decompression using coblation (nucleoplasty) in the treatment of chronic discogenic pain. *Pain Physician* 5(3):250-259, 2002.

193. Zhang Y et al: Clinical diagnosis for discogenic low back pain. *Int J Biol Sci* 5:647-648, 2009.

2 Establishing the Diagnosis of Discogenic Back Pain: An Evidence-Based Algorithmic Approach

Farshad M. Ahadian and Mark S. Wallace

CHAPTER OVERVIEW

Chapter Synopsis: Discogenic back pain represents one of the most challenging conditions to patients and pain clinicians. The condition is particularly difficult to diagnose accurately. Completely accurate diagnosis, which is not attainable for any condition, requires 100% sensitivity (in which all cases are detected) and 100% specificity (in which no false positives are included). To approach this ideal, clinicians seek out a definitive diagnostic test. Such a definitive test arguably does not exist for discogenic pain. Tissue confirmation may not be possible in living patients, and even when available may not provide a gold standard of diagnosis. Imaging studies may be misleading in the diagnosis of discogenic pain because anatomical criteria often do not correlate with pain. Diagnostic tests and interventions have proven more useful in spinal pain conditions. This chapter presents an algorithmic approach to diagnosing discogenic pain that makes use of multiple clinical components, including history, physical examination, laboratory studies, imaging, and diagnostic interventions. Effective communication with the patient may represent the most critical component to arriving at a correct diagnosis and therefore effective treatment.

Important Points:
- Discogenic pain is among the most common and most challenging diagnosis the pain physician faces.
- No single test or intervention can accurately establish the diagnosis of discogenic pain.
- The predictive value of modalities used to diagnose discogenic pain depends directly on the pretest probability of the disease.
- With proper patient selection and standardized diagnostic criteria, discography has a high degree of predictive value for discogenic pain.

Clinical Pearls:
- Effective communication is the key to success with diagnostic interventions.
- Identify patient's usual pain distribution and character immediately before the procedure.
- Educate the patient in advance about the nature and process of the diagnostic intervention that he or she is going to have.
- Educate the patient in advance on the proper use of the numerical rating scale (NRS) by providing specific examples of mild, moderate, and severe pain ratings.

Clinical Pitfalls:
- Avoid excessive sedation when performing diagnostic interventions because it may lead to increased false-negative or false-positive responses and an increased complication rate.
- Instruct patients to continue their usual analgesic and anxiolytic regimen before diagnostic interventions to avoid withdrawal and increased false-positive responses.

Discogenic Pain: A Diagnostic Challenge

The concept of pain arising from the intervertebral disc (IVD) dates back to the 1940s.[1] Discogenic pain is among the most common and most challenging of the diagnoses that the pain physician must confront. This premise remains as true today as it did in 1970 when Crock[2] first described internal disc disruption (IDD) characterized by radial fissures or tears through the annulus fibrosis (AF) despite a normal or near-normal disc contour. The term *discogenic pain* refers to pain arising from the disc itself in contrast to nerve root pain caused by disc protrusion.

Many factors contribute to the complexity of this condition. These include the numerous sources of pain in the spine that cause symptoms similar in distribution and character, confounding psychosocial factors, the subjective nature of pain itself, and the limitations of available diagnostic tools. To further complicate the picture there are a wide variety of diagnostic and therapeutic approaches among different specialties that deal with spine pain, leading to a lack of consensus.

This chapter presents an algorithmic approach to evaluation of discogenic pain. This systematic approach provides a step-by-step process that assists the clinician to more reliably distinguish discogenic pain from other potential sources of spine pain. To deal effectively with the vast body of evidence and debate on the topic of discogenic pain, this chapter begins with a review of the nomenclature and principles of diagnostic testing and medical decision making that has been referred to so often in this literature. The role and relative contribution of each component of the evaluation process for discogenic pain is then discussed, including history, physical examination, laboratory studies, imaging, and diagnostic interventions. The algorithms presented are based on the current evidence, published guidelines, strengths and limitations of diagnostic tools, and risks and benefits of potential diagnostic and therapeutic interventions.

General Principles of Diagnostic Testing

Diagnostic tests used in evaluation of spine pain may be assessed using the general principles that apply to all medical diagnostic testing. These principles are referred to frequently in the medical literature to discuss diagnostic spine interventions and are the basis of clinical decision making. It is important for physicians dealing with spine disorders to be acquainted with this nomenclature. The desirable features of diagnostic medical tests include accuracy, reproducibility, and safety.

Sensitivity and specificity are parameters used to describe accuracy. Sensitivity is a measure of false-negative rates. Specificity is a measure of false-positive rates. **Fig. 2-1** demonstrates the relationship among the parameters used to measure accuracy of laboratory tests. A test that is 100% sensitive would detect all cases in which the disease may be present. A test that is 100% specific would detect only those cases in which the disease is certain to be present and exclude all cases in which the disease is absent. In reality, diagnostic medical tests never reach this ideal level of accuracy, leaving some degree of uncertainty regarding the diagnostic information.[3]

The gold standard is defined as a diagnostic test or benchmark that is regarded as definitive. A gold standard allows for determination of true positive results when a given diagnosis is present and true negative results when the diagnosis is absent. The specificity and sensitivity of a given diagnostic test may then be calculated accordingly. The most commonly accepted gold standard in various medical disciplines is tissue confirmation. However, it is frequently not possible to apply a gold standard test to each patient. The gold standard may be impossible to perform in a living patient, or may carry an unacceptable level of risk such as a biopsy or surgical confirmation. In the absence of a true gold standard, the term *criterion standard* has been coined and is now the preferred term for a number of publications. The Journal of the American Medical Association defines criterion standard as a method having established or widely accepted accuracy for determining a diagnosis, providing a standard to which a new screening or diagnostic test can be compared.

Spine disorders pose yet another barrier to determination of accuracy of diagnostic tests. There is a range of anatomical features in spinal structures and a lack of correlation of these features to painful states. Therefore, even when possible, tissue or surgical confirmation may not serve as a reliable gold standard when pain is the primary outcome measure. Not surprising, diagnosis of spinal pain disorders relies far more on pain-provoking or pain-relieving interventions than laboratory or imaging studies.

Principles of Medical Decision Making

Despite the limitations in determining their accuracy, diagnostic tests and interventions serve a valuable purpose. When viewed from the perspective of probability, these tests and interventions help the clinician deal with the inherent uncertainty of clinical decision making.[4-6] The probability that the results of a diagnostic test are valid may be influenced by factors inherent to the test such as sensitivity and specificity and the clinical setting in which the test is applied. Bayes' theorem is a mathematical expression of conditional probability and a governing principle of diagnostic testing (**Fig. 2-2**). According to Bayes' theorem, the posttest odds of a test result are directly proportional to the pretest odds multiplied by the likelihood ratio for the test result, which is a function of the prevalence of the disease. In clinical terms the prevalence of a disease process directly affects the degree of meaning of the test results. When the prevalence is high, there is a higher probability that a positive result indicates the presence of the disease.[7] Conversely, interpretation of a test result in a population in which the prevalence is low has limited value.

The positive predictive value (PPV) is the proportion of patients with positive test results who are correctly diagnosed.[8] PPV indicates the probability that a positive test reflects the underlying condition being tested for and is the most important measure of a diagnostic method. However, its value does depend on the

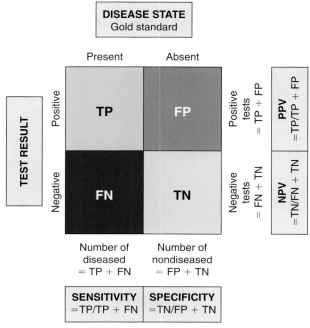

Fig. 2-1 Accuracy parameters of diagnostic tests. *FP,* False positive; *NPV,* negative predictive value; *PPV,* positive predictive value; *TN,* true negative; *TP,* true positive.

$$\text{Posttest odds} = \text{Pretest odds} \times \text{Likelihood ratio}$$

$$\text{Odds} = \frac{\text{Probability}}{1 - \text{Probability}} \qquad \text{Probability} = \frac{\text{Odds}}{1 + \text{Odds}}$$

$$\text{Likelihood ratio} = \frac{\text{Probability of result in diseased person}}{\text{Probability of result in nondiseased person}}$$

Fig. 2-2 Bayes' theorem.

prevalence of the disease, which may vary. Therefore results of diagnostic tests are not absolute. They must be interpreted in the context of the specific clinical conditions where the test is applied.

The various measures of accuracy and reliability of diagnostic tests may be expressed in terms of validity or the soundness of diagnostic interventions. Many types of validity have been described, but the terms are not necessarily defined in a consistent manner among all practitioners. Concept validity examines the theoretical basis of a test such as the anatomical or physiological basis of an intervention. Diagnostic blocks have concept validity because a pain generator may be identified based on anatomical and physiological basis. In effect, the structure may be anesthetized, resulting in pain relief. Content validity requires that a test or intervention be clearly and accurately defined. For an intervention to have content validity the clinician must adhere to the accepted definition. This allows for a valid comparison of results both within and between various samples. Face validity requires that an intervention actually achieves its intended goal on an anatomical and physiological basis. Face validity may be established on a statistical basis using a large-scale study by demonstrating that, if content validity is achieved, a specific result may be expected by all practitioners. Face validity may also be demonstrated on an individual basis. For example, in case of diagnostic blocks, administration of contrast medium under fluoroscopic imaging may demonstrate selective spread of contrast at the target site and avoidance of spread to adjacent structures. Construct validity measures the extent to which a test correctly distinguishes the presence or absence of the condition that the test is designed to detect. Construct validity is measured using the principles of diagnostic testing and clinical decision making described previously. Face validity and construct validity are critical features of any diagnostic intervention. Finally, predictive validity is a measure of the ability of a diagnostic intervention to predict successful treatment outcome. This constitutes the therapeutic use of the diagnostic intervention.[9]

Sources of Pain in the Spine

Because of the multiple pain-producing structures in the spine, it may be difficult to determine the exact source of back pain (**Box 2-1**). Often discogenic pain is a diagnosis of exclusion when other areas of the spine have been ruled out as potential causes. Many structures in the spine are known or have a high likelihood of producing pain. This section discusses the different pain-producing structures implicated in the production of spine pain to aid in the differential diagnosis (**Box 2-2**).

Zygapophyseal Joint Pain

Morphological studies on humans[10-12] have demonstrated neuropeptides and nerve endings in the facet joint capsule. Although it remains controversial, pathology within these joints appears to

result in significant back pain, which should be ruled out before diagnosing discogenic pain.

Because the joints are deep structures, pain that arises from them radiate to other deep structures of the body via sclerotomes and myotomes, which results in a poorly localized pain pattern similar to that of discogenic pain. These referral patterns may result in secondary zones of reflex muscle spasm and resultant trigger points.

Sacroiliac Joint

As with the facet joint, there has been controversy about the sacroiliac joint (SIJ) (**Fig. 2-3**) as a cause of low back pain (LBP). However, many clinicians believe that the potential for this joint to

---

Box 2-2: Differential Diagnosis of Spine Pain

- Internal disc disruption
- Disc protrusion
- Radiculopathy
- Facet dysfunction
- Sacroiliac dysfunction
- Vertebral body fracture
- Spondylolysis
- Spondylolisthesis
- Scoliosis
- Spinal enthesopathy
- Nerve entrapment syndrome
- Epidural lipomatosis
- Diffuse idiopathic skeletal hyperostosis
- Rheumatological disorders
- Infection
- Malignancy
- Visceral pathology
- Gastrointestinal
- Genitourinary
- Vascular

Box 2-1: Sources of Pain in the Spine

- Nerve roots
- Discs
- Facet joints
- Sacroiliac joints
- Vertebral bodies
- Ligaments
- Soft tissues
- Dura

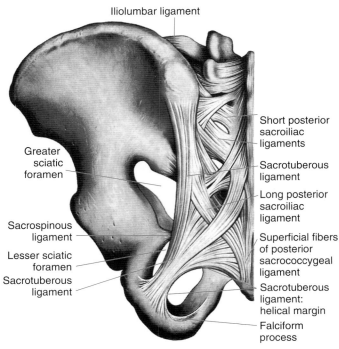

Fig. 2-3 Ligaments on the posterior aspect of the left half of the pelvis and the fifth lumbar vertebra. From Standring et al, editors: *Gray's anatomy: the anatomical basis of clinical practice*, ed 39, 2005, Elsevier Churchill Livingstone: New York, pp 762.

cause pain is underestimated.[13-17] The SIJ is classified as a diarthrodial joint; however, with age the joint develops fibrous adhesions, which restrict movement.[18,19] This restriction of movement decreases the buffering capacity of the joint, which may lead to chronic pain. Like the facet joints, the SIJ is richly innervated with both free nerve endings and mechanoreceptors. The innervation has been extensively described and supports the belief that this joint is a pain-sensitive structure.[20-22]

Intervertebral Disc

Nerve endings capable of transmitting pain impulses are abundant in the outer one third of the AF in the IVD.[23-26] In addition, nerves within the IVD contain neuropeptides, which are involved in pain transmission.[27] Injuries in the AF may result in pain while the external appearance of the disc remains normal, with no direct or obvious nerve root involvement. [28]

Ligaments of the Spine

Many ligamentous structures in the spine are innervated with free nerve endings. However, the density of this innervation varies. Of all of the ligamentous structures, the posterior longitudinal ligament appears to be the most heavily innervated with free nerve endings,[29-31] and the ligamentum flavum the least innervated.[32]

Degenerative changes within these ligaments may result in sensitization of free nerve endings, leading to chronic pain. In addition, the close proximity of the anterior and posterior longitudinal ligaments to the discs makes these structures susceptible to exposure to the disc contents in the event of disc rupture (see Chapter 1, **Fig. 1-5**). The disc contents may induce an inflammatory process in these ligaments, leading to pain.

Nerve Root

The nerve root is innervated by the sinuvertebral nerve, which branches from the segmental nerve and travels backward into the neural foramen. The arachnoidal covering of the nerve root is heavily innervated and a source of pain (**Fig. 2-4**). Mechanical compression or irritation of these structures can lead to pain in the extremities that is associated with neurological changes. The nerve root may be stimulated mechanically by disc herniation, osteophyte formation, foraminal narrowing caused by degenerative disc disease (DDD), or tumor invasion. In addition, it has been postulated that both the disc and facet joint contents may induce an arachnoiditis; however, Haughton, Nguyen, and Ho[33] showed this only to be true for the disc contents.

Clinical Evaluation of the Patient with Discogenic Pain

Targeted History

History and physical examination have limited specificity for discogenic pain. However, they serve two critical functions that make the clinical evaluation the foundation for establishing the diagnosis of discogenic pain. The first and most important role of the clinical evaluation is identification of "red flags" that may indicate presence of sinister pathology. Second, it is through a careful and detailed history and physical evaluation that the clinician identifies the population of patients with a high pretest probability for discogenic pain. Red flags that require immediate attention include recent trauma, mild trauma or strain with a history of osteoporosis, unexplained weight loss, history of cancer, fever, pain worse at night, bowel or bladder dysfunction, intravenous drug use, and

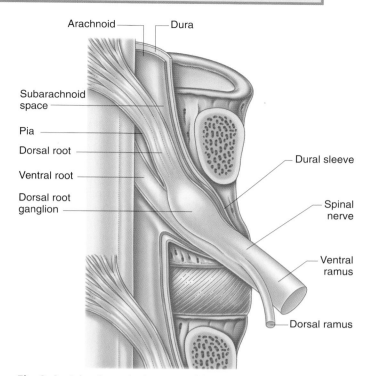

Fig. 2-4 A lumbar spinal nerve and its roots and meningeal coverings. From Standring et al, editors: *Gray's anatomy: the anatomical basis of clinical practice*, ed 39, 2005, Elsevier Churchill Livingstone: New York, p 782.

pain that is not relieved in the supine position or that awakens the patient from sleep.[34]

The history should look for signs of nondiscogenic pain. Although the signs taken in isolation are not very valuable, together with the physical examination and diagnostic testing they can prove to be helpful. Lumbar facet pain is worse in the morning and with inactivity and is aggravated by extension, rotation, and side bending of the spine to the diseased side. Pain from the SIJ is usually referred to the buttocks, groin, posterior thigh, and occasionally below the knee.[35-38] The pain worsens with bending and prolonged sitting and improves with walking or standing.[35,39]

Symptoms that tend to be more associated with discogenic pain include increased pain with sitting, flexion, coughing, sneezing, or activities that increase intradiscal pressure such as straining. A case report of a subject demonstrated that disc pressures progressively increased with the following positions: supine < lateral decubitus < standing < sitting < standing with forward flexion < sitting with forward flexion < standing with forward flexion against resistance < sitting with forward flexion against resistance.[40] There are no studies that correlate these positions with the diagnosis of discogenic pain. The symptoms described in the history should not be taken at face value but rather used as a whole with physical findings and diagnostic tests.

Physical Examination

Like the history, the physical examination is most valuable in identifying potentially serious or harmful pathology. As such, a comprehensive physical examination must be documented before proceeding with advanced interventional modalities.

Physical examination findings have limited specificity for diagnosis of discogenic pain. In the absence of neural compromise, the neurological examination of patients with LBP is usually normal. The most common presentation on musculoskeletal examination is axial pain reproduction associated with decreased range of motion of the spine, especially with flexion. Palpation usually reveals midline tenderness near the affected segments. There may also be evidence for increased tension in the paravertebral musculature and active trigger points. A number of provocational maneuvers and examinations may help distinguish various causes of axial spine pain and increase the pretest probability of discogenic pain.

Lumbar facet pain rarely produces true radicular pain into the extremity; but, because of the close association of the facet joint with the nerve root, true radicular symptoms can occur with facet joint disease (i.e., synovial cysts, facet hypertrophy, or osteophytes).[41] Therefore a neurological examination should be performed, especially for pain radiating below the knee, to look for nerve root compression. If side bending results in pain on the opposite side, soft tissue pain should be entertained. Because of the anatomical location of the facet joints, the physical examination of facet pain appears to be nonspecific, and the diagnosis relies more on symptomatology and diagnostic blockade.

Because of the anatomical location of the SIJ, this structure is difficult to examine; and many of the provocative tests may result in false-positive responses and inter-tester variability.[42,43] However, there are several provocation tests that are easy to interpret and reliable.[44,45] Gillet's test notes the change in relationship of the upper sacral spinous process and the posterior superior iliac spine (PSIS). When the patient is standing, these processes are located on the same plane. When the patient is asked to lift one leg, under normal conditions the ipsilateral PSIS moves inferiorly relative to the spinous process. In a patient with sacroiliac dysfunction the PSIS remains at the same level or moves superiorly. Patrick's test is performed with the patient in the supine position. The patient is asked to cross one leg with the ankle placed just above the opposite knee. The examiner then pushes the knee of the crossed leg toward the floor. This test stresses the hip and the SIJ. If hip pathology is present, pain is produced in the lateral hip and groin. If SIJ pathology is present, pain is produced over the sacroiliac junction. Gaenslen's test is performed with the patient in the supine position. This test is performed by maximally flexing the hip on one side and maximally extending the hip on the opposite side. This test stresses both joints simultaneously and is positive if pain is produced over the sacroiliac junction. Yeoman's test is performed with the patient in the prone position. The hip is maximally extended by lifting it off the table. A positive test produces pain over the sacroiliac junction. This test may also stress the lumbar facet joints, and pain produced over the lower back is positive for facet pain. The sacroiliac shear test is performed with the patient in the prone position. The palm of the hand is placed over the posterior part of the ilium and thrust anteriorly. If positive, this test produces pain over the sacroiliac junction. The hip rotation test evaluates the integrity of the musculature surrounding the SIJ. If SIJ pain is present, reflex muscle spasms may limit its mobility. Under normal conditions external rotation of the leg lengthens the leg, and internal rotation shortens the leg. If SIJ pain is present, this lengthening and shortening does not occur.

Two additional examinations have been proposed to be more specific for detection of discogenic pain: centralization phenomenon (CP) and the bony vibration test (BVT). CP is the report of migration of pain toward the midline of the spine with repeated maneuvers of the spine in flexion-extension or side bending. This pain pattern is thought to arise because of the central location of the disc, which is perceived as midline pain when stressed, compared to facet and SIJ pain, which tend to cause more lateral pain.

The specificity of this test has been reported to range from 70% to 100% with a sensitivity of 64%.[46-49] However, the time and training required for proper performance of this test limits its usefulness in most clinical settings and as a single physical examination maneuver; most experts agree that it is of low value and should be used together with diagnostic testing to make the diagnosis of discogenic pain. BVT involves applying a blunt electric vibrator over the spinous processes of the vertebrae. If the patient reports pain, it suggests discogenic LBP. The sensitivity and specificity of this test are controversial; studies are inconclusive because of questionable patient selection.[50-52] Nonetheless, like the CP, it should be used together with the patient's history and diagnostic testing to make the diagnosis of discogenic LBP.

Imaging and Discogenic Pain

Imaging studies used in evaluation of painful spinal disorders may include plain radiographs, nuclear medicine scans, magnetic resonance imaging (MRI), computed tomography (CT), myelography, CT myelography, and single-photon emission computed tomography (SPECT). Plain radiographs may help detect spinal instability, bony malalignment or deformity, and the presence of degenerative disease. Nuclear medicine scans are useful in detection of tumors, fractures, and infection. SPECT scans may play a limited role in identifying a subset of patients with facet disease.[53]

Before advances in MRI, myelography and CT with and without myelography were commonly used, although not without controversy, in diagnosis and management of disc protrusion, stenotic lesions, and other deformities of the spine.[54-56] Currently, however, MRI is the first line imaging of choice for painful spinal disorders, thanks to its high degree of spatial resolution and the best soft tissue contrast of all the imaging modalities. All of these imaging studies have a high degree of PPV when radiculopathy, nerve root compression, and spinal deformities are the target diagnoses. However, when diagnosing the causes of axial spinal pain, these imaging modalities fail to provide a reasonable PPV; rather their greatest value is to rule out sinister pathology.[3,57-60]

Plain Radiographs

Most agree that plain radiographs in two views (anteroposterior and lateral) should be the first image of choice. Plain films demonstrate lumbar alignment, bone density, and the presence of fractures and osteophytes. Addition of flexion and extension views should be considered before interventional disc treatments are recommended. This will serve to rule out segmental instability. Ideally images should be obtained in the upright weight-bearing posture. The disadvantages of plain radiographs are their inability to provide any information about the integrity of the discs and significant radiation exposure. Digital fluoroscopic video assessment of the spine in the sagittal view has been proposed as an alternative to static end-range flexion and extension images for evaluation of segmental instability. At this time there are insufficient data to support the use of this technology.

Magnetic Resonance Imaging

The MRI provides details of the spinal cord, cauda equina, disc, and paraspinal soft tissue. It is the best image test to evaluate the discs. Three changes detected on MRI may signal discogenic pain: low signal intensity of the disc on T2 weighting, high intensity zone (HIZ), and endplate changes.

Age-related disc degeneration results in reduced water content, resulting in a low signal intensity, or "black disc," on T2 weighting. Although this finding is associated with disc degeneration, most agree that it is poorly correlated with discogenic pain. A study on healthy discs showed that 17% of the discs had low-intensity signals and concluded that this finding has almost a 100% sensitivity but a very low specificity for discogenic LBP.[61,62] The MRI hallmark of internal disc disruption is the HIZ. The HIZ is associated with annular fissures; however, the correlation of the HIZ with discogenic low back pain is controversial. The HIZ is thought to result from inflammation caused by the annular disruption, which leads to stimulation of pain fibers. The correlation of the HIZ to discogenic pain has a sensitivity that ranges from 81% to 92.5%, a specificity that ranges from 26.7% to 89%, and a PPV that ranges from 87% to 90%.[63-65] With grade III tears it has been suggested that the HIZ has a 100% sensitivity and specificity for discogenic pain.[66] Although there is evidence that supports the predictive value of the HIZ for discogenic pain, HIZ is present in a large number of asymptomatic discs (incidence ranging from 25% to 39%), putting into question its predictive value for discogenic pain.[67-70]

DDD often leads to changes in the vertebral endplate, which can be detected on MRI. These endplate changes are classified as Modic I-III changes.[71,72] Modic I changes, known as the inflammatory phase, are characterized by low signal intensity on T1W and high signal intensity on T2W imaging. Modic II changes, known as the fat deposition phase, is characterized by high signal intensity on T1W and an equivalent or mildly high signal on T2W imaging. Modic III changes, known as the bone sclerosis phase, is characterized by low signal intensity in T1W and T2W imaging. Modic changes appear to be more prevalent in patients with LBP than asymptomatic patients.[70,73] Multiple studies have shown a strong correlation between Modic changes, particularly type I, with chronic LBP and positive discography.[74-79] Modic changes appear to have a high sensitivity but low specificity for discogenic pain.[62]

Electrodiagnostics

Electrodiagnostic testing (EDT) is an extension of the history and physical examination. Although EDT does not diagnose discogenic LBP, it can be useful in identifying a radiculopathy as a cause of the pain. In addition, there is overlap between discogenic low back pain and radiculopathy. Most patients with radiculopathy start with discogenic pain. Because nondiscogenic causes of LBP can refer pain into the lower extremity, EDT can be useful in differentiating referred pain from radicular pain. Although EDT is useful in diagnosing lumbar radiculopathy, sensitivity is limited.[80] EDT combined with MRI is much better in diagnosing discogenic LBP than either modality alone.[81,82]

Diagnostic Interventions

Considering the lack of predictive value of available diagnostic imaging and EDT, it is not surprising that diagnostic interventions are relied on so heavily for diagnosis of axial spinal pain. In the absence of correlation between objective data and subjective findings, diagnostic interventions rely on pain provocation or pain relief as a means of identifying the cause.[83] These diagnostic interventions are best conceptualized as an extension of the physical examination and not simply as imaging or laboratory tests performed in clinical medicine. The presence and level of pain ultimately remain subjective parameters and cannot be confirmed or refuted definitively, unlike typical laboratory studies that may be compared to a gold standard. Therefore there is an inherent limitation in application of the principles of diagnostic testing to these interventions. Caution is advised when interpreting measures of sensitivity, specificity, or predictive values for diagnostic interventions.[84] However, this should not be cause for alarm. When viewed from the perspective of probability, with proper application of the principles of medical decision making, and when placed in the proper context of a comprehensive medical evaluation, including history, physical examination, and diagnostic imaging, the results of diagnostic interventions are valuable tools that allow the clinician and patient to select the appropriate course of therapy for painful spinal disorders.[3,4,85]

Diagnostic interventions have a favorable risk-benefit safety profile. Reports of adverse events have been limited to case reports of soft tissue infection.[86] Although extremely rare, high spinal blockade is possible with cervical and possibly thoracic medial branch blockade (MBB). Other adverse events most commonly reported include vasovagal response and headache.[87]

Diagnostic Neural Blockade

Once sinister and nonspinal causes have been ruled out, chronic benign spine pain may be broadly divided into three categories: neuropathic, somatic, and discogenic. The facet joints, SIJs, and IVDs are common causes of somatic and discogenic pain, respectively.[88-98] The combination of the comprehensive medical evaluation, imaging, and neurophysiological testing generally allows for accurate identification of neuropathic causes of spine pain. However, discrimination between somatic and discogenic pain poses a greater challenge. It has been estimated that, in the absence of disc contour abnormalities and associated neurological findings, the comprehensive medical evaluation, diagnostic imaging, neurophysiological testing, and psychological assessment may identify the cause of LBP in as few as 15% of patients.[99-101] In contrast, diagnostic neural blockade may determine the cause of spine pain and help with selection of appropriate treatment options in as many as 85% of patients.[95,96,102] Diagnostic neural blockade may be indicated before therapeutic interventions or surgery.

However, diagnostic blocks are not indicated if the results will not have an impact on future treatment options or if the possible therapeutic options are contraindicated for other reasons. Potential treatment options should be discussed with the patient before proceeding with diagnostic blockade.

Facet Blocks

The predictive value of lumbar MBB has been validated. With adherence to proper technique, local anesthetic blockade of the medial branch of the dorsal primary ramus does not affect adjacent spinal structures that may confound patient responses.[103] Anesthetizing the facet joints using MBB prevents experimentally induced facet joint pain in healthy volunteers.[104] Positive response to MBB reliably predicts successful outcome following medial branch neurotomy.[105] The validity of cervical MBB has also been demonstrated. A small volume of solution injected at the centroid of the cervical articular pillar remains in that location without spread to adjacent spinal structures.[106] Cervical MBB predicts successful outcome from cervical medial branch radiofrequency neurotomy.[107,108] False-negative responses to MBB caused by undetected intravascular injection of the local anesthetic are possible, but they may be eliminated by administration of contrast medium under continuous fluoroscopic examination before local anesthetic administration, leading to a sensitivity approaching 100%. Therefore the face validity and construct validity for these blocks has been well established. Facet joint block may also be accomplished by intraarticular local anesthetic injection. Two main limitations to this approach are failure to place the needle within the joint space and extravasation of local anesthetic outside the joint space because of defects or rupture of the joint capsule. With proper technique, intraarticular injections and MBB are of equal value in diagnostic blockade of the facet joints.[109]

Sacroiliac Blocks

Diagnostic blockade of the SIJ is most commonly achieved by intraarticular injection of local anesthetics. However, this method may lack specificity. Local anesthetics injected in the joint space may spread to adjacent soft tissue and neural structures through defects in the ventral and dorsal capsule.[38,110] Intraarticular injection of local anesthetics may also fail to anesthetize the interosseous or dorsal sacroiliac ligaments, an alternate source of SIJ pain.[111-113] This may lead to false-negative responses.

An alternative to intraarticular SIJ injections is blockade of its neural innervation using local anesthetics. The SIJ is well innervated posteriorly by the medial branch of the L5 dorsal ramus and the lateral branches of the sacral dorsal rami.[114,115] But controversy regarding innervation to the ventral aspect of the joint has not been fully resolved.[116,117] The face validity of lateral branch blocks (LBBs) of the sacral dorsal primary rami was assessed in an anatomical study by a multisite, multidepth injection technique demonstrating successful staining of 91% of target nerves.[118] This is a substantial improvement compared to previously described single-site, single-depth injection technique yielding a 36% success rate. A subsequent placebo controlled study in healthy volunteers demonstrated that 70% of subjects undergoing active local anesthetic blockade were protected from experimentally evoked pain from the interosseous and dorsal sacroiliac ligaments and SIJ puncture. In comparison, only 10% of subjects in the placebo group were protected from evoked pain in the interosseous ligament, and none of the subjects were protected from pain in the dorsal sacroiliac ligament or with SIJ puncture. Interestingly, LBBs did not protect the subjects from pain evoked by SIJ distention. This finding supports the possibility of ventral innervation of the SIJ and addresses prior concerns regarding distinction between intraarticular SIJ pathology vs. extraarticular ligamentous structures.[119]

These findings are consistent with clinical observations. Of patients treated with radiofrequency treatment of the dorsal innervation of the SIJ, 60% to 89% experience relief of pain.[120-122] However, a smaller subset of patients respond well to intraarticular local anesthetic and corticosteroid injections but do not respond to radiofrequency neurotomy. Recent data demonstrate validity of controlled blocks of the L5 medial branch and the sacral lateral branches as a predictor of radiofrequency neurotomy for the SIJ; whereas intraarticular SIJ pathology is best assessed using intraarticular injections. The two diagnostic tests should be used systematically to assess the SIJ complex.[118]

Provocation Discography

Lindblom in 1948[123] and Hirsch in 1949[124] are credited with the first reports of diagnostic puncture of the IVDs in an attempt to diagnose the level of a disc lesion in the context of radiculopathy. The diagnostic value of discography to reproduce back and referred pain in patients with or without evidence of disc protrusion or nerve root compression was noted subsequently by other investigators.[2,125-132] In 1968 Holt's seminal study of discography in asymptomatic volunteers[133] claimed an unacceptably high false-positive rate of 37%. Since then discography has been the subject of controversy and debate.

To a great extent this controversy was related to the changing role of discography. Thanks to the establishment of well-defined techniques and standardized criteria, much of the controversy has been resolved. The specificity and sensitivity of discography as an imaging study for detection of disc degeneration and disc contour abnormalities are high.[58,134-136] Indeed, discography was originally pioneered as a morphological test to replace or add information to myelography. This is in stark contrast to the contemporary role of discography as a physiological, prevocational, diagnostic tool. The debate over discography is regarding its accuracy for diagnosis of discogenic pain. As with other diagnostic interventions, the primary hurdle is the absence of a gold standard. Pathological confirmation or surgical exposure may confirm presence of degenerative disc changes, but the presence or absence of discogenic pain cannot be determined by these techniques.

Twenty years after its publication, Holt's data[133] were subjected to reanalysis using contemporary criteria. The paper has been refuted on methodological grounds and the establishment of new standards that constitute positive discography.[137] Since then several systematic studies have been instrumental in development of criterion standards for diagnosis of discogenic pain. The characteristic pathological feature of IDD is the presence of radial fissures within the AF. The Dallas discogram scale may be used to categorize these radiographic findings. There is a strong correlation between pain on discography and fissures that reach the innervated outer third of the AF.[56] In a controlled prospective study in normal volunteers, Walsh and associates[138] demonstrated that, using standardized uniform criteria, discography is 100% specific as a physiological tool to determine if a disc is painful. Application of the new criteria to Holt's[133] original data resulted in a 3.7% false-positive rate per disc, a marked reduction compared to the original 37%.

In a series of studies Carragee and associates[139,140] reported higher false-positive rates of discography in subjects with nonspine-related chronic pain and subjects with abnormal psychometric profile. These studies underscore the importance of the principles of diagnostic testing in interpretation of results (see **Fig. 2-2**). If diagnostic testing is performed in a population with extremely low prevalence of discogenic pain, by definition the PPV of a positive response is very low. Furthermore, when the contemporary standardized criteria of Walsh[138] are strictly applied to the data, the false-positive rates are observed at 7.1% per disc and 12.5% per patient, in contrast to 28.5% per disc and 50% per patient concluded by the study.[3,141]

These studies raise an important caveat. Presence of overlap in segmental innervation and nociceptive receptor field between the intervertebral disc and adjacent structures may be a confounding factor, causing an increase in false-positive rate of discography. Performance of discography on subjects with prior history of iliac crest bone graft harvest is such an example. The innervation of the iliac crest and superior gluteal region is derived from T12-L3 dorsal rami.[142] However, the sensory innervation of the lumbar IVD may also originate from the upper lumbar dorsal root ganglia (DRGs).[143-145] Clinicians must be aware of other possible sources of pain in patients undergoing discography. These sources may mimic concordant pain on discography.

False-positive rates of lumbar provocation discography in asymptomatic subjects and subjects with chronic pain not related to the lumbar spine were recently subjected to systematic review and meta-analysis.[141] Using the International Spine Intervention Society (ISIS)/International Association for the Study of Pain (IASP)[146] criteria, the false-positive rate for asymptomatic subjects was demonstrated to be 2.1% per disc tested and 3% per patient. For subjects with chronic pain of nonspine origin, the false-positive rate increased slightly to 3.85% per disc and 5.6% per patient.

The impact of chronic LBP on the predictive value of discography was examined by Derby and associates.[147] This study compared discs with grade 3 annular tears in patients with discogenic LBP to grade 3 discs in asymptomatic controls. There was no statistical difference in the pain intensity at increasing pressures between control discs in patients with LBP vs. asymptomatic controls. In contrast, the difference between positive discs and controls in the LBP group was substantial and easily distinguishable by patients. For example, at 50 psi above opening pressure (a.o.) the mean pain scores were as follows: asymptomatic volunteers 1.6/10, control disc in LBP group 1.1/10, and positive discs in LBP group 8.7/10 (p < 0.001). Therefore with standardized criteria discography may reliably distinguish asymptomatic discs among morphologically abnormal discs in patients with chronic LBP.

The effect of abnormal psychometric profiles on discography in patients with chronic LBP has also been studied by Derby and associates.[148] In this study 81 patients with chronic LBP underwent psychometric testing before discography using the Distress and Risk Assessment Method (DRAM).[149-153] Subjects were divided into four groups: normal, at risk, distressed-depressive, and distressed-somatic. There was no statistically significant difference among the psychometric groups with regard to the following measures: (1) Rate of positive discograms; (2) mean pain scores at 15, 30, and 50 psi a.o.; (3) mean pressure at initial pain response; and (4) mean volume at initial pain response. Therefore in patients with chronic LBP abnormal psychometric profiles do not appear to result in increased false-positive rates.

Somatization disorder is a particularly challenging co-morbidity in diagnosis and management of chronic LBP. Manchikanti and associates[154] studied the effect of somatization disorder and other psychiatric co-morbidities on discography in a prospective clinical trial of patients with chronic LBP. All subjects underwent psychological testing using the Millon Clinical Multiaxial Inventory-III (MCMI-III). The study found no difference in positive discography rates between subjects without psychiatric abnormalities compared to those with somatization disorder, depression, generalized anxiety disorder, and combinations thereof. Current evidence supports use of discography as a reliable diagnostic tool in patients with somatization disorder and chronic LBP. Despite this, caution is advised. Patients with somatization disorder are likely to have high rates of recurrence of pain, pseudoneurological symptoms, excessive medication use, and iatrogenic illnesses.[155] This group of patients are also hospitalized and undergo surgery three times as often as depressed patients.[156] Data regarding the predictive value of discography in patients with prior spinal surgery are limited. Carragee[139] reported a false-positive discography rate of 35% per patient in the postsurgical discs of 20 asymptomatic volunteers. The implications of this study are uncertain. Although discectomy may provide symptomatic relief or remission by structural or functional alterations within the disc, there is currently no evidence that after surgical decompression the disc becomes pain free on subsequent provocation discography. Therefore the fundamental premise of the study may not be valid. From a statistical standpoint, in this subgroup the pretest probability of IDD is very high since the subjects have known disease. Therefore the posttest probability of disease and the PPV of the test are also high, and the high discography rate may represent true presence of disease. Further research in this population is indicated.

Provocation discography is not a stand-alone measure for diagnosis of discogenic pain. When applied indiscriminately it has limited predictive value and clinical value. However, in a population with a high pretest probability of discogenic pain as determined by history, physical examination, diagnostic imaging, and appropriate laboratory studies to rule out sinister pathology and identify other potential sources of pain, discography has been demonstrated to have a high degree of PPV for identification of discogenic pain. It is important that clinicians familiarize themselves with clinical risk factors that may lead to increased false-positive results on discography. It is equally important that clinicians use standardized diagnostic criteria and techniques while performing discography to further reduce the false-positive responses.

An Algorithmic Approach to Discogenic Pain

An algorithm may be defined as an explicit protocol with well-defined rules to be followed in solving a complex problem. Algorithms are useful ways of exploring and communicating evidence-based medicine. However, although complex problems in medicine abound, the clinical solutions to those problems are rarely well defined or explicit. Patients rarely present with single, well-defined pathological findings; and, in the case of spine pain, coexistence of multiple pain generators is the rule and not the exception. Therefore no algorithm is able to replace sound clinical judgment, and each individual patient will likely require a unique treatment plan. In this section four sets of algorithms are explored, each addressing a component of the medical decision-making process. Together these algorithms guide the clinician from the initial presentation of axial spine pain through comprehensive patient evaluation and ultimately establishment of the diagnosis of discogenic pain.

Chronic Pain Algorithm

Fig. 2-5 summarizes the general algorithm for evaluation of the patient with persistent chronic pain. As with any chronic pain condition, chronic LBP, especially discogenic pain, should be evaluated in the context of a multidisciplinary model. The algorithm starts with a thorough history and physical examination. The history and physical examination specific to discogenic LBP was discussed previously. The provider must first search for "red flags" that require immediate attention or specialty evaluation. In addition, physical functioning, litigation or secondary gain, and any inconsistencies in the patient's reported mechanism of injury and complaints must be thoroughly assessed. After a thorough history and physical examination, a differential diagnosis can be established that then guides the diagnostic pathway to be taken. After the diagnosis of discogenic LBP has been made, a multidisciplinary approach to management is often required since single-modality physical treatments are often not enough to address the problem. This is especially true for patients who are severely deconditioned or have litigation or coexisting psychosocial issues. If interventional therapies are recommended for the treatment of the discogenic pain, other concomitant therapies such as medication management, behavioral therapies, and physical therapies should be considered.

Frequent reevaluation may be required during the treatment of discogenic LBP since the patient responses are highly variable. For patients with persistent pain, the history and physical examination should be performed again, and the algorithm revisited.

Chronic Low Back Pain Algorithm

Fig. 2-6 summarizes the initial approach to the patient with spine pain. As discussed previously, the first step in evaluation of the patient with spine pain is comprehensive history and physical examination. The first question the clinician must answer is whether sinister pathology is present. Once the differential diagnosis is narrowed, the spinal causes of pain may be explored systematically. History, physical examination, imaging, and EDT are

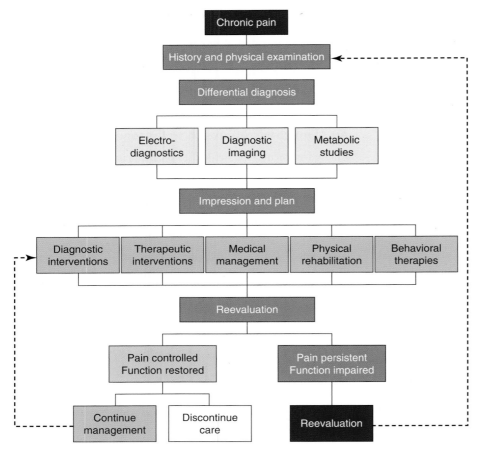

Fig. 2-5 Chronic pain algorithm.

highly sensitive and specific for identification of radiculopathy, with a very favorable risk-benefit profile for treatment. Therefore identification and treatment of radicular symptoms is the first step in management of spinal pain. Next attention is diverted to possible somatic causes of spine pain such as facet and SIJ disease. As previously mentioned, other potential sources of pain in the axial region should also be identified since they may mimic concordant discogenic pain. Only when radicular and somatic causes have been ruled out or treated is attention focused on discogenic pain. This approach allows the clinician to select a population of patients with the highest pretest probability of discogenic pain, leading to a high rate of success. This approach also ensures that more conservative lower-risk and less expensive modalities appropriate to the care of the patient are used first.

Discogenic Pain Algorithm

Once patients with a high pretest probability of discogenic pain have been identified, two questions are raised:

1. Is this patient an appropriate candidate for provocation discography?
2. Will discography results have a meaningful impact on potential treatment options? Alternatively stated, is the patient an appropriate candidate for specific treatment options that would follow diagnostic discography? If no such treatment option exists, discography should not be performed since it has no intrinsic therapeutic value.

Fig. 2-7 explores the discogenic pain algorithm. Dynamic imaging of the spine with flexion and extension radiographs in the upright weight-bearing position should be performed early in

the decision-making process to rule out segmental instability that may preclude the patient from percutaneous disc treatments and shift the care toward surgical intervention. Low-grade degenerative spondylolisthesis without evidence of dynamic instability does not automatically preclude patients from percutaneous treatment options but may have a negative prognostic impact and affect the treatment options. For example, electrothermal annuloplasty may be relatively contraindicated in this instance, but treatment options with no impact on integrity of the AF may be well tolerated. Evidence is lacking to assist the clinician in this decision process, and caution is advised.

Next, advanced imaging should be evaluated, most commonly MRI. Patients with single-level minimal-to-moderate DDD, good disc height preservation, and minimal-to-no evidence of a stenotic lesion are the ideal candidates for provocation discography and potential percutaneous disc treatments. Patients with three or more levels of DDD, sequestered or extruded discs, 60% or greater loss of disc height, severe degenerative changes, and high-grade stenotic lesions are poor candidates for percutaneous disc treatments. In these situations discography is not routinely recommended but may be appropriate in individual cases to help determine potential treatment options. For example, confirmation of single-level discogenic pain in association with spondylolisthesis with absence of pain from adjacent discs may reduce a potential multilevel spinal fusion with instrumentation (based on diagnostic imaging alone) to a single-level procedure with improved outcome. Alternatively, in selected cases a two-step staged treatment plan may be indicated with percutaneous disc decompression at one level followed by surgical stabilization of an adjacent level in 3 to 6 months.

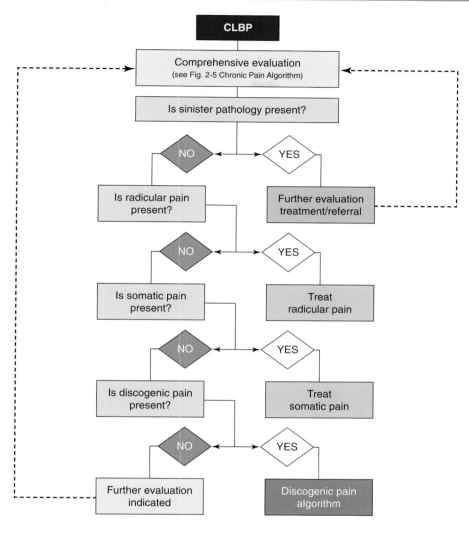

Fig. 2-6 Chronic low back pain (CLBP) algorithm.

Discography Algorithm

Even in experienced hands, discography is a painful and anxiety-provoking intervention. Patient preparation, establishment of a therapeutic relationship, and effective communication are important keys to obtaining accurate and reliable test results and a satisfied patient despite significant intraoperative and postoperative discomfort. Adherence to standardized criteria is critical to minimize the false-positive rate and maximize the PPV of discography. The algorithm for provocation discography is summarized in **Fig. 2-8.** Ideal predictors for discogenic pain include concordant pain ≥7/10 provoked at an intradiscal pressure of ≤50 psi a.o. in conjunction with radiographic findings of grade 3 annular tear and the presence of a radiographically normal control disc with 0/10 pain. Failure to meet these criteria may contribute to increased false-positive rates and decreased predictive value of discography. Presence of a grade 5 annular tear with extravasation of contrast medium outside the disc margin poses a special challenge. These discs may be very difficult to adequately pressurize with the usual volumes and rates of contrast administration. This may result in a higher false-negative rate and the risk of missing the diagnosis. Higher volumes and rates of contrast injection may be necessary during discography to adequately test these discs. Identification of grade 5 tears serves another important function of discography. Presence of full-thickness tears is a risk factor for development of neurological deficit after thermal disc lesions. Discography is mandatory before thermal disc treatments.

> **Box 2-3: Recommendations for Improved Accuracy and Success with Discography**
>
> - Communicate effectively (consider interpreter).
> - Identify patient's usual pain distribution and character in advance.
> - Educate patient about discography.
> - Educate patient in advance on proper use of the pain numerical rating scale.
> - Avoid excessive sedation.
> - Insert needles on the least symptomatic side.
> - Validate each pain response by confirmatory pressurization.
> - Keep the volume of contrast ≤3.5 mL for grade 0 to 4 discs.
> - Increased rate and volume of contrast may be necessary for grade 5 tears or endplate fractures to reach 50 psi a.o.
> - Continue patient's usual analgesics before discography to avoid withdrawal and increased false-positive rates.
>
> *a.o.,* Above opening pressure.

Box 2-3 provides a list of other recommendations for improved accuracy and success with discography. Discography involves interpretation of subjective information. As such, all impediments to effective communication must be eliminated in advance. Consider the use of a qualified medical interpreter in case of a language barrier. The patient's usual pain distribution and characteristics must be discussed immediately before the start of the procedure

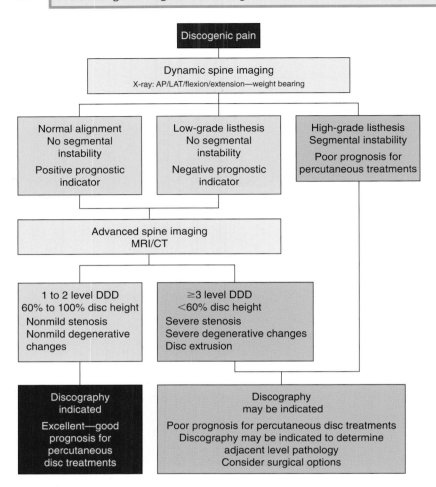

Fig. 2-7 Discogenic pain algorithm. *AP*, Anteroposterior; *CT*, computed tomography; *DDD*, degenerative disc disease; *MRI*, magnetic resonance imaging.

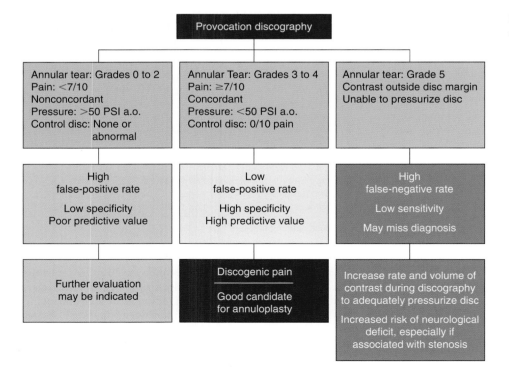

Fig. 2-8 Discography algorithm. *a.o.*, Above opening pressure.

and before administration of sedatives or analgesics so the concordance of symptoms may be confirmed clearly during the test. The patient must be educated in detail about what to expect at every stage of the procedure and proper use of the numerical rating scale (NRS). Consider educating the patient about specific clinical examples of mild, moderate, and severe pain and their corresponding numbers on the NRS. Other recommendations include avoiding excessive levels of sedation during the procedure, which may result in false-negative responses. Excessive sedation may also lead to increased risk of injury during interventional therapies. Alternatively, in selected patients prone to emotional disinhibition, use of benzodiazepines is best avoided. Patients on chronic analgesics should be instructed to continue their usual medications. This helps to avoid a state of early withdrawal immediately before the procedure and the potential for false-positive responses. It is recommended that needles be inserted on the asymptomatic or least symptomatic side of the patient's spine. Once an initial pain response is provoked, consider validating the response by further confirmatory pressurization of the disc, especially when the initial pain response is sudden and short-lived. The volume of contrast administered should be kept below 3.5 mL. Increased volumes may result in false-positive responses. However, for discs with grade 5 annual tears or endplate fractures, increased volume and rate of contrast administration may be necessary to achieve adequate pressurization of the disc and pain reproduction.[157]

Conclusion

Holt's contentious publication in 1968[133] catapulted the topic of discogenic pain into decades of debate and controversy. However, thanks to a multitude of contributions over the last two decades from experts in both camps, we now have a far greater understanding of this condition. With an estimated prevalence of 26% to 39% among those with chronic LBP, discogenic pain is of major medical and economic concern. For many individuals with chronic LBP, the controversy and lack of understanding has led to years of unnecessary suffering, misdiagnosis, and maltreatment. As a result of the complexity of this condition, no single test or intervention can accurately establish the diagnosis of discogenic pain. Rather, a comprehensive and systematic investigation must be undertaken that begins with a targeted history and physical examination followed by diagnostic and therapeutic interventions and ultimately, for selected individuals, culminating in discography to confirm the diagnosis and level of disease. An integral part of this systematic approach is strict adherence to patient selection guidelines, standardized diagnostic criteria for discography, and proper technique.

The journey toward full understanding and effective treatment of discogenic pain is not yet complete. The algorithms presented here should not only serve individual clinicians through this systematic evaluation process but also establish a unified approach among the various specialties dealing with discogenic pain. It is through this standardized approach that understanding of this challenging condition will continue to expand.

References

1. Inman VT, Saunders JB: Anatomicophysiological aspects of injuries to the intervertebral disc. *J Bone Joint Surg [Am]* 29:461-475, 1947.
2. Crock HV: A reappraisal of intervertebral disc lesions. *Med J Aust* 1:983-989, 1970.
3. Saal JS: General principles of diagnostic testing as related to painful lumbar spine disorders: a critical appraisal of current diagnostic techniques, *Spine* 27:2538-2545; discussion 2546, 2002.
4. Lurie JD, Sox HC: Principles of medical decision making. *Spine* 24:493-498, 1999.
5. Kong A, Barnett GO, Mosteller F, et al: How medical professionals evaluate expressions of probability. *N Engl J Med* 315:740-744 1986.
6. Mazur DJ, Hickam DH: Patients' interpretations of probability terms. *J Gen Intern Med* 6:237-240, 1991.
7. Andersson GB, Deyo RA: History and physical examination in patients with herniated lumbar discs. *Spine* 21:10S-18S, 1996.
8. Altman DG, Bland JM: Diagnostic tests 2: predictive values. *Br Med J* 309:102, 1994.
9. Bogduk N: Principles of diagnostic blocks, interventional spine. In Slip CW, editor: *An Algorithmic Approach*, ed 1, Philadelphia, 2008, Saunders, pp 187-188.
10. Videman T, Nurminen M, Troup J: Lumbar spinal pathology in cadaveric material in relation to history of back pain, occupation, and physical loading. *Spine* 15:728-740, 1990.
11. Ashton I et al: Morphological basis for back pain: the demonstration of nerve fibers and neuropeptides in the lumbar facet joint capsule but not in the ligamentum flavum. *J Orthop Res* 10:72, 1992.
12. Giles L: Pathoanatomic studies and clinical significance of lumbosacral zygapophyseal (facet) joints. *J Manip Physiol Ther* 15:36-40, 1992.
13. Cassidy J: The pathoanatomy and clinical significance of the sacroiliac joints. *J Manip Physiol Ther* 15:41-42, 1992.
14. Daum W: The sacroiliac joint: an underappreciated pain generator. *Am J Orthop* 24:475-478, 1995.
15. Don Tigny R: Anterior dysfunction of the sacroiliac joint as a major factor in the etiology of idiopathic low back pain syndrome. *Phys Ther* 70:250-265, 1990.
16. Jajic I, Jajic Z: The prevalence of osteoarthritis of the sacroiliac joints in an urban population. *Clin Rheum* 6:39-41, 1987.
17. Walker J: The sacroiliac joint: a critical review. *Phys Ther* 72:903-916, 1992.
18. Bowen V, Cassidy J: Macroscopic and microscopic anatomy of the sacroiliac joint from embryonic life until the eighth decade. *Spine* 6:620-628, 1981.
19. Walker J: Age-related differences in the human sacroiliac joint: a histological study: implications of therapy. *J Orthop Sports Phys Ther* 7:325-334, 1986.
20. Bogduk N: The innervation of the lumbar spine. *Spine* 8:286, 1983.
21. Bogduk N, Wilson A, Tynan W: The human lumbar dorsal rami. *J Anat* 134:383-397, 1982.
22. Ikeda R: Innervation of the sacroiliac joint: macroscopic and histological studies. *J Nippon Med School* 58:587-596, 1991.
23. Groen G, Baljet B, Drukker J: Nerves and nerve plexuses of the human vertebral column. *Am J Anat* 188:282, 1990.
24. Malinsky J: The ontogenetic development of nerve terminations in the intravertebral discs of man. *Acta Anat* 38:96-113, 1959.
25. Yamashita T et al: Mechanosensitive afferent units in the lumbar intervertebral disc and adjacent muscle. *Spine* 18:2252-2256, 1993.
26. Yashizawa H et al: The neuropathology of intervertebral discs removed for low-back pain. *J Pathol* 132:95-104, 1980.
27. Weinstein J, Claverie W, Gibson S: The pain of discography. *Spine* 13:1344-1348, 1988.
28. Bogduk N, Twomey L, editors: *Clinical anatomy of the lumbar spine*, Melbourne, 1991, Churchill Livingstone.
29. Gronblad M, Weinstein J, Santavirta S: Immunohistochemical observations on spinal tissue innervation: a review of hypothetical mechanisms of back pain. *Acta Orthop Scand* 2:614-622, 1991.
30. Pionchon H et al: Study of the innervation of the spinal ligaments at the lumbar level. *Bull de L Assoc des Anat* 70:63-67, 1986.
31. Yahia H, Newman N: A light and electron microscopic study of spinal ligament innervation. *Zeitschrift fur Mikroskopisch-Anatomische Forschung* 03:664-674, 1989.
32. Rhalmi A et al: Immunohistochemical study of nerves in lumbar spine ligaments. *Spine* 18:264-267, 1993.
33. Haughton V, Nguyen C, Ho K: The etiology of focal spinal arachnoiditis: an experimental study. *Spine* 18:1193-1198, 1993.

34. Dorsi M, Belzberg A: Low back pain. In Wallace M, editor: *Just the facts*, New York, 2005, McGraw Hill, pp 141-146.

35. Bernard T, Cassidy J: The sacroiliac joint syndrome: pathophysiology, diagnosis, and management. In Frymoyer J, editor: *The adult spine: principles and practice*, New York, 1991, Raven Press, p 2107.

36. Fortin J et al: Sacroiliac joint: pain referral maps upon applying a new injection/arthrography technique. Part II. Clinical evaluation. *Spine* 19:1483-1489, 1994.

37. Fortin J et al: Sacroiliac joint: pain referral maps upon applying a new injection/arthrography technique. Part I: asymptomatic volunteers, *Spine* 19:1475-1482, 1994.

38. Schwarzer AC, Aprill CN, Bogduk N: The sacroiliac joint in chronic low back pain. *Spine* 20:31-37, 1995.

39. Jajic Z et al: Analysis of the location of pain related to sacroiliitis in ankylosing spondylitis. *Reumatizam* 41:1-3, 1994.

40. Nachemson A: The effect of forward leaning on lumbar intradiscal pressure. *Acta Orthop Scand* 35:314-328, 1965.

41. Wilde G, Szypryt E, Mulholland R: Unilateral lumbar facet joint hypertrophy causing nerve root irritation. *Ann Royal Coll Surg Eng* 70:307-310, 1988.

42. Dreyfuss P et al: Positive sacroiliac screening tests in asymptomatic adults. *Spine* 19:1138-1143, 1994.

43. Potter N, Rothstein J: Intertester reliability for selected clinical tests of the sacroiliac joint. *Phys Ther* 65:1671-1675, 1985.

44. Bernard T, Kirkaldy-Willis W: Recognizing specific characteristics of nonspecific low back pain. *Clin Orthop Relat Res* 217:266-280, 1987.

45. Laslett M, William M: The reliability of selected pain provocation tests for sacroiliac joint pathology. *Spine* 19:1243-1249, 1994.

46. Donelson R et al: A prospective study of centralization of lumbar and referred pain: a predictor of symptomatic discs and anular competence. *Spine* 22:1115-1122, 1997.

47. Berthelot J et al: Contributions of centralization phenomenon to the diagnosis, prognosis, and treatment of diskogenic low back pain. *Joint Bone Spin* 74:319-323, 2007.

48. Yountg S, April C, Laslett M: Correlation of clinical examination characteristics with three sources of chronic low back pain. *Spine* 3:460-465, 2003.

49. Laslett M et al: Centralization as a predictor of provocation discography results in chronic low back pain and the influence of disability and distress on diagnostic power. *Spine* 5:370-380, 2005.

50. Yrjama M, Vanharanta H: Bony vibration stimulation: a new non-invasive method for examining intradiscal pain, *Eur Spine* 3:233-235, 1994.

51. Yrjama M, Tervonen O, Vanharanta H: Ultrasonic imaging of lumbar discs combined with vibration pain provocation compared with discography in the diagnosis of internal annular fissures of the lumbar spine. *Spine* 21:571-575, 1997.

52. Yrjama M et al: Bony vibration stimulation test combined with magnetic resonance imaging: Can discography be replaced? *Spine* 22:808-813, 1997.

53. Dolan AL et al: The value of SPECT scans in identifying back pain likely to benefit from facet joint injection. *Br J Rheumatol* 35:1269-1273, 1994.

54. Antti-Poika I et al: Clinical relevance of discography combined with CT scanning: a study of 100 patients. *J Bone Joint Surg [Br]* 72:480-485, 1990.

55. Jackson RP et al: The neuroradiographic diagnosis of lumbar herniated nucleus pulposus. I. A comparison of computed tomography (CT), myelography, CT-myelography, discography, and CT-discography. *Spine* 14:1356-1361, 1989.

56. Vanharanta H et al: A comparison of CT/discography, pain response and radiographic disc height. *Spine* 13:321-324, 1988.

57. Jensen MC et al: Magnetic resonance imaging of the lumbar spine in people without back pain. *N Engl J Med* 331:69-73, 1994.

58. Milette PC et al: Differentiating lumbar disc protrusions, disc bulges, and discs with normal contour but abnormal signal intensity: magnetic resonance imaging with discographic correlations. *Spine* 24:44-53, 1999.

59. Smith BM et al: Interobserver reliability of detecting lumbar intervertebral disc high-intensity zone on magnetic resonance imaging and association of high-intensity zone with pain and anular disruption. *Spine* 23:2074-2080, 1998.

60. Hicks GE, Morone N, Weiner DK: Degenerative lumbar disc and facet joint disease in older adults: prevalence and clinical correlates. *Spine* 34:1301-1306, 2009.

61. Collins C et al: The role of discography in lumbar disc disease: a comparative study of magnetic resonance imaging and discography. *Clin Radiol* 4:252-257, 1990.

62. Zhang Y-G et al: Clinical diagnosis of discogenic low back pain. *Int J Biol Sci* 6:647-658, 2009.

63. April C, Bodguk N: High-intensity zone: a diagnostic sign of painful lumbar disc on magnetic resonance imaging. *Br J Radiol* 773:361-369, 1992.

64. Saifuddin A et al: The value of lumbar spine magnetic resonance imaging in the demonstration of annular tears. *Spine* 23:453-457, 1998.

65. Lam K, Carlin D, Mulholland R: Lumbar disc high-intensity zone: the value and significance of provocative discography in the determination of the discogenic pain source. *Eur Spine* 9(1):36-41, 2000.

66. Peng B et al: The pathogenesis and clinical significance of a high-intensity zone (HIZ) of lumbar intervertebral disc on MR imaging in the patient with discogenic low back pain. *Eur Spine* 15:583-587, 2006.

67. Carragee E, Paragioudakis S, Khurana S: Lumbar high-intensity zone and discography in subjects without low back problems. *Spine* 25:2987-2992, 2000.

68. Carragee E et al: A gold standard evaluation of the "discogenic pain" diagnosis as determined by provocative discography. *Spine* 31:2115-2123, 2006.

69. Boden S et al: Abnormal magnetic-resonance scans of the lumbar spine in asymptomatic subjects: a prospective investigation. *J Bone Joint Surg [Am]* 72:403-408, 1990.

70. Mitra D, Cassar-Pullicino V, McCall I: Longitudinal study of vertebral type-1 end plate changes on MR of the lumbar spine. *Eur Radiol* 14:1574-1581, 2004.

71. Modic M et al: Imaging of degenerative disk disease. *Radiology* 168:177-186, 1988.

72. Modic M, Steinberg P, Ross J, et al: Degenerative disk disease: assessment of changes in vertebral body marrow with MR imaging. *Radiology* 166:193-199, 1988.

73. Karchevsky M et al: Reactive endplate marrow changes: a systematic morphologic and epidemiologic evaluation. *Skeletal Radiol* 34:125-129, 2005.

74. Albert H, Manniche C: Modic changes following lumbar disc herniation. *Eur Spine* 16:977-982, 2007.

75. Kjaer P et al: Modic changes and their associations with clinical findings. *Eur Spine* 15:1312-1319, 2006.

76. Kjaer P et al: Magnestic resonance imaging and low back pain in adults: a diagnostic imaging study of 40 year old men and women. *Spine* 30:1173-1180, 2005.

77. Marshman L et al: Reverse transformation of Modic type 2 changes to Modic type 1 changes during sustained chronic low back pain severity: report of two cases and review of literature. *J Neurosurg Spine* 6:152-155, 2007.

78. Braithwaite I et al: Vertebral end plate (Modic) changes on lumbar spine MRI: correlation with pain reproduction at lumbar discography. *Eur Spine* 7:363-368, 1998.

79. Buttermann G: The effect of spinal steroid injections for degenerative disc disease. *Spine J* 4:495-505, 2004.

80. Dillingham T: Electrodiagnostic approach to patients with suspected radiculopathy. *Phys Med Rehabil Clin North Am* 13:567, 2002.

81. McDonald C et al: Magnetic resonance imaging of denervated muscle: comparison to electromyography. *Muscle Nerve* 23:1431, 2000.

82. Nardin R et al: Electromyography and magnetic resonance imaging in the evaluation of radiculopathy. *Muscle Nerve* 22:151, 1999.

83. Ito M et al: Predictive signs of discogenic lumbar pain on magnetic resonance imaging with discography correlation. *Spine* 23:1252-1258; discussion 1259-1260, 1998.

84. Nicoll D, Pignone M: Basic principles of diagnostic test use and interpretation. In Nicoll D: *Pocket guide to diagnostic tests*, ed 3, New York, 2001, McGraw-Hill, pp 1-21.

85. Griner PF et al: Selection and interpretation of diagnostic tests and procedures: principles and applications. *Ann Intern Med* 94:557-592, 1981.

86. Cook NJ, Hanrahan P, Song S: Paraspinal abscess following facet joint injection. *Clin Rheumatol* 18:52-53, 1999.

87. Zhou Y, Thompson S: Quality assurance for interventional pain management procedures in private practice. *Pain Physician* 11:43-55, 2008.

88. Bogduk N, editor: *Clinical anatomy of lumbar spine and sacrum*, New York, 2005, Churchill Livingstone, pp 183-216.

89. van Tulder MW et al: Spinal radiographic findings and nonspecific low back pain: a systematic review of observational studies. *Spine* 22:427-434, 1997.

90. Hancock MJ et al: Systematic review of tests to identify the disc, SIJ, or facet joint as the source of low back pain. *Eur Spine J* 16:1539-1550, 2007.

91. Schwarzer AC et al: The value of the provocation response in lumbar zygapophyseal joint injections. *Clin J Pain* 10:309-313, 1994.

92. Schwarzer AC et al: Pain from the lumbar zygapophyseal joints: a test of two models. *J Spinal Disord* 7:331-336, 1994.

93. Laslett M et al: Clinical predictors of screening lumbar zygapophyseal joint blocks: development of clinical prediction rules. *Spine J* 6:370-379, 2006.

94. Schwarzer AC et al: The ability of computed tomography to identify a painful zygapophyseal joint in patients with chronic low back pain. *Spine* 20:907-912, 1995.

95. Pang WW et al: Application of spinal pain mapping in the diagnosis of low back pain: analysis of 104 cases. *Acta Anaesthesiol Sin* 36:71-74, 1998.

96. Manchikanti L et al: Evaluation of the relative contributions of various structures in chronic low back pain. *Pain Physician* 4:308-316, 2001.

97. Kuslich SD, Ulstrom CL, Michael CJ: The tissue origin of low back pain and sciatica: a report of pain response to tissue stimulation during operations on the lumbar spine using local anesthesia. *Orthop Clin North Am* 22:181-187, 1991.

98. Bogduk N: International Spinal Injection Society guidelines for the performance of spinal injection procedures. Part 1: Zygapophyseal joint blocks. *Clin J Pain* 13:285-302, 1997.

99. Bogduk N, McGuirk B: Causes and sources of chronic low back pain. In Bogduk N, editor: *Medical management of acute and chronic low back pain: an evidence-based approach: pain research and clinical management*, Amsterdam, 2002, Elsevier Science BV, pp 115-126.

100. Bogduk N, McGuirk B: An algorithm for precision diagnosis. In Bogduk N, editor: *Medical management of acute and chronic low back pain: an evidence-based approach: pain research and clinical management*, Amsterdam, 2002, Elsevier Science BV, pp 177-186.

101. Deyo RA, Rainville J, Kent DL: What can the history and physical examination tell us about low back pain? *JAMA* 268:760-765, 1992.

102. Yin W, Bogduk N: The nature of neck pain in a private pain clinic in the United States. *Pain Med* 9:196-203, 2008.

103. Dreyfuss P et al: Specificity of lumbar medial branch and L5 dorsal ramus blocks: a computed tomography study. *Spine* 22:895-902, 1997.

104. Kaplan M et al: The ability of lumbar medial branch blocks to anesthetize the zygapophysial joint: a physiologic challenge. *Spine* 23:1847-1852, 1998.

105. Dreyfuss P et al: Efficacy and validity of radiofrequency neurotomy for chronic lumbar zygapophysial joint pain. *Spine* 25:1270-1277, 2000.

106. Barnsley L, Bogduk N: Medial branch blocks are specific for the diagnosis of cervical zygapophyseal joint pain. *Reg Anesth* 18:343-350, 1993.

107. Lord SM et al: Percutaneous radio-frequency neurotomy for chronic cervical zygapophyseal-joint pain. *N Engl J Med* 335:1721-1726, 1996.

108. McDonald GJ, Lord SM, Bogduk N: Long-term follow-up of patients treated with cervical radiofrequency neurotomy for chronic neck pain. *Neurosurgery* 45:61-67; discussion 67-68, 1999.

109. Marks RC, Houston T, Thulbourne T: Facet joint injection and facet nerve block: a randomised comparison in 86 patients with chronic low back pain. *Pain* 49:325-328, 1992.

110. Fortin JD, Washington WJ, Falco FJ: Three pathways between the sacroiliac joint and neural structures. *Am J Neuroradiol* 20:1429-1434, 1999.

111. Szadek KM et al: Nociceptive nerve fibers in the sacroiliac joint in humans. *Reg Anesth Pain Med* 33:36-43, 2008.

112. Vilensky JA et al: Histologic analysis of neural elements in the human sacroiliac joint. *Spine* 27:1202-1207, 2002.

113. McGrath MC, Zhang M: Lateral branches of dorsal sacral nerve plexus and the long posterior sacroiliac ligament. *Surg Radiol Anat* 27:327-330, 2005.

114. Fortin JD et al: Sacroiliac joint innervation and pain. *Am J Orthop* 28:687-690, 1999.

115. Grob KR, Neuhuber WL, Kissling RO: Innervation of the sacroiliac joint of the human. *Z Rheumatol* 54:117-122, 1995.

116. Ikeda R: Innervation of the sacroiliac joint: Macroscopical and histological studies. *Nippon Ika Daigaku Zasshi* 58:587-596, 1991.

117. Solonen KA: The sacroiliac joint in the light of anatomical, roentgenological and clinical studies. *Acta Orthop Scand* 27(suppl):1-127, 1957.

118. Dreyfuss P et al: The ability of multi-site, multi-depth sacral lateral branch blocks to anesthetize the sacroiliac joint complex. *Pain Med* 10:679-688, 2009.

119. Laslett M: The value of the physical examination in diagnosis of painful sacroiliac joint pathologies. *Spine* 23:962-964, 1998.

120. Vallejo R et al: Pulsed radiofrequency denervation for the treatment of sacroiliac joint syndrome. *Pain Med* 7:429-434, 2006.

121. Yin W et al: Sensory stimulation-guided sacroiliac joint radiofrequency neurotomy: technique based on neuroanatomy of the dorsal sacral plexus. *Spine* 28:2419-2425, 2003.

122. Cohen SP, Abdi S: Lateral branch blocks as a treatment for sacroiliac joint pain: a pilot study. *Reg Anesth Pain Med* 28:113-119, 2003.

123. Lindblom K: Diagnostic puncture of intervertebral disks in sciatica. *Acta Orthop Scand* 17:231-239, 1948.

124. Hirsch C: An attempt to diagnose the level of a disc lesion clinically by disc puncture. *Acta Orthop Scand* 18:132-140, 1949.

125. Friedman J, Goldner MZ: Discography in evaluation of lumbar disk lesions. *Radiology 1955*; 65:653-662, 1955.

126. Keck C: Discography: technique and interpretation. *Arch Surg* 80:580-585, 1960.

127. Butt WP: Lumbar discography. *J Can Assoc Radiol* 14:172-181, 1963.

128. Feinberg SB: The place of diskography in radiology as based on 2,320 cases. *Am J Roentgenol Radium Ther Nucl Med* 92:1275-1281, 1964.

129. Wiley JJ, Macnab I, Wortzman G: Lumbar discography and its clinical applications. *Can J Surg* 11:280-289, 1968.

130. Wilson DH, MacCarty WC: Discography: its role in the diagnosis of lumbar disc protrusion. *J Neurosurg* 31:520-523, 1969.

131. Patrick BS: Lumbar discography: a five-year study. *Surg Neurol* 1:267-273, 1973.

132. Simmons EH, Segil CM: An evaluation of discography in the localization of symptomatic levels in discogenic disease of the spine. *Clin Orthop Relat Res* 57-69, 1975.

133. Holt EP, Jr.: The question of lumbar discography. *J Bone Joint Surg [Am]* 50:720-726, 1968.

134. Haueisen DC et al: The diagnostic accuracy of spinal nerve injection studies: their role in the evaluation of recurrent sciatica. *Clin Orthop Relat Res* 179-183, 1985.

135. Vanharanta H et al: Disc deterioration in low-back syndromes: a prospective, multi-center CT/discography study. *Spine* 13:1349-1351, 1988.

136. Schellhas KP et al: Lumbar disc high-intensity zone. correlation of magnetic resonance imaging and discography. *Spine* 21:79-86, 1996.

137. Simmons JW, Aprill CN, Dwyer AP, et al: A reassessment of Holt's data on: "the question of lumbar discography." *Clin Orthop Relat Res* 237:120-124, 1988.

138. Walsh TR et al: Lumbar discography in normal subjects: a controlled, prospective study. *J Bone Joint Surg [Am]* 72:1081-1088, 1990.

139. Carragee EJ et al: False-positive findings on lumbar discography: reliability of subjective concordance assessment during provocative disc injection. *Spine* 24:2542-2547, 1999.

140. Carragee EJ et al: The rates of false-positive lumbar discography in select patients without low back symptoms. *Spine* 25:1373-1380; discussion 1381, 2000.

141. Wolfer LR et al: Systematic review of lumbar provocation discography in asymptomatic subjects with a meta-analysis of false-positive rates. *Pain Physician* 11:513-538, 2008.

142. Maigne JY, Doursounian L: Entrapment neuropathy of the medial superior cluneal nerve: nineteen cases surgically treated, with a minimum of 2 years' follow-up. *Spine* 22:1156-1159, 1997.

143. Morinaga T et al: Sensory innervation to the anterior portion of lumbar intervertebral disc. *Spine* 21:1848-1851, 1996.

144. Aoki Y et al: Sensory innervation of the lateral portion of the lumbar intervertebral disc in rats. *Spine J* 4:275-280, 2004.

145. Ohtori S et al: Sensory innervation of the dorsal portion of the lumbar intervertebral discs in rats. *Spine* 26:946-950, 2001.

146. Bogduk N: Lumbar disc stimulation. In Bogduk N, editor: *Practice guidelines for spinal diagnostic and treatment procedures*, San Francisco, 2004, International Spine Intervention Society, pp 20-46.

147. Derby R et al: Comparison of discographic findings in asymptomatic subject discs and the negative discs of chronic LBP patients: can discography distinguish asymptomatic discs among morphologically abnormal discs? *Spine J* 5:389-394, 2005.

148. Derby R et al: The influence of psychologic factors on diskography in patients with chronic axial low back pain. *Arch Phys Med Rehabil* 89:1300-1304, 2008.

149. Main CJ et al: The distress and risk assessment method: a simple patient classification to identify distress and evaluate the risk of poor outcome. *Spine* 17:42-52, 1992.

150. Main CJ: The modified somatic perception questionnaire (MSPQ). *J Psychosom Res* 27:503-514, 1983.

151. Mannion AF, Dolan P, Adams MA: Psychological questionnaires: do "abnormal" scores precede or follow first-time low back pain? *Spine* 21:2603-2611, 1996.

152. Wand BM, Bird C, McAuley JH, et al: Early intervention for the management of acute low back pain: a single-blind randomized controlled trial of biopsychosocial education, manual therapy, and exercise. *Spine* 29:2350-2356, 2004.

153. Waddell G et al: Chronic low-back pain, psychologic distress, and illness behavior. *Spine* 9:209-213, 1984.

154. Manchikanti L et al: Provocative discography in low back pain patients with or without somatization disorder: a randomized prospective evaluation. *Pain Physician* 4:227-239, 2001.

155. Ketterer MW, Buckholtz CD: Somatization disorder. *J Am Osteopath Assoc* 89:489-490, 495-499, 1989.

156. Zoccolillo MS, Cloninger CR: Excess medical care of women with somatization disorder. *South Med J* 79:532-535, 1986.

157. Landers MH et al: Lumbar spinal neuraxial procedures. In Raj PP, editor: *Interventional pain management: image guided procedures*, ed 2, Philadelphia, 2008, Saunders Elsevier, pp 322-367.

3 Imaging for Discogenic Pain

Timothy P. Maus and David P. Martin

CHAPTER OVERVIEW

Chapter Synopsis: Utilization of imaging studies for the diagnosis of back pain has increased significantly in recent years; the critical question is whether this improves patient outcomes This chapter will initially look to the literature to assess the sensitivity, specificity, risks, and benefits of imaging the back pain patient. It will then summarize the existing literature on the identification of discogenic pain by noninvasive imaging. The primary role of imaging in the back pain patient is the detection of underlying systemic disease, a very uncommon occurrence. Imaging does incur risk. Exposure to radiation can accrue with multiple imaging procedures. Imaging is costly and may inappropriately label the patient as suffering from a degenerative process, which may lead to fear-avoidance behaviors with subsequent deconditioning and/or depression. When imaging studies are performed, the likelihood of minimally invasive procedures and surgery, which carry their own risks, increases dramatically. Finally, imaging techniques for spinal pain (and discogenic pain in particular) have limited specificity and sensitivity, which may lead to false-negative or false-positive diagnoses.

There is extensive literature addressing identification of discogenic pain on imaging studies, and its correlation with provocation discography. Distilling this to a coherent set of interpretive guidelines requires a careful, critical analysis, which we undertake and present to the reader.

Important Points:
- The decision to image patients with possible discogenic pain should carefully weigh risk and cost against possible benefit.
- The primary role of imaging is the detection of underlying systemic disease.
- Degenerative changes on all imaging studies are common and frequently asymptomatic.

Clinical Pearls:
Imaging diagnosis of discogenic pain is problematic, but available literature suggests:
- Severe nuclear signal loss (black disc) or severe loss of disc space height strongly predicts a painful disc.
- Normal nuclear signal virtually excludes a painful disc.
- When nuclear signal is intermediate, the inflammatory markers of the high intensity zone (HIZ) and endplate marrow change come into play.
- A truly *high* intensity zone is infrequent, but strongly predicts a painful disc.
- When an HIZ is seen in combination with a disc protrusion, it very strongly predicts a painful disc.
- Marrow endplate change of type I or type II involving greater than 25% of the vertebral body is uncommon but very strongly predicts a painful disc.

Clinical Pitfalls:
- All spine imaging studies have a major specificity fault: asymptomatic degenerative phenomena on imaging studies are common, and increase with advancing age.
- Spine imaging may be insensitive to dynamic lesions.
- Imaging carries risk: cost, radiation exposure, labeling the patient as suffering from a degenerative process, and prompting unwarranted minimally invasive and surgical interventions.
- Evaluation of the efficacy of imaging, as well as provocation and anesthetic procedures, is confounded by the lack of a pathological or surgical gold standard.

Introduction

Axial back pain, of which discogenic pain is a subset, is extremely common in Western societies. It is the most common and expensive cause of work disability in the United States.[1] Recent data suggest that approximately 26% of U.S. citizens have experienced low back pain within the previous 3 months.[2] The use of advanced imaging in the evaluation of back pain has dramatically increased in recent years; lumbar spine magnetic resonance imaging (MRI) scanning (measured by Medicare use) increased 307% in the 12-year interval 1994 to 2005.[3] In the year 2002, the number of physician office visits related to back pain in the United States amounted to 890 million.[2] This increasing use of imaging often provides little if any value to the patient. The inconsistent and often incoherent use of imaging is manifest in the large regional variations in the intensity of spine imaging across the United States; from one third to two thirds of all spine computed tomography (CT) and MRI studies are judged to be inappropriate when measured against established guidelines.[3] The purpose of this chapter is to examine the existing literature regarding the imaging evaluation of the patient with suspected discogenic pain, in part with the hope that the unreasoned use of imaging may be curtailed. It is only when the literature underpinning the interpretation and significance of imaging is well understood that the clinician

Table 3-1: Differential Diagnosis of Low Back Pain

Mechanical Low Back or Leg Pain (97%)	Nonmechanical Spine Conditions (1%)	Visceral Disease (2%)
Lumbar strain or sprain (70%)	Neoplasia (0.7%)	Pelvic organ involvement
Degenerative process of disc and facets	Multiple myeloma	Prostatitis
(usually related to age) (10%)	Metastatic carcinoma	Endometriosis
Herniated disc (4%)	Lymphoma and leukemia	Chronic pelvic inflammatory disease
Spinal stenosis (3%)	Spinal cord tumors	Renal involvement
Osteoporotic compression fracture (4%)	Retroperitoneal tumors	Nephrolithiasis
Spondylolisthesis (2%)	Primary vertebral tumors	Pyelonephritis
Traumatic fractures (<1%)	Infection (0.01%)	Perinephric abscess
Congenital disease (<1%)	Osteomyelitis	Aortic aneurysm
Severe kyphosis	Septic discitis	Gastrointestinal involvement
Severe scoliosis	Paraspinous abscess	Pancreatitis
Transitional vertebrae	Epidural abscess	Cholecystitis
Spondylolysis	Shingles	Penetrating ulcer
Internal disc disruption or discogenic back pain	Inflammatory arthritis	
Presumed instability	(often HLA-B27 associated)(0.3%)	
	Ankylosing spondylitis	
	Psoriatic spondylitis	
	Reiter syndrome	
	Inflammatory bowel disease	
	Scheuermann disease (osteochondrosis)	
	Paget disease	

From Jarvik JG, Deyo RA: Diagnostic evaluation of low back pain with emphasis on imaging, *Ann Intern Med* 137(7), 2002.

can effectively incorporate imaging into his or her diagnostic armamentarium.

This task is complicated by the poorly defined nature of discogenic pain and the lack of a pathological or surgical gold standard. Although extensive literature regarding imaging findings purports to identify discogenic pain, comparing and collating numerous studies is confounded by shifting definitions and fixed preconceptions among authors. One must examine this literature critically since in many instances the unstated motivation in validating imaging findings of discogenic pain is the performance of therapeutic interventions. The existing evidence lent itself to diametrically opposed interpretations by different physician groups and societies, illustrating the importance of perspective and motivation.

It must also be remembered that most back pain is benign and self-limiting and benefits neither from imaging nor intervention. A generation ago, it was thought that acute low back pain was almost exclusively self limiting, with 90% of low back pain resolving within 2 months.[4] More recent literature is less optimistic, but a benign course still dominates. A study by Von Korff and associates[5] evaluated patients with a recent history of low back pain and found that 6 months from onset 21% of patients had no pain and 55% had mild pain with low disability. Only 14% had significant disability with moderate-to-severe limitation of function. A Dutch study[6] found that, although 70% of acute patients with low back pain have persistent pain 4 weeks from onset, at 12 weeks only 35% experience persistent discomfort, and at 1 year only 10%

have persistent pain. Many of these episodes of low back pain are thought to result from muscular strains, ligamentous sprains, or nonspecific degenerative phenomenon, which elude specific diagnosis in up to 85% of cases.[1]

In this context the primary role of imaging is to detect underlying systemic disease, which presents as low back pain. Such disease is uncommon, as detailed in the differential diagnosis of back pain compiled by Jarvik and Deyo in **Table 3-1**.[1] In patients presenting to a primary care setting with back pain, approximately 0.7% have metastatic neoplasm as the underlying cause. Spine infections, including spondylodiscitis and epidural abscess, account for only 0.01%. Osteoporotic compression fractures are relatively common at 4%, whereas inflammatory spondyloarthropathies account for 0.3%. Characterization of neurological impairment that requires intervention is also a primary goal of imaging, typically because of disc herniation or central canal compromise. This typically presents as radicular pain, radiculopathy, or the syndrome of spinal stenosis; confusion with discogenic pain is unlikely. Although the use of imaging to identify axial pain generators is much discussed and often initiated, it rests on a far less firm foundation than its primary functions of identifying systemic disease and characterizing neurological impairment.

We initiate our examination of imaging in the patient with potential discogenic pain by reviewing basic imaging principles that apply broadly to the evaluation of all pain of spinal origin. This includes the use of radiographs and advanced imaging in the acute presentation of low back or leg pain, including existing recommendations of professional societies. The decision to initiate imaging of the patient with back pain is examined in a risk-benefit context, as befits any medical test. Specificity and sensitivity shortcomings of all spine imaging are addressed. The bulk of the chapter then examines specific imaging findings that may be predictive of discogenic pain.

Basic Imaging Principles

It is well established that there is no role for imaging in the patient who presents with acute back and/or leg pain in the absence of signs of systemic disease or neurological impairment that may require intervention. Chou and associates[7] performed a meta-analysis of all randomized controlled trials comparing immediate imaging (radiographs, CT, MRI) vs. clinically directed care in the acute back pain patient. There were six qualifying trials; the analysis showed no significant differences in pain or function in imaged vs. nonimaged patients in either the short term (3 months) or long term (6 to 12 months). They concluded that "lumbar imaging for low back pain without indications of serious underlying conditions does not improve clinical outcomes".[7] In addition to being ineffective, early use of imaging is costly; a cost-effectiveness analysis performed by Liang and Komaroff[8] demonstrated that simply performing radiographs at the initial presentation of back pain results in a cost of $2000 (1982 dollars) to alleviate a single day of pain. The lack of utility of imaging in the acute setting was also well illustrated by a 5-year prospective observational study performed by Carragee and colleagues.[9] A large cohort of asymptomatic persons who were at risk for developing back pain as a result of physically intensive vocations underwent MRI scanning. This cohort was followed periodically over 5 years; a subset ultimately presented to a physician with back or leg pain, at which time a second MRI was performed. Less than 5% of the MRI scans obtained at the time of acute presentation with back or leg pain showed clinically relevant new findings; virtually all of the "abnormalities" noted on the scans obtained at presentation with back pain had been present on imaging obtained when the patient was asymptomatic. Only direct evidence of neural compression in patients with a corresponding radicular pain syndrome was assessed to be useful imaging information. Psychosocial factors, not the morphology seen by imaging, were the primary predictors of the degree of disability caused by back pain.[9]

Analysis of such data has resulted in recommendations against the use of imaging in the patient who presents with acute back pain. The imaging recommendations of the American College of Radiology were recently restated by Bradley.[10] Imaging in the patient who presents with acute low back pain is not indicated except in the presence of "red flag" features, which include recent significant trauma, minor trauma in a patient older than 50, weight loss, fever, immunosuppression, history of neoplasm, steroid use or osteoporosis, age greater than 70, known intravenous drug abuse, or a progressive neurological deficit with intractable symptoms. Similarly, a joint recommendation from the American College of Physicians and the American Pain Society in 2007 stated that imaging should not be obtained in patients with nonspecific low back pain.[11] Imaging should only be performed when severe or progressive neurological deficits are present or when serious underlying systemic disease is suspected. Furthermore, patients with signs or symptoms of radiculopathy or spinal stenosis should be imaged only if they are candidates for surgery or epidural steroid injection. These recommendations emphasize the primary role of imaging as a means of detecting underlying systemic disease, typically neoplasm, infection, or unsuspected traumatic injury.

Risks and Benefits of Imaging for Back Pain

In the absence of signs of systemic disease or neurological deficit, a physician managing a patient with low back pain may choose to initiate imaging when the pain remains intractable despite clinically directed conservative management. Certainly there are benefits that accrue from spine imaging. It may lead to the diagnosis of previously unsuspected systemic disease. In the absence of sinister findings on imaging, the patient should be reassured, providing this is appropriately conveyed by the supervising physician. In some patients imaging may identify the structural basis of a chronic pain syndrome such as discogenic pain or pain generated by sacroiliac dysfunction of facet inflammation. This may then lead to successful therapeutic interventions or, at a minimum, establish a diagnosis, resulting in cessation of further workup.

However, there are risks associated with imaging, which include the labeling effect, radiation exposure, cost, and provocation of intervention. The labeling effect refers to patient self-identification as suffering from a degenerative process. Degenerative phenomena are inevitably identified on any imaging study, as we discuss further regarding specificity of imaging. Unless appropriately educated to the contrary, patients may perceive this as representing the start of an inevitable downward spiral of spine degeneration. This may lead to fear-avoidance behaviors with diminished activity, deconditioning, and depression. A recent Cochrane database review established the effectiveness of active patient education, particularly in the setting of acute low back pain.[12] The irrelevance of degenerative findings on imaging studies and the importance of maintaining core muscle strength and high activity levels must be reinforced at every patient encounter.

Exposure to radiation from radiographs or CT generates a cumulative risk. Effective absorbed radiation dose is measured by the sievert (Sv); the average annual natural background exposure in North America is approximately 3 mSv.[13] A frontal and lateral chest radiograph may be considered the common currency of radiation exposure; it incurs a dose of 0.1 mSv.[13] A three-view lumbar spine radiographic series is worth 1.5 mSv, or 15 chest radiographic series.[13] A dose of 6 mSv is typical for a lumbar spine CT scan (60 chest radiographs). A technetium bone scan has a similar dose of 6.3 mSv.[13] For context, an abdomen and pelvis CT study incurs 14 mSv.[13] All radiation exposure cumulates over the patient's lifetime and contributes to a risk of radiation-induced neoplasm. Radiograph-based imaging studies must be used with careful consideration of risk and anticipated benefit.

Imaging is costly. In the United States the medical imaging community incurs more than $100 billion of societal cost per year. The 2009 Medicare reimbursements for lumbar spine imaging studies were radiographs: $41; noncontrast CT: $264; myelogram: $506; noncontrast MRI: $439; whole body positron emission tomography (PET)/CT: $1183; bone scan with single photon emission computed tomography (SPECT): $261.[14] Nominal fees are typically three to five times the Medicare reimbursements. It is easy to appreciate how quickly imaging costs can accrue.

Finally, and perhaps most important, imaging the spine increases the likelihood that there will be minimally invasive or surgical intervention. Jarvik and associates[15] showed that early MRI imaging leads to more surgical interventions despite equivalent pain and disability profiles when compared with nonimaged patients. Similarly, Lurie, Birkmeyer, and Weinstein[16] noted that the large regional variations (twelvefold) in surgical rates for spinal stenosis can be directly explained by the frequency of CT and MRI use. When we image, we intervene. This is particularly significant in the realm of discogenic pain, in which we have no well-validated therapies, whether surgical or minimally invasive. A recent meta-analysis of surgical fusion for axial back pain noted that three of the four randomized controlled trials in the literature showed no benefit for fusion when compared with structured conservative care.[17] The only randomized study showing minimal benefit for fusion had no organized conservative care as the control arm. Similarly, none of the numerous device-based image-guided interventions that have entered (and left) the marketplace in the United States in the last two decades have shown substantial benefit in randomized trials. Most of the procedures have never even undergone rigorous evaluation with a randomized controlled trial. In a highly imperfect medical marketplace, imaging frequently leads to interventions that have little or no evidence of efficacy, only demonstrable risk and cost.

Sensitivity and Specificity of Spine Imaging

Having weighed the risks and benefits of imaging and chosen to proceed, it is imperative to understand the sensitivity and specificity shortcomings that are common to all spine imaging modalities. We first consider specificity. Imaging findings of degenerative phenomenon in both the anterior and posterior columns of the spine are commonly seen in asymptomatic populations and cannot be considered causal of an individual patient's pain syndrome. In adult populations without low back pain, the prevalence of degenerative changes is significant, with 56% to 72% of asymptomatic adults showing evidence of disc degeneration, 20% to 81% demonstrating disc bulges, 27% to 33% having disc protrusions, 0% to 18% demonstrating disc extrusions, 6% to 56% having annular fissures or high intensity zones, and 2% to 7% demonstrating endplate marrow changes (**Table 3-2**).[1]

More recently studies have addressed the prevalence of degenerative findings in younger populations, primarily in Scandinavian countries, using MRI. These were population-based studies without respect to symptomatology. Kjaer and associates,[29] studying children age 13, found a 21% prevalence of disc degeneration. In a study of adolescents, Salminen and colleagues[30] found a 31% prevalence of disc degeneration in 15-year-olds, which rose to 42% in 18-year-olds. Takatalo and associates[31] evaluated 558 young adults ages 20 to 22.[31] Using the five-point Pfirrmann classification of disc degeneration, they noted disc degeneration of grade 3 or higher in 47% of these young adults. There was a higher prevalence in males (54%) than in females (42%). Multilevel degeneration was identified in 17%.

These studies illustrate that imaging evidence of disc degenerative is widespread, even in asymptomatic and very young populations. The prevalence of such findings in asymptomatic populations increases with age. We subsequently address several of these findings, specifically in regard to discogenic pain; but it is clear that there is a general lack of specificity inherent in all imaging findings of degenerative phenomena.

There is also a basic sensitivity fault present in all spine imaging modalities. This applies most significantly to neuroclaudicatory processes in which compression of neural structures results in radicular pain or neural dysfunction. It is well demonstrated that pain caused by neural compressive processes is exacerbated by extension positioning and axial load. The cross-sectional area of the lumbar central canal, lateral recesses, and foramina are known to diminish with extension and axial load.[32] Advanced imaging performed in a supine, psoas relaxed position may be insensitive to dynamic neural compressive lesions. This can be overcome by imaging with axial loading devices in conventional CT or MRI scanners,[33] or by imaging with MRI scanners that allow standing or seated positions.[34] The imaging trade-off is that such MRI scanners are of low field strength and produce limited image quality.

Regarding discogenic pain, imaging is primarily limited to static morphology. It is largely unknown whether there may be dynamic structural processes that only become evident with extension and axial load that may serve as markers for painful discs. Looking at imaging more broadly, the ability to quantitatively or qualitatively detect inflammatory cytokines or other biochemical mediators of the pain generation process and map them to specific spatial locations may be what is ultimately necessary to truly localize discogenic pain.

Table 3-2: Imaging Abnormalities in Asymptomatic Subjects								
Test	**Author**	**Pts (N)**	**Age (mean)**	**Disc Herniation (%)**	**Disc Bulge (%)**	**Disc Degeneration (%)**	**Central Canal Stenosis (%)**	**Annular Fissure (%)**
X-ray	Hult,[18] 1954	1200	40-44 55-59			56 95		
X-ray	Hellstrom and colleagues,[19] 1990	143	14-25			20		
Myelogram	Hitselberger and Witten,[20] 1968	300	(51)	31				
CT	Wiesel and associates,[21] 1984	51	(40)	20			3.4	
MRI	Weinreb and colleagues,[22] 1989	86	(28)	9	44			
MRI	Boden and associates,[23] 1990	53	<60 ≥60	22 36	54 79	46 93	1 21	
MRI	Jensen and associates,[24] 1994	98	(42)	28	52		7	
MRI	Boos and associates,[25] 1995	46	(36)	76	51	85		
MRI	Stadnik and associates,[26] 1998	36	(42)	33	81	56		56
MRI	Weishaupt and colleagues,[27] 1998	60	(35)	60	28	72		20
MRI	Jarvik and colleagues,[28] 2001	148	(54)	38	64	91	10	38

From Jarvik JG, Deyo RA: Diagnostic evaluation of low back pain with emphasis on imaging, *Ann Intern Med* 137(7), 2002.
CT, Computed tomography; *MRI*, magnetic resonance imaging.

Having considered recommendations for imaging in the patient with acute back pain, the risks and benefits of imaging, and the specificity and sensitivity shortcomings common to all spine imaging, we focus more specifically on the patient with suspected discogenic pain. The pathophysiology of discogenic pain and discography is discussed in greater detail elsewhere in this volume. We revisit these themes only as they bear on noninvasive imaging findings.

Imaging Findings Predictive of Discogenic Pain

The changes seen in the intervertebral disc with aging in the asymptomatic person and in the patient with low back pain are of multifactorial origin. Mechanical, traumatic, nutritional, and genetic factors are involved. For purposes of this discussion, the term *degenerative* encompasses both normal aging and the similar but more rapidly progressive pathological process. Such phenomena are ubiquitous, with 85% to 95% of adults over the age of 50 showing evidence of degenerative disc changes at autopsy.[4] The consensus terminology agreed on by multiple spine imaging medical and surgical societies uses the term *spondylosis deformans*, originally introduced by Schmorl and Junghanns, to describe normal aging phenomenon; this primarily reflects changes in the annulus fibrosis and adjacent vertebral apophyses resulting in anterior and lateral endplate osteophytes.[35] Such osteophytes are present in 100% of skeletons of individuals over 40 years of age.[36] *Intervertebral osteochondrosis* is the term used to describe pathological (although not necessarily symptomatic) degeneration; it involves failure of the nucleus pulposus to effectively disperse axial load with concurrent changes in the vertebral endplates and extensive fissuring in the annulus fibrosis.[35] Pathological changes in this process include posterior vertebral osteophytes, endplate erosions, extensive annular fissuring, and reactive bone marrow changes.

When the disc-endplate complex undergoes degeneration with annular failure, disc contour alteration (i.e., herniation) may occur. Discussion of disc herniation requires a brief commentary on nomenclature. Description of disc herniation has historically been chaotic, with no common terminology among various medical and surgical specialties. This was resolved by a combined task force of the North American Spine Society (NASS), American Society of Spine Radiology (ASSR), and the American Society of Neuroradiology (ASNR), whose recommendations were published in 2001.[35] This imaging lexicon should allow us to communicate better across specialty and regional lines; it is depicted in **Fig. 3-1.** *Herniation* is the broad term describing displacement of disc material beyond its normal intervertebral disc space. If the extent of the herniation is greater than 50% of the circumference of the disc, it may be considered a bulge. A localized herniation is defined as involving less than 50% of the disc circumference. Localized herniations may be further divided into broad-based herniations, which encompass 25% to 50% of the disc circumference, and focal herniations, which constitute less than 25% of the circumference. The distinction between protrusion and extrusion is one of shape. In a protrusion the width of displaced disc material in any plane does not exceed the width of its base or the aperture through which the disc material had left its normal position. In an extrusion the width of the displaced disc material exceeds its base or aperture in any plane. The presence of an extrusion shape suggests that there has been complete disruption of the outer annulus and disc material has entered the epidural space. *Sequestration* is the term for loss of continuity of a disc fragment with the parent disc from which it arose. Displacement of disc material away from the parent disc is termed *migration*.

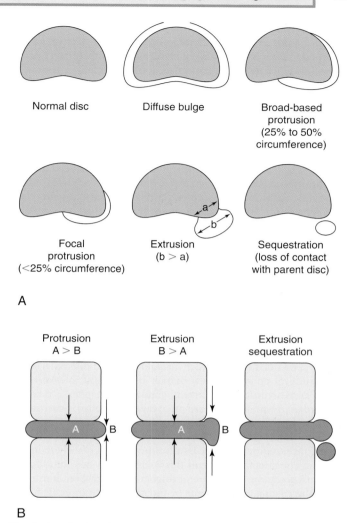

Fig. 3-1 Disc herniations. **A,** Disc herniation configurations in the axial plane. **B,** Disc herniation configurations in the sagittal plane.

Imaging findings that potentially predict discogenic pain may include those observable with x-ray–based studies (radiographs, CT) such as vertebral osteophytes, endplate sclerosis, loss of disc space height, vacuum phenomenon (nitrogen gas) within the disc, and soft tissue findings that are only observable with MRI, including alterations in disc contour (bulges, protrusions, extrusions), T2 signal loss within the disc, high T2 intensity annular fissures (high-intensity zone [HIZ]), and changes in the sub-endplate marrow (Modic change).

The existing literature that seeks to identify imaging findings predictive of discogenic pain deals primarily with MRI findings, which is the focus of our discussion. The findings to be evaluated include (1) loss of disc space height, (2) alterations of disc contour, (3) generalized alterations in T2 signal within the disc, (4) endplate marrow changes, and (5) the presence of HIZs or fissures within the posterior disc annulus. These imaging features are examined initially as independent variables with subsequent discussion of the more limited literature in which they are combined in a multivariate analysis. A significant portion of the presented data was drawn from a systematic review of imaging and clinical markers of axial pain generators in the lumbar spine performed by Hancock and colleagues.[37] Additional studies not included in that report or published subsequent to it have been added. A common set of measures was compiled from the numerous studies: sensitivity, specificity, positive predictive value, negative predictive value, and likelihood ratios. When imaging features were quantified (e.g., T2 signal loss in the disc was reported as normal, moderate, or severe), a threshold was used. Original data were combined and recalculated to reflect setting a detection threshold as moderate (including moderate and severe cases) or severe only. Since the diagnosis of discogenic pain may provoke therapeutic interventions (most of which carry risk and have unproven efficacy), emphasis is placed on those measurements that inform us about false-positive results: specificity (true negatives/true negatives + false positives) and positive predictive value (true positives/true positives + false positives). These measures can be conflicting when class sizes vary and depend on the prevalence of the condition being studied.[38] Likelihood ratios (LRs) are prevalence independent, given by sensitivity/(1 − specificity). The higher the positive LRs (+LR), the more likely it is that a patient with a positive test does have the disease, here discogenic pain. When the +LR exceeds 2, the finding is considered useful when the confidence interval does not cross 1. The lower a negative likelihood ratio (−LR), the more likely a patient with a negative test does not have the disease. When the −LR is less than 0.5, the finding is considered informative when the confidence interval does not include 1.

Before proceeding with examination of individual imaging findings, we must first consider the gold standard dilemma. There is no surgical or pathological marker of a painful intervertebral disc. The most restrictive current standard for a painful disc is a concordant response to manometrically controlled provocation discography with nonpainful control levels as defined by the practice guidelines of the International Spine Intervention Society (ISIS).[39] Discography is discussed in more detail elsewhere in this volume. The target audience of this volume likely advocates for, or is at least accepting of, the use of discography. However, it must be remembered that examination of the same body of evidence by different physician societies regarding the validity of discography has resulted in diametrically opposed recommendations regarding its use. The ISIS,[39] the North American Spine Society (NASS),[40] and the International Association for the Study of Pain (IASP)[41] accept discography as a useful diagnostic tool in the patient with back pain and recommend its use. The American Pain Society rejects discography as a diagnostically useful test.[42] A comprehensive review of discography in the journal of the American Society of Regional Anesthesia and Pain Medicine notes that, although CT discography is the gold standard for the assessment of structural disc degeneration, there is no convincing evidence that the use of discography as a selection tool improves surgical outcomes.[43] Thus any analysis of imaging findings in the discogenic pain patient remains based on a reference standard (provocation discography) that is ultimately unproven. This is further confounded by evolution of the criteria for a positive discogram within the past decade. The literature evaluating imaging findings with discography as a reference often uses varying or unstated criteria for a positive discogram and must be read critically. For the purposes of this discussion, only concordant pain responses were considered to represent a positive discogram. A significant concordant pain response without specification of pain intensity or use of manometry is defined as *Walsh criteria*[44] for the remainder of this chapter. Including the requirement for a normal control disc elevates the criteria to that of IASP.[41] None of the studies presented meaningfully used manometric control nor met the ISIS criteria for positive discography.[39]

Loss of Disc Height

The reports of Ito and associates,[45] O'Neill and associates,[46] and Lim and associates[47] studied loss of disc space height as an imaging finding that may correlate with positive provocation discography; data are summarized in **Table 3-3**. Ito and associates[45] studied 101 discs in 39 patients of mean age 37 years; duration and prior therapy for back pain were not included in the report. Loss of disc space height was graded as normal, moderate, or severe. Discography was performed without manometry or specification of the intensity of pain produced; pain provocation was scored as absent, nonconcordant, or concordant. Concordant pain only was accepted as a positive discogram (Walsh criteria). In **Table 3-3** Ito's data are presented for severe disc space narrowing and recalculated for the threshold of moderate narrowing (combined moderate and severe categories). Severe disc space narrowing was uncommon in Ito and associates' series (9% prevalence) but had a very high specificity (97%) and a high positive predictive value (PPV = 78%). Among nonpainful discs, very few are severely narrowed, and most severely narrowed discs are painful, supported by the +LR of 11.9. Relaxing the criteria to moderate narrowing reduces the specificity and PPV (**Fig. 3-2**).

O'Neill and colleagues[46] included disc narrowing among a number of variables studied both individually and in a

Author, Date	Discogram Criteria	Height Loss Criteria	Prevalence (%)	Sensitivity (%)	Specificity (%)	PPV (%)	NPV (%)	+LR (CI)	−LR (CI)
Ito and associates,[45] 1998	Walsh	Moderate + severe	44	87	69	46	95	2.8 (2.0-4.1)	0.2 (0.1-0.6)
		Severe	9	30	97	78	83	11.9 (2.7-53.3)	0.7 (0.5-0.9)
Lim and associates,[47] 2004	Walsh	Reduced?	22	30	82	48	68	1.7 (0.8-3.5)	0.9 (0.7-1.1)
O'Neill and associates,[46] 2008	IASP	Moderate + severe	47	73	81	81	74	3.9 (3.0-5.2)	0.3 (0.3-0.4)
		Severe	10	18	98	90	52	8.0 (3.2-19.7)	0.8 (0.8-0.9)

Table 3-3: Loss of Disc Height

CI, Confidence interval; IASP, International Association for the Study of Pain; +LR, positive likelihood ratio; −LR, negative likelihood ratio; NPV, negative predictive value; PPV, positive predictive value.

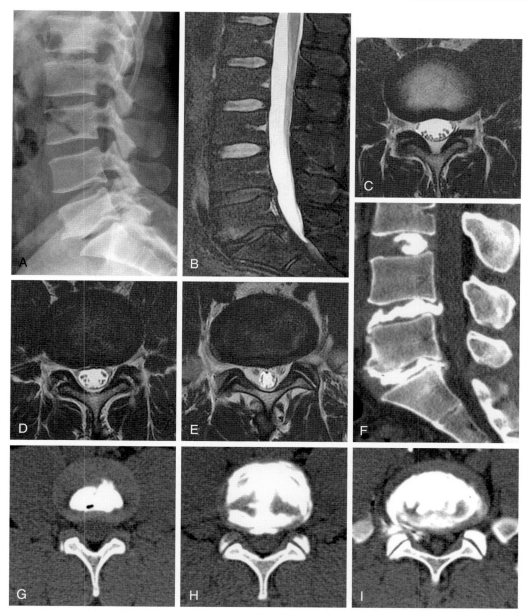

Fig. 3-2 Disc height and signal loss. **A,** Lateral radiograph of a 50-year-old male with intractable axial pain. Note loss of height of lumbosacral disc, which contains gas, indicative of degeneration. There is slight retrolisthesis of L4 on L5 and L5 on S1. Sagittal fat-saturated T2 weighted MRI **(B)** shows loss of T2 signal in L4 and L5 discs with normal upper lumbar discs. Axial T2 weighted images at L3 **(C)**, L4 **(D)**, and L5 **(E)** demonstrate normal L3 disc, loss of T2 signal in L4 with a small central herniation, and a broad bulge at L5. Sagittal CT discogram **(F)** and axial images at L3 **(G)**, L4 **(H)**, and L5 **(I)** show normal L3 disc and extensive annular disruption at L4 and L5 with leak of contrast from the right posterolateral annulus at L5. Patient had concordant axial pain at L4 and L5 with a normal control disc at L3.

multivariate analysis. They studied 460 discs in 143 patients (mean age of 43 years) with at least 6 months of low back pain. Disc height was again categorized in a three-part scale: normal (0% to 10% loss of expected height), moderate (10% to 50% loss of expected height), and severe (greater than 50% loss of expected height). Discography was done with manometric control, but there was no specification as to how this influenced the diagnosis. Discograms were considered positive when pain was concordant at ≥6/10 intensity with a negative control level, most closely approaching the IASP criteria. Severe disc space narrowing again had a low prevalence (10%) but a very high specificity (98%), a high PPV (90%), and very high +LR (8). In O'Neill and associates' data, lowering the threshold to moderate and severe narrowing

retained moderate specificity (81%) and PPV (81%) and a strong +LR of 3.9 while raising the sensitivity for a positive discogram to 73%. In the multivariate analysis loss of disc space height, loss of nuclear signal and disc contour abnormalities had strong interdependence; there was no statistical significance between these variables in their area under receiver operating characteristic (ROC) curves.

The study by Lim and associates[47] was less supportive, with specificity of 82%, PPV of 48%, and +LR of 1.7. They studied 97 discs in 47 patients with low back pain. Disc height was considered normal if it equaled the height of the next supra-adjacent disc. Discography used Walsh criteria with no requirement for negative control discs.

Table 3-4: Disc Contour Abnormality

Author, Date	Discogram Criteria	Disc Contour	Prevalence (%)	Sensitivity (%)	Specificity (%)	PPV (%)	NPV (%)	+LR (CI)	−LR (CI)
O'Neill and associates,[46] 2008	IASP	Bulge	23	38	93	85	58	5.3 (3.2-8.7)	0.7 (0.6-0.7)
O'Neill and associates	IASP	Protrusion	18	29	93	82	55	4.3 (2.5-7.2)	0.8 (0.7-0.8)
O'Neill and associates	IASP	Extrusion	5	7	98	76	49	3.0 (1.1-7.9)	0.9 (0.9-0)
Kang and associates,[48] 2009	IASP	Focal + broad-based protrusion	32	68	81	54	89	3.51 (2.4-5.2)	0.4 (0.3-0.6)

CI, Confidence interval; IASP, International Association for the Study of Pain; +LR, positive likelihood ratio; −LR, negative likelihood ratio; NPV, negative predictive value; PPV, positive predictive value.

Alterations of Disc Contour

The studies of O'Neill and colleagues[46] and Kang and associates[48] included data correlating disc contour abnormalities and discography; data are summarized in **Table 3-4**. Kang and associates studied 178 discs in 62 consecutive patients with low back pain (mean age 46 years) who had failed 6 months of conservative therapy. Contour abnormality definitions were those of Fardon and Milette.[35] The criteria for a positive discogram included reproduction of concordant pain at or greater then 6/10 in intensity, with a normal control disc, most closely resembling the IASP criteria. No manometric control was described. The prevalence of painful discs at discography in this data set was 25%. These authors compared discography findings to disc contour abnormalities, disc degeneration, presence of high intensity zones, presence of endplate marrow signal change (Modic change), and combinations of these findings. Data regarding contour abnormalities combined focal and broad based protrusions. The presence of a disc protrusion was significantly associated with positive discography (p < 0.01). Prevalence of disc protrusion was 32% in this data set, with a specificity of 81% but a PPV of only 54%. The presence of a contour abnormality alone was not deemed to be a useful finding by the authors, although analysis of their data does reveal a +LR of 3.5. As will be described in the section on multivariate analysis, when disc protrusion was combined with the presence of an HIZ, the specificity and PPV rose to 98% and 87% respectively (**Fig. 3-3**).

The basic structure of O'Neill and associates' study is summarized in the previous paragraph.[46] Disc contour was described as normal, bulge, protrusion, or extrusion, using the definitions of Fardon and Milette.[35] There were strong correlations between disc height loss, disc signal, and disc contour abnormalities. There was a statistically significant correlation between disc contour abnormality and discography.[46] As **Table 3-4** demonstrates, all contour abnormalities had informative likelihood ratios; disc bulge was most useful, with a +LR of 5.3. The multivariate analysis is presented in the following paragraphs.

Disc Degeneration (T2 Signal Loss)

Studies addressing the correlation between MRI evidence of disc degeneration and discogenic pain identified by discography reach back nearly 20 years. The several publications are summarized in **Table 3-5**. The definition of disc degeneration varies and is described for each study; most classifications rely primarily on loss of T2 nuclear signal in association with loss of the boundary between nucleus and annulus and loss of disc space height. The studies of Osti and Fraser[49] and Horton and Daftari[50] were published in 1992. Osti and Fraser evaluated 114 discs in 33 consecutive patients with low back pain of mean age 35 years. Disc degeneration was evaluated using midsagittal T2 weighted images, with nuclear signal intensity classified as normal, reduced, or absent. Disc height was not considered. Statistics were calculated from their data using severe degeneration and moderate plus severe degeneration as the MRI variables. In this study, discography was performed with notation of absent, atypical, or typical pain; only typical pain reproduction was considered as a positive discogram (Walsh criteria, no control discs). The presence of severe T2 signal loss was uncommon (prevalence = 13%) but quite specific for a painful disc (specificity 92%, +LR of 2.8). Using the threshold of moderate signal loss as degeneration, any usefulness fell away.

The 1992 study of Horton and Daftari[50] encompassed 59 discs in 25 consecutive patients who had failed 6 weeks of conservative therapy for low back pain without radiculopathy. Disc degeneration was evaluated on midsagittal T2 weighted images using a three part classification: hyperintense white signal (normal), speckled dark and light signal (intermediate), and dark signal (severe degeneration). Provocation discography was considered positive when patients reported concordant pain that was either moderate or severe in intensity (vs. mild or absent) in the presence of a morphologically abnormal disc (Walsh criteria). There was no requirement for a normal control disc or manometery. Statistics in **Table 3-6** were calculated from their data for both dark signal (severe degeneration) on MRI and dark or speckled signal (moderate and severe degeneration). Similar to Osti and Fraser's study,[49] severe degeneration has fairly high specificity (88%) but a low PPV (58%). A threshold of moderate degeneration was not useful. However, its negative predictive value was 94% with an informative −LR; therefore it is highly unlikely that discs with normal nuclear signal will be painful. These authors also combined the disc signal abnormality parameters with a three-part contour abnormality assessment: normal, bulge, or disruption of the posterior annulus/posterior longitudinal ligamentous (PLL) complex. There were no protrusion or extrusion categories, and assessment was limited to sagittal images. The validity of this assessment on MRI images of this era is questionable. It is worth noting that all cases of dark discs with apparent disruption of the posterior annulus/PLL were painful, but this was a very infrequent finding (3 of 59 discs).

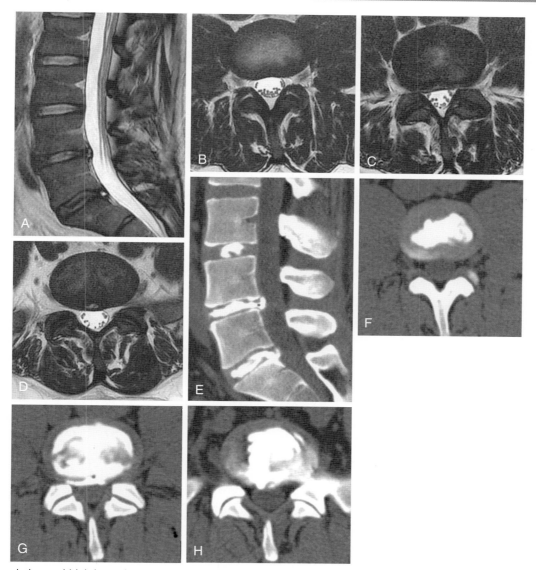

Fig. 3-3   Disc herniation and high intensity zone (HIZ). **A,** Patient with axial back pain; sagittal T2 weighted MRI shows disc degeneration and herniations at L4 and L5 with HIZ at L5. Axial T2 images show a normal L3 disc **(B),** broad-based protrusion at L4 **(C),** and small central extrusion at L5 with caudal migration of disc material **(D).** Sagittal computed tomography discogram **(E)** and axial images at L3 **(F),** L4 **(G),** and L5 **(H)** show a normal L3 disc; diffuse, complex fissure with protrusion at L4; and more focal radial fissure leading to a small extrusion at L5. There was concordant pain at L4 and L5 at low pressures of injection (<20 psi above opening pressure); L3 was a normal control disc.

Ito and associates' 1998 study[45] has been described previously; the Walsh discography criteria were used. Much like the prior studies, disc degeneration was assessed with a three-part (normal, moderate T2 signal loss, severe signal loss) scale of signal loss without consideration of loss of disc space height. The results in **Table 3-6** tell a similar tale; severe degeneration is very informative, with a +LR of 5.7 but with a low prevalence as an imaging finding and a modest PPV (64%). The negative predictive value of the moderate-plus-severe signal loss category (i.e., a normal nuclear signal disc) is again very high (97%).

In 2001 Weishaupt and colleagues[51] studied 116 discs in 50 consecutive patients with chronic (at least 6 weeks) low back pain without radicular leg pain. Disc degeneration was among the parameters evaluated; the 5-grade classification of Pearce and associates[52] was used, which combines T2 signal loss with loss of disc space height and loss of nuclear-annular boundary. Grades 1 and

2 were considered normal and specify hyperintense T2 nuclear signal, normal disc height, and a normal nuclear-annular boundary, with a dark intranuclear cleft appearing in grade 2 discs. Grades 3 to 5, with progressive loss of nuclear signal, boundary zone blurring, and loss of height, were all considered degenerated discs resulting in a binary classification. Discography evaluation used IASP criteria, including the requirement for a normal control disc. This classification of disc degeneration resulted in a very high negative predictive value (97%) and informative −LR for normal nuclear signal with or without intranuclear cleft. Only one disc that was normal by MRI criteria was painful. Disc degeneration had a modest specificity (59%) and positive predictive value (64%), which are not useful.

A study by Lim and associates in 2005[47] examined 97 discs in 47 patients of mean age 43 years with low back pain with or without leg pain. It is not stated if these represented consecutive

Table 3-5: Disc Degeneration (T2 Signal Loss)

Author, Date	Discogram Criteria	T2 Signal Criteria	Prevalence (%)	Sensitivity (%)	Specificity (%)	PPV (%)	NPV (%)	+LR (CI)	−LR (CI)
Osti and Fraser,[49] 1992	Walsh	Moderate + severe	47	70	64	50	80	1.9 (1.3-2.7)	0.49 (0.3-0.8)
		Severe only	13	23	92	60	70	2.8 (1.1-7.0)	0.83 (0.7-1.0)
Horton and Daftari,[50] 1992	Walsh	Moderate + severe	69	95	43	44	94	1.6 (1.2-2.2)	0.18 (0.04-0.9)
		Severe only	20	37	88	58	74	2.8 (1.1-7.3)	0.72 (0.5-1.0)
Ito and associates,[45] 1998	Walsh	Moderate + severe	63	96	46	34	97	1.7 (1.4-2.2)	0.14 (0.03-0.6)
		Severe only	25	70	89	64	91	5.7 (3.0-11.0)	0.36 (0.2-0.7)
Weishaupt and colleagues,[51] 2001	IASP	3-5 of grade-5 Pearce	65	98	59	64	98	2.3 (1.8-3.1)	0.05 (0.01-0.3)
Lim and associates,[47] 2005	Walsh	4 and 5 of grade-5 Pearce	62	88	52	50	89	1.8 (1.4-2.4)	0.25 (0.1-0.6)
Lei and associates,[53] 2008	IASP	3 and 4 of 4-point Woodward	57	94	77	78	94	4.0 (2.5-6.4)	0.07 (0.02-0.2)
O'Neill and associates,[46] 2008	IASP	Moderate + severe	62	90	67	75	86	2.7 (2.2-3.3)	0.16 (0.1-0.2)
		Severe only	15	24	96	87	54	6.0 (3.0-11.7)	0.79 (0.7-0.9)
Kang and associates,[48] 2009	IASP	3, 4, and 5 on Pfirrmann 5-point scale	70	95	39	34	96	1.6 (1.3-1.8)	0.12 (0.03-0.5)

CI, Confidence interval; *IASP*, International Association for the Study of Pain; *+LR*, positive likelihood ratio; *−LR*, negative likelihood ratio; *NPV*, negative predictive value; *PPV*, positive predictive value.

patients. Disc degeneration was quantified using the 5-grade classification of Pearce and associates[52]; results were reported with grades 4 and 5 grouped together as degenerative discs. Discography was performed using Walsh criteria. Concordant pain production at discography was significantly ($p < 0.05$) associated with grade 4 or 5 disc degeneration in this series. Sensitivity for this definition of disc degeneration was 88%, specificity only 52% with a PPV of 50% and a negative predictive value (NPV) of 89%. Only the −LR was informative. Raw data were not presented to allow calculation of other definitions of degeneration.

Lei and associates studied 131 discs in 55 consecutive patients with disabling low back pain for at least 6 months.[53] Disc degeneration was scored using a four-part system encompassing nuclear signal, disc height, and annular tears: grade 1, white nuclear signal, normal height, no tears; grade 2, speckled nuclear signal, <10% height reduction, small tears not reaching the PLL; grade 3, speckled or dark nucleus, height reduced by 10% to 50%, annular tears up to or including PLL; grade 4, dark nucleus, height >50% reduced, ± complex tears. The analysis grouped grades 3 and 4 discs with grade 2 discs having tears to the outer third of the annulus as degenerated discs; grades 1 and 2 discs without peripheral tears were considered normal. Discography used the IASP criteria without manometry but with the requirement of a negative control disc. Again, the negative predictive value of a normal disc by these

criteria was very high (94%), and the −LR very informative. Specificity and positive predictive value of a degenerated disc as defined in this study was 77% and 78%, respectively, with a very informative +LR of 4.

O'Neill and associates' study[46] (described previously) also evaluated disc degeneration manifested by T2 signal loss. Disc height and contour abnormalities were separately tabulated. Nuclear signal loss was classified by a three-part scale similar to that of Ito and associates[45]: normal (white signal), severe (homogeneous black signal), and intermediate (all expressions between normal and severe). The data were again recalculated to evaluate thresholds. Disc signal abnormality had the highest correlation with discogenic pain of all individual MRI parameters studied by O'Neill and colleagues. The results of the multivariate analysis are discussed in the following paragraphs. Severe signal loss was a highly specific finding (specificity = 96%) with a PPV of 87%. The NPV of a normal disc signal was 86%.

Finally the study by Kang and associates[48] (described previously) categorized disc degeneration via the five-part Pfirrmann scale.[54] It uses midsagittal T2 weighted images: grade 1: homogeneous bright T2 nuclear signal; grade 2: inhomogeneous bright T2 nuclear signal, preservation of disc height and nuclear-annular boundary; grade 3: inhomogeneous intermediate gray nuclear signal, nuclear-annular boundary indistinct, disc height normal or

Table 3-6: Endplate (Modic) Changes

Author, Date	Discogram Criteria	Modic Type	Prevalence per Disc (%)	Sensitivity (%)	Specificity (%)	PPV (%)	NPV (5)	+LR (CI)	−LR (CI)
Braithwaite and associates,[63] 1998	Walsh	I + II	25 imaged 15 tested	24	96	91	47	6.0 (1.7-21.2)	0.80 (0.7-0.9)
		I	4 tested	5	100	100	42	7.4 (0.4-131)	0.95 (0.9-1.0)
		II	12 tested	18	96	89	48	4.4 (1.2-16.1)	0.86 (0.8-0.9)
Ito and associates,[45] 1998	Walsh	I + II + III?	9	23	94	56	80	4.0 (1.3-12.8)	0.82 (0.7-1.0)
Weishaupt and associates,[51] 2001	IASP	I	14	29	97	88	66	9.9 (2.4-41.6)	0.73 (0.6-0.9)
		II	9	19	99	90	63	12.75 (1.7-97.3)	0.83 (0.7-0.9)
		I + II	22	48	96	88	72	10.86 (3.5-34.1)	0.55 (0.4-0.7)
		I + II Moderate + severe	16	38	100	100	69	52.1 (3.2-844)	0.63 (0.5-0.8)
Kokkonen and associates,[64] 2002	Walsh	I	17	19	85	41	65	1.25 (0.5-3.0)	0.96 (0.8-1.2)
		II	19	19	80	35	64	0.96 (0.4-2.2)	1.0 (0.8-1.2)
		I + II	36	38	65	38	65	1.1 (0.6-1.8)	0.95 (0.7-1.3)
Lim and associates,[47] 2005	Walsh	I + II	14	9	83	21	62	0.6 (0.2-1.7)	1.1 (0.9-1.3)
Lei and associates,[53] 2008	IASP	I + II?	14	32	98	94	62	19.25 (2.7-140)	0.69 (0.6-0.8)
O'Neill and associates,[46] 2008	IASP	I	4	6	99	88	49	6.94 (1.6-29.9)	0.95 (0.9-1.0)
		II	4	7	99	90	50	8.32 (1.9-35.5)	0.93 (0.9-1.0)
		I + II	8	14	98	89	51	7.63 (2.8-21.2)	0.88 (0.8-0.9)
Kang and associates,[48] 2009	IASP	I + II	13	14	87	26	76	1.08 (0.5-2.6)	0.99 (0.9-1.1)

CI, Confidence interval; IASP, International Association for the Study of Pain; +LR, positive likelihood ratio; −LR, negative likelihood ratio; NPV, negative predictive value; PPV, positive predictive value.

slightly decreased; grade 4: inhomogeneous dark gray signal, nuclear-annular boundary lost, normal to moderately reduced disc height; grade 5: inhomogeneous dark signal, no nuclear-annular boundary, disc space collapse. Grades 1 and 2 were grouped together as normal; grades 3 to 5 were grouped together as degenerative. There was also a logistic regression analysis performed on grades 3, 4, and 5 individually. A normal disc (grades 1 and 2) had a 96% NPV for concordant pain at provocation discography. There was a statistically significant difference in pain production for normal vs. all degenerated discs; this significance fell away when each individual grade of degeneration was compared to normal discs. Specificity for this definition of disc degeneration for pain production was only 39% with a PPV of 34%.

The difficulty in drawing conclusions from the existing literature regarding the usefulness of imaging parameters in predicting discogenic pain at provocation discography is well illustrated by these summarized studies. The definitions of disc degeneration on MRI are inconsistent. The discographic criteria for discogenic pain have evolved significantly over the 18-year span bridged by these studies. The even greater challenge of the uncertain validity of discography as a gold standard for discogenic pain lurks unpleasantly in the background.

Acknowledging these shortcomings, some general conclusions can be advanced. The negative predictive value of discs of normal nuclear signal is uniformly high and −LRs are highly informative; discs of normal nuclear signal are rarely painful. Severe disc degeneration, manifest as uniformly dark T2 signal with or without loss of disc space height, is a finding of high specificity (88% to 96% in studies using a three-part classification system) and strongly informative +LR. Discs with severe T2 signal loss are very rarely nonpainful. The usefulness of this finding is reduced by its low prevalence (it is found in 13% to 25% of discs undergoing discography in patients with discogenic pain) and low sensitivity (23%, 24%, 37%, and 70% in the studies with a three-part classification system). Discs with intermediate signal loss may be painful but with less certainty.

Endplate and Subchondral Marrow (Modic) Changes

The functional unity of the disc and the cartilaginous endplate is manifest in signal changes within the endplate and adjacent subchondral marrow that accompany disc degeneration (**Fig. 3-4**). Endplate marrow changes were originally classified by Modic and associates in 1988.[55] Type I change represents ingrowth of vascularized granulation tissue into subendplate marrow; it exhibits hypointense T1 and hyperintense T2 signal on MRI and may enhance with gadolinium. Type II change exhibits elevated T1 and T2 signal and reflects fatty infiltration of subendplate marrow. Type III change is hypointense on T1 and T2; it correlates with bony sclerosis. Type I change is thought to represent an active inflammatory state, with type II being more quiescent, and type III postinflammatory. Ohtori and associates[56] noted elevated levels of protein gene product (PGP) 9.5 immunoreactive nerve fibers and tumor necrosis factor (TNF) immunoreactive cells in the cartilaginous endplates of patients with Modic changes.[56] The immunoreactive nerve ingrowth was seen exclusively in patients with the discogenic low back pain. TNF immunoreactive cells were more common in type I endplate changes.

Modic endplate changes do carry an association with low back pain, particularly type I change. Toyone and colleagues[57] found that 73% of patients with type I change had low back pain as opposed to 11% of type II patients.[7] Likewise, Albert and Maniche[58] reported low back pain in 60% of patients with Modic changes but in only

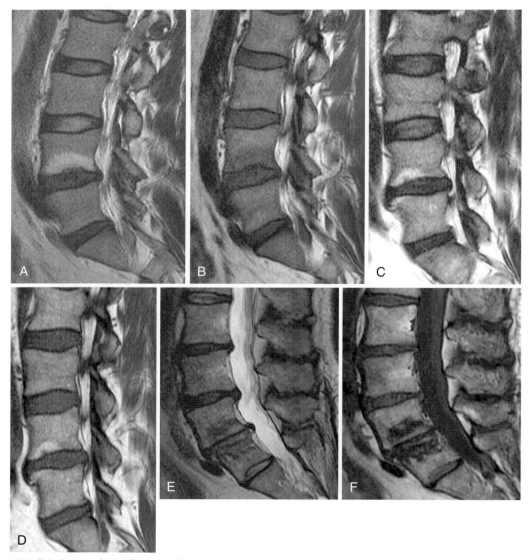

Fig. 3-4 Endplate (Modic) change. **A** and **B,** T2 and T1 weighted MRI images, respectively, show high T2 and low T1 signal at L4 inferior endplate consistent with the vascularized granulation tissue of type I endplate change. **C** and **D,** T2 and T1 weighted MRI images in another patient demonstrate elevated T1 and T2 signal about the L4 interspace, reflecting the fatty infiltration of type 2 endplate change. **E** and **F,** T2 and T1 weighted MRI images show low T2 and T1 signal about the L4 interspace, indicative of type 3 endplate change.

20% for those without Modic change. Type I change was more strongly associated with low back pain than type 2 change. Modic type I change may also be associated with segmental instability; in the study of Toyone and associates,[57] 70% of patients with type I change were found to have segmental hypermobility (greater than 3-mm translation on flexion-extension films). Hypermobility was seen in only 16% of those with type II change. Similarly, in postfusion patients the studies of Butterman and colleagues[59] and Lang and colleagues[60] showed persistent type I change in patients ultimately shown to have pseudarthroses. Patients with solid fusions tend to have type II change or resolution of all Modic changes. The studies of Chataigner, Onimus, and Polette[61] and Esposito and associates[62] evaluated Modic change as a predictor of fusion outcome; patients with type I change at the operative level on preprocedure imaging tended to have much better outcomes than patients operated on with isolated disc degeneration or disc generation plus type II endplate change.

The studies that have compared endplate changes to provocation discography are summarized in **Table 3-6**. Endplate marrow change as a predictor of discogenic pain at provocation discography was initially described by Braithwaite and colleagues in 1998.[63] They studied 152 discs in 58 consecutive patients being evaluated for back and/or leg pain of mean age 42 years. Sagittal T1 and T2 weighted images were used to assess Modic changes of type I, II, or III; marrow changes associated with Schmorl's nodes were discounted. The presence of an HIZ was also noted as discussed in the following paragraphs. Discography used the Walsh criteria. Evaluating all the MRI imaged levels (not all of which underwent discography), Modic change was present in 48% of patients, 11% of all discs imaged, and 24% of degenerated discs. Modic change was only seen in association with disc degeneration; there were no discs with normal nuclear signal and adjacent Modic change. The vast majority (84%) of Modic change occurred about the L4 and L5 interspace levels. There were 31 interspaces exhibiting Modic change; type II change was present at 21 levels (68%); only 6 levels had Modic I change. Modic type III change was rare and only seen in combination with type I or II change. The presence of Modic change (any type) was significantly associated with pain production at discography ($p < 0.00004$). Of the 23 levels that exhibited Modic change and underwent discography, 21 were painful; the two nonpainful discs had type II change. Combining Modic I and II change yields a specificity of 97%, a PPV of 91%, and a strongly informative positive likelihood ratio of 6. All type I discs were painful although present in only 4% of the levels that underwent discography.

Ito and associates' 1998 report[45] included evaluation of endplate changes.[45] Although not explicitly stated, it appears that all marrow change types (I, II, and III) were grouped together. Marrow changes were infrequent (prevalence = 9% of tested discs) but exhibited high specificity (95%) and a +LR of 4. Weishaupt and colleagues[51] reported on endplate abnormalities correlated with discography in 2001; the study parameters were described previously. Regarding endplate abnormalities, they noted the three Modic types; but, when two types coexisted in a given endplate, only one was reported based on a priority of type I > II > III. This study also classified severity of the marrow change based on the percentage of the vertebrae height involved: minimal, 0% to 25% of vertebral height; moderate, 25% to 50%; severe, >50%. When the involvement on either side of the disc differed, the most severe was recorded. For types I and II changes considered together, the specificity was 96%, and the PPV was 88% when all levels of severity of marrow change were included. When only moderate and severe endplate changes of both types I and II were considered (marrow change involving

>25% of the vertebral body height), the specificity and PPV were both 100%; all discs in these categories were painful at discography with no false-positive cases. Positive likelihood ratios are strongly informative for all types of Modic change.

In contrast to the studies of Braithwaite and associates,[63] Ito and associates,[45] and Weishaupt and colleagues,[51] the 2002 study of Kokkonen and colleagues[64] showed no significant association between endplate degeneration and pain provocation at discography. This study involved 36 patients, mean age 40, with greater than 1 year of low back pain; average length of symptoms was 2.5 years. One hundred three discs were examined with MRI and discography. MRI images were classified by Modic type. Discographic technique is not described in detail and is presumed to follow that of Walsh. The prevalence of endplate degeneration was considerably higher than in the prior series at 36% per disc. As expected, there were strong correlations between endplate change and disc degeneration on MRI and CT discography but no correlation with pain provocation. The values in **Table 3-6** were not presented in the paper but calculated from the presented data. The specificity of endplate degeneration was much lower than in prior reports, with 23 out of 27 discs exhibiting either type I or type II endplate change provoking no pain (19) or nonconcordant pain (4) at discography. PPV was only 38%, and the likelihood ratios suggest that the information is not helpful. The authors offer no explanation for the discordance between their results and those previously published. It is worthy to note that the patients in this study appear to have had a significantly longer duration of symptoms than in the earlier reports. The much higher prevalence of endplate changes in this series also raises questions as to whether minimal alterations in endplate signal, below the reporting threshold in other publications, may have been included in this report. The report by Lim and associates[47] in 2005 also found no correlation between endplate changes and painful discs.

In 2008 Lei and colleagues[53] tabulated endplate changes but did not describe type or severity. Presumably types I, II, and III are reported together as endplate changes. Their data closely matched that of Braithwaite and associates,[63] Ito and associates,[45] and Weishaupt and colleagues,[51] with a 14% prevalence of endplate changes, a specificity of 98%, PPV of 94%, and informative +LR. O'Neill and associate' 2008 series[46] reported type I and type II endplate change in relationship to provocation discography. Endplate change had a significant correlation with discography outcome but with lesser correlation than nuclear signal, disc height, disc contour, or HIZ. Type I, type II, and the combination of I + II had very high specificity (98%, 99%, 98%, respectively) and PPV (88%, 90%, 89%, respectively). Prevalence of the finding was at the low end of the reported spectrum, with type I + II discs accounting for only 8% of the discs evaluated.

Finally the Kang and associates' study[48] tabulated endplate change by Modic definitions without grading their severity. Modic changes were present in 13% of discs, with Modic type II most common. No statistically significant correlation could be identified between endplate changes and discogenic pain. Specificity was high (87%), but false positives outnumbered true positives with a PPV of only 26%. It is unclear why the false-positive rate was so high in this study.

Again we are left with disparate data in considering the value of Modic type endplate changes as predictors of discogenic pain. The studies of Braithwaite and associates,[63] Weishaupt and associates,[51] Lei and colleagues,[63] and O'Neill and colleagues[46] had very few false positives (i.e., discs with adjacent type I or type II endplate changes that were nonpainful). The specificity, PPV, and +LRs in these studies were very high. The usefulness of the MRI finding is only limited by its infrequency. However, the studies of Kokkonen and colleagues,[64] Lim and associates,[47] and Kang and colleagues[48] showed no association between endplate and discogenic pain, with significant numbers of false positives. The Kokkonen and associates'[64] and Lim and associates'[47] papers provide scant description of the discography technique, which raises concerns. However, the paper by Kang and colleagues[48] describes appropriate technique in detail. The compelling results presented by Weishaupt suggest a threshold for marrow change to be significant; with a threshold at 25% of vertebral body height, there were no false positives in this study. A reasonable conclusion may be that Modic type I or II marrow change of 25% vertebral height will be an infrequent but highly specific finding, with a high PPV for discogenic pain.

High Intensity Zone

In 1992 Aprill and Bogduk[65] described the HIZ (Fig. 3-5) as an imaging marker of a painful disc at provocation discography. Their definition of the HIZ is as follows: "high-intensity signal (bright white) located in the substance of the posterior annulus fibrosis, clearly dissociated from the signal of the nucleus pulposus in that it is surrounded superiorly, inferiorly, posteriorly, and anteriorly by the low intensity (black) signal of the annulus fibrosis and is appreciably brighter than that of the nucleus pulposus." This finding was identified on a midsagittal T2 weighted image; it may

occur centrally in an otherwise normal annulus or a bulging annulus or be located superiorly or inferiorly behind the edge of the vertebral body in a severely bulging annulus. The prevalence of this finding was assessed in the MRI examinations of 500 consecutive patients. The per-patient prevalence was 29%; the per-disc prevalence of an HIZ was 6%. There was excellent reliability in identification of this finding, with independent observers in agreement on the presence or absence of an HIZ in 411/412 discs. The finding was best demonstrated on spin-echo T2 weighted images and not well demonstrated on gradient-echo images. The vast majority of HIZs were present at the L4 and L5 disc levels, confirmed on later studies.

The relationship of the HIZ to pain production was evaluated in a subset of 41 patients selected for the presence of an HIZ on prediscography MRI. Discography was performed using IASP criteria with the requirement of a nonpainful control disc for a diagnosis of discogenic pain. Pain responses were tabulated both as "exact" reproduction of pain and "similar pain." Correlation of pain provocation at discography with the HIZ is seen in **Table 3-7**. In the 41 patients 118 discs were tested; the per-disc prevalence of the HIZ was 34%, reflecting the selection bias in this nonconsecutive series. In detecting exact pain, the HIZ had a sensitivity of 82% and specificity of 89%, a 70% PPV, and a +LR of 7.3. When the discographic criteria were relaxed to exact or similar pain, the

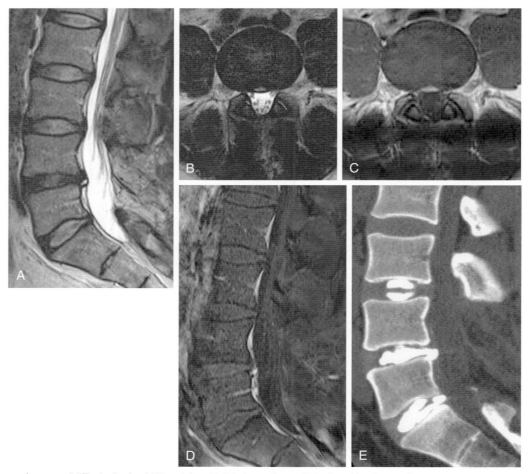

Fig. 3-5 High intensity zone (HIZ). **A,** Sagittal T2 weighted MRI shows loss of T2 signal in the L4 disc with an HIZ in the posterior annulus. **B,** Axial T2 weighted MRI at L4 interspace demonstrates the HIZ in the posterior annulus. **C,** Axial enhanced T1 weighted MRI image showing enhancement in the HIZ, also demonstrated in the sagittal fat-saturated T1 image **(D)**. **E,** Sagittal postdiscogram computed tomography demonstrates annular fissure at L4 leading to HIZ.

Table 3-7: High Intensity Zone

Author, Date	Discogram Criteria	HIZ Criteria	Prevalence per disc (%)	Sensitivity (%)	Specificity (%)	PPV (%)	NPV	+LR (CI)	−LR (CI)
Aprill and Bogduk,[65] 1992	IASP Exact pain	Aprill	34*	82	89	78	91	7.3 (3.9-13.7)	0.21 (0.1-0.4)
	Exact or similar pain	Aprill		63	97	95	72	18.4 (4.6-72.7)	0.38 (0.3-0.5)
Schellhas and associates,[66] 1996	IASP	Schellhas[†]	60*	97	83	87	97	5.7 (3.5-9.3)	0.03 (0.01-0.11)
Ricketson, Simmons, and Hauser,[67] 1996	Walsh	Aprill	9	12	92	57	54	1.5 (0.4-5.6)	0.96 (0.8-1.1)
Saifuddin and associates,[69] 1998	Walsh	Aprill	18	27	94	89	47	4.8 (1.7-14.2)	0.77 (0.7-0.9)
Ito and associates,[45] 1998	Walsh	Aprill	20	52	89	60	87	4.8 (2.3-10.2)	0.54 (0.4-0.8)
Smith and associates,[68] 1998	Walsh	Aprill	13	27	90	40	80	2.6 (1.2-5.6)	0.82 (0.7-1.0)
Carragee, Paragioudakis, and Khurana,[70] 2000	Walsh	Carragee[‡]	30	45	84	73	62	2.8 (1.5-5.5)	0.7 (0.5-0.9)
Weishaupt and associates,[51] 2001	IASP	Aprill	20	27	85	56	62	1.8 (0.8-3.7)	0.86 (0.7-1.0)
Peng, Hou, and Wu,[71] 2006	Walsh	Aprill	12	NC	NC	100	NC	NC	NC
Lei and associates,[53] 2008	Walsh	Aprill	19	25	87	62	57	1.8 (0.8-4.1)	0.87 (0.7-1.1)
O'Neill and associates,[46] 2008	IASP	O'Neill[§] 1 + 2 + 3 intensity grades	28	44	89	82	60	4.1 (2.7-6.1)	0.62 (0.5-0.7)
		2 + 3	16	26	95	86	54	5.7 (3.0-10.9)	0.78 (0.7-0.8)
		3	9	15	98	86	52	6.8 (2.7-17.1)	0.87 (0.8-0.9)
Kang,[47] 2009	IASP	Aprill	26	57	84	53	86	3.46 (2.2-5.5)	0.52 (0.4-0.7)

CI, Confidence interval; HIZ, high intensity zone; IASP, International Association for the Study of Pain; +LR, positive likelihood ratio; −LR, negative likelihood ratio; NPV, negative predictive value; PPV, positive predictive value.
*Nonconsecutive series with presence of an HIZ as an inclusion criteria. Sensitivity and prevalence values are not meaningful because of this selection bias.
[†]Includes lesions with thin line of T2 hyperintensity within annulus or connecting nucleus to HIZ.
[‡]Includes posterolateral lesions, HIZ signal intensity within 10% of cerebrospinal fluid T2 signal.
[§]Schellhas criteria plus posterolateral and lateral lesions.

specificity rose to 97% with a positive predictive value of 95%; there were only two false-positive cases in which a disc bearing an HIZ was nonpainful. The authors postulated that the HIZ represents a complex grade 4 fissure (Dallas discography scale) where the nuclear material has been trapped within the lamellae of the annulus fibrosis and become inflamed, accounting for the T2 signal intensity, which is brighter than that of the parent nucleus. They advanced the HIZ finding as pathognomonic of a symptomatic disc. The publication of these findings elicited considerable interest and numerous subsequent studies attempting to verify or refute these conclusions.

Schellhas and colleagues[66] performed a retrospective analysis of patients who had undergone MRI evaluation and provocation discography; the inclusion criteria included at least one each HIZ disc.

The definition of an HIZ was relaxed to include cases in which a thin line of high T2 signal was present on the posterior annulus or connected the HIZ to the nucleus. The series consisted of 100 HIZ discs in 63 adult patients. Discography was performed with notation of the intensity and concordance of pain. A nonpainful or nonconcordant control disc was confirmed in every case. Of the 100 discs bearing an HIZ, 87 were concordantly painful, 77 with a pain intensity of seven or greater on a 10-point scale. All 87 concordantly painful discs showed grades 3 to 5 annular tears on CT discography. The authors also performed MRI scans on 17 asymptomatic subjects and identified only one HIZ disc among the 85 lumbar levels evaluated. They concluded that the HIZ is a reliable marker for painful annular disruption in individuals with low back pain. They also noted the presence of HIZ-like signal abnormality in the posterolateral aspects of the disc and suggested expanding the definition beyond a midsagittal location.

This optimistic review of the HIZ as a marker of discogenic pain was challenged by Ricketson and colleagues, also in 1996.[67] They studied 80 discs in 29 consecutive patients with low back pain with or without radiculopathy. Discography was performed using Walsh criteria. No significant correlation ($p < 0.05$) was identified between a concordant pain response and the presence of an HIZ. From their data, a contingency table was constructed, and statistics calculated (see **Table 3-7**). The HIZ was an uncommon finding in this series, with a prevalence of 9% per disc. The HIZ finding showed high specificity (93%) but low positive predictive value (57%) and an uninformative likelihood ratio. The 1998 study of Smith and colleagues[68] was also less supportive of the HIZ as a useful marker for discogenic pain. They evaluated the reliability of the HIZ imaging finding as defined by Aprill and Bogduk[65] in 432 discs and showed only a fair-to-good agreement between two evaluating neuroradiologists. Correlation with provocation discography was performed on 152 discs in 55 patients. Discography was performed with Walsh criteria. Prevalence of HIZ discs was 13%. An HIZ disc had high specificity (90%) but low PPV (40%) for a concord of a painful disc. Of the 20 HIZ discs identified, only eight were associated with a concordant pain response.

Saifuddin and colleagues[69] studied 152 discs in 58 consecutive patients, also in 1998. The criteria of Aprill and Bogduk[65] for the HIZ finding were used. Discography used Walsh criteria. There were 27 HIZ discs identified; 24 had a concordant pain response. There was a statistically significant ($p < 0.0004$, Fisher) association between an HIZ disc and concordant pain at discography. HIZ discs were present with 18% prevalence per disc, a 95% specificity, 89% PPV, and +LR of 4.8 for concordant pain at discography. The 1998 study by Ito and colleagues has been described previously.[45] The definition of April and Bogduk[65] for HIZ was used. HIZ discs were present with 20% prevalence; the HIZ finding exhibited a 90% specificity, a PPV of 60%, and a +LR of 4.8.

In 2000 Carragee, Paragioudakis, and Khurana[70] evaluated the presence and significance of the HIZ in both symptomatic and asymptomatic subjects. The definition of HIZ was expanded to include bright signal in the posterolateral quadrants of the annulus rather than only those seen on the midsagittal images as originally described. Quantitated signal intensity was required to be within 10% of that exhibited by cerebrospinal fluid (CSF) to be considered an HIZ; areas of elevated but less intense signal were classified as medium intensity zones. Discography was performed with Walsh criteria, requiring 3/5 intensity concordant pain. The methods section states that pressure measurements occurred, but no statement is made regarding how this altered diagnostic criteria, nor are any data presented. Forty-two symptomatic patients (109 discs) and 54 asymptomatic subjects (143 discs) were studied. In the symptomatic group 59% of patients had HIZ discs, whereas in the asymptomatic group only 24% had HIZ discs (significant, $p = 0.001$). In symptomatic patients 30% of discs had an HIZ; only 9% of discs in asymptomatic subjects contained an HIZ (significant, $p < 0.0001$). The statistics for the symptomatic group are presented in **Table 3-7**; an HIZ disc has an 84% specificity, a 73% PPV, and a +LR of 2.8 for discogenic pain. These data support the HIZ as a useful marker for the painful disc. However, the authors point out that the presence of an HIZ disc strongly predicted a positive pain response at discography in both the symptomatic (73%) and asymptomatic (69%) groups. The asymptomatic group had also been stratified by psychometric evaluation; in participants with either chronic pain or abnormal psychometric studies, all HIZ discs produced pain with pressurization. The authors contend that the similar painful response rate of HIZ discs in symptomatic and asymptomatic subjects devalues the HIZ as a useful finding since the total weight of diagnosis depends on concordance vs. non-concordance of pain response. The "medium intensity zone" did not predict discogenic pain, suggesting a threshold effect for the significance of the HIZ, as had been noted in the original description.

The Weishaupt study of 2001[51] evaluated 116 discs in 50 patients. The discography has been previously described; they used the original Aprill and Bogduk HIZ criteria.[65] In their series the HIZ had a 20% per disc prevalence with 85% specificity but only 56% PPV for discogenic pain. Of the 23 HIZ discs identified, only 13 were concordantly painful at discography. Peng and associates[71] reported on 142 discs in 52 consecutive low back pain patients without radicular features (mean age 39 years). They used the original Aprill and Bogduk HIZ standard. The discography methodology is incompletely described but appears to approximate Walsh criteria. Contingency table data were not presented; they stated that all 17 discs with an HIZ produced concordant pain at discography. This would imply a 100% specificity and PPV, but the number of false negatives cannot be determined. Of the 17 HIV discs, 11 were ultimately excised during posterior interbody fusion procedures. Histological study showed disruption of the lamellar structure of the annulus with vascularized granulation tissue at the site of the HIZ. The presence of vascularized granulation tissue explains the gadolinium enhancement frequently demonstrated on enhanced MRI. Lei and associates' 2008 study[53] used the original Aprill and Bogduk criteria. The 18 patients who reported noncordant pain on discography were excluded from the analysis of endplate changes and the HIZ; it would have been more consistent with the Walsh discographic criteria to consider these negative responses. Within the 113 discs evaluated, there were 21 HIZ discs; 13 produced concordant pain on pressurization, and 8 produced no pain. Sensitivity was 25%, specificity 87%, and PPV 62%. The results section states that there were 25 HIZ discs; this would imply that there were 4 HIZ discs with nonconcordant pain. Properly including these as false positives would reduce the PPV to 52%.

O'Neill and associates' study of 2008[46] modified the Aprill and Bogduk criteria to include HIZ lesions connected to the nuclear compartment by a thin line of high T2 signal or consisted only of a thin horizontal line of high T2 signal within the annulus. They also included posterior, posterolateral, and lateral lesions. HIZ lesions were further segregated by intensity of T2 signal on a three-part scale (mild, moderate, and markedly hyperintense). Contingency tables were constructed from the published data, and the statistics calculated for three thresholds of HIZ detection: markedly intense cases, markedly and moderately intense cases, and combining all three (see **Table 3-7**). As the threshold tightened, the specificity and +LR rose; the PPV remained high for all three threshold levels. For only markedly hyperintense HIZs the specificity was 98%, the PPV 86%, and the +LR 6.8. This would support Bogduk's comments that "low intensity zones may well occur in asymptomatic volunteers, but that when activated (ostensibly inflamed), these fissures become painful and assume a higher signal intensity."[38] Finally the Kang and associates' study[48] evaluated the HIZ using the original Aprill definition both as an independent variable and in combination with other findings. Prevalence of HIZs was 26% per disc. As an independent variable, the HIZ exhibited 84% specificity with a PPV of 53%.

Again, general conclusions are confounded by alterations in the definition of the parameter under study (HIZ) by various authors, and significant variability of the gold standard test, provocation discography. The Aprill and Bogduk,[65] Schellhas and associates,[66]

Weishaupt and associates,[51] O'Neill and associates,[46] and Kang and associates[48] studies used IASP criteria with a negative control disc; the remaining studies did not. No studies used ISIS criteria with manometry. Schelhas and associates[66]; Carragee, Paragioudakis, and Khurana[70]; and O'Neill and associates[46] expanded the definition of the HIZ. The data of O'Neill and associates suggest a threshold effect, with higher levels of T2 signal having greater specificity and PPV for pain production. It is reasonable to conclude from the several studies that the HIZ is a finding of modest frequency in patients being investigated for discogenic pain, with a per-patient prevalence approaching 30%. When present, the preponderance of data would suggest that it predicts a painful disc with high specificity, positive predictive value, and +LR. There is likely a threshold effect for signal intensity.

Multivariate Analysis

The studies of Kang and associates[48] and O'Neill and associates[46] included multivariate analyses. The study parameters were described previously. O'Neill and associates showed that the disc degenerative findings (i.e., loss of disc height, loss of nuclear signal, and disc contour abnormalities) correlated strongly with each other; the inflammatory findings, HIZ, and endplate change did not, with the exception of HIZ and disc contour abnormality. The rank correlations of the MRI findings with a positive discogram were signal abnormality > disc height > disc contour > HIZ > endplate change. Disc signal change alone was as accurate as other individual parameters or combinations thereof. This was most evident at the two extremes of the ROC curve: when disc signal is normal, it is highly unlikely that the disc will be painful, regardless of other findings; and when there is severe signal loss, the disc is highly likely to be painful. Other parameters become useful when disc signal is intermediate. The authors noted that disc bulge was most helpful when signal loss was intermediate, resulting in a sensitivity of 80% and a specificity of 79%. In the presence of intermediate signal loss, the findings of moderate loss of disc space height or presence of an HIZ boosted the specificity further at the cost of sensitivity.

Kang and colleagues[48] introduced a new MRI classification system combining the findings that have been previously addressed as independent variables: class 1, normal or bulging disc without an HIZ; class 2, normal or bulging disc with an HIZ; class 3, disc protrusion without HIZ; class 4, disc protrusion with HIZ. Disc extrusions and sequestrations were excluded from the analysis. Logistic regression analysis showed that class 4, disc protrusion with HIZ, had the strongest correlation with concordant pain at discography. This combination had a specificity of 87% and a PPV of 98%. This finding had a prevalence of 13% and a sensitivity of 45%.

Conclusions

Identifying painful discs with diagnostic imaging is challenging because of the following:

1. There is no pathological or surgical gold standard.
2. The existing standard of comparison, provocation discography, is ultimately unproven, subjective in its interpretation, and has evolved over time in its criteria for a positive test—none of the studies reviewed here used the most current and restrictive criteria, those of ISIS.
3. The imaging findings likely have threshold effects in which only a significant expression of the finding (intensity of an HIZ, extent of marrow change) is a useful predictor of discogenic pain. Most studies do not account for this.

4. Imaging findings are likely technique dependent to an unknown degree, and imaging techniques are evolving.

An HIZ may be seen with greater conspicuity on thinner slices than thicker ones; it was originally described with spin-echo T2 weighted sequences, whereas most current T2 weighted imaging uses fast spin-echo (FSE) or turbo spin-echo (TSE) sequences. Is a bright signal in the posterior annulus on a short tau inversion recovery (STIR) or fat-saturated FSE equivalent to the original description? Will marrow edema be better seen on a T1 fluid attenuated inversion recovery (FLAIR) sequence or a conventional spin-echo sequence? These questions are unanswered.

Although it is tempting to succumb under the weight of these uncertainties, there are also evolving reasons to press the cause of noninvasive imaging. Discography has until recently been considered a minimally invasive but nondestructive test. There is now in vitro and in vivo evidence suggesting that disc puncture or discography may contribute to disc dysfunction and degeneration. Korecki, Costi, and Iatridis[72] noted that in a bovine disc model, single punctures with a 25-gauge needle resulted in biomechanical degradation of disc function with cyclic loading. Carragee and associates[73] demonstrated on 10-year follow-up MRI imaging that asymptomatic subjects who had undergone investigational discography showed more degenerative phenomena than matched control subjects. Although the clinical significance of these reports remains uncertain, it would seem clear that noninvasive diagnosis is preferable.

From the thicket of data, useful patterns do emerge. This is what we believe can be concluded from existing research:

1. The disc degenerative markers (i.e., loss of disc space height, loss of nuclear T2 signal, and disc herniation) correlate strongly with one another; loss of nuclear signal is most significant.
2. Severe nuclear signal loss (black disc) or severe loss of disc space height strongly predicts a painful disc.
3. Normal nuclear signal virtually excludes a painful disc.
4. When nuclear signal is intermediate, the inflammatory markers of the HIZ and endplate marrow change come into play.
5. A truly *high* intensity zone is infrequent but strongly predicts a painful disc.
6. When an HIZ is seen in combination with a disc protrusion, it very strongly predicts a painful disc.
7. Marrow endplate change of type I or type II involving greater than 25% of the vertebral body is uncommon but very strongly predicts a painful disc.

On the horizon are glimmers of light, advanced MRI imaging that may allow better characterization of disc degeneration. Watanabe and colleagues[74] used three Tesla MR images to generate axial T2 maps of the intervertebral disc, which may allow earlier detection of disc degeneration. Johannessen and associates[75] used a novel pulse sequence, T1ρ relaxation, to study degenerated discs in human cadavers; this was performed on a standard 1.5 Tesla imager. Their work showed a strong correlation between T1ρ signal and sulfated glycosaminoglycan content in the nucleus. Sodium (as opposed to proton) MRI has also been reported as a means of quantification of the proteoglycan content in the nuclear compartment of the disc.[76] These studies demonstrate the future—to be ultimately valuable in the diagnosis of discogenic pain, imaging must move beyond macroscopic descriptions of morphology to the realm of biochemical imaging, quantifying the change in nuclear constituents over time. In addition to biochemical degradation, imaging will also need to more precisely identify inflammatory mediators in the disc and adjacent cartilaginous endplate. Perhaps then we will truly be capable of the noninvasive diagnosis of discogenic pain.

Acknowledgement: The authors gratefully acknowledge the assistance of Dr. Rickey Carter, PhD (Mayo Biomedical Statistics) in performing statistical calculations from original data.

References

1. Jarvik JG, Deyo R: Diagnostic evaluation of low back pain with emphasis on imaging. *Ann Intern Med* 137:586-597, 2002.

2. Deyo RA, Mirza SK, Martin BI: Back pain prevalence and visit rates: estimates from US national surveys, 2002. *Spine* 31:2724-2727, 2006.

3. Deyo R, Mirza S, Turner Y: Overtreating chronic back pain: time to back off? *JABFM* 22(1):62-68, 2009.

4. Quinet RJ, Hadler NM: Diagnosis and treatment of backache. *Semin Arthr Rheum* 8(4):261-287, 1979.

5. Von Korff M et al: Back pain in primary care: outcomes at 1 year. *Spine* 18:855-862, 1993.

6. Van den Hoogen HJ, Koes BW, van Eijk JT et al: On the course of low back pain in general practice: a one-year follow-up study. *Ann Rheum Dis* 57:13-19, 1998.

7. Chou R et al: Imaging strategies for low-back pain: systematic review and metaanalysis. *Lancet* 373:463-472, 2009.

8. Liang M, Komaroff AL: Roentgenograms in primary care patients with acute low back pain: a cost-effective analysis. *Arch Intern Med* 142: 1108-1112, 1982.

9. Carragee E et al: Are first-time episodes of serious LBP associated with new MRI findings? *Spine J* 6:624-635, 2006.

10. Bradley W: Low back pain. *Am J Neuroradiol* 28(5):990-992, 2007.

11. Chou R et al: Diagnosis and treatment of low back pain: a joint clinical practice guideline from the American College of Physicians and the American Pain Society. *Ann Intern Med* 147:478-491, 2007.

12. Engers A et al: Individual patient education for low back pain, *Cochrane Database of Systematic Reviews*; Art. No. CD004057 DOI: 10.1002/14651858.CD004057. Pub 3, 2008.

13. Mettler FA et al: Effective doses in radiology and diagnostic nuclear medicine: a catalog. *Radiology* 48:254-263, 2008.

14. E-publication 2009 Centers for Medicare & Medicaid Services. http://www.cms.hhs.gov/. Accessed November 2009.

15. Jarvik JG et al: Rapid magnetic resonance imaging vs radiographs for patients with low back pain. *JAMA* 289:2810-2818, 2003.

16. Lurie JD, Birkmeyer NJ, Weinstein JN: Rates of advanced spinal imaging and spine surgery. *Spine* 28:616-620, 2003.

17. Mirza S, Deyo R: Systematic review of randomized trials comparing lumbar fusion surgery to nonoperative care for treatment of chronic back pain. *Spine* 1:32(7):816-823, 2007.

18. Hult L: Cervical, dorsal and lumbar spinal syndromes. *Acta Orthop Scand* 17(suppl):1-102, 1954.

19. Hellstrom M et al: Radiologic abnormalities of the thoracolumbar spine in athletes. *Acta Radiol* 31:127-132, 1990.

20. Hitselberger WE, Witten RM: Abnormal myelograms in asymptomatic patients. *J Neurosurg* 28:204-206, 1968.

21. Wiesel SW et al: A study of computer-assisted tomography. I. The incidence of positive CAT scans in an asymptomatic group of patients. *Spine* 9:549-551, 1984.

22. Weinreb JC et al: Prevalence of lumbosacral intervertebral disc abnormalities on MR images in pregnant and asymptomatic nonpregnant women. *Radiology* 170:125-128, 1989.

23. Boden SD et al: Abnormal magnetic-resonance scans of the cervical spine in asymptomatic subjects: a prospective investigation. *J Bone Joint Surg [Am]* 72(8):1178-1184, 1990.

24. Jensen MC et al: Magnetic resonance imaging of the lumbar spine in people without back pain. *N Engl J Med* 331:69-73, 1994.

25. Boos N et al: 1995 Volvo Award in Clinical Sciences: the diagnostic accuracy of magnetic resonance imaging, work perception, and psychosocial factors in identifying symptomatic disc herniation. *Spine* 20:2613-2625, 1995.

26. Stadnik TW et al: annular tears and disc herniation: prevalence and contrast enhancement on MR images in the absence of low back pain or sciatica. *Radiology* 206(1):49-55, 1998.

27. Weishaupt D et al: MR Imaging of the lumbar spine: prevalence of intervertebral disc extrusion and sequestration, nerve root compression, endplate abnormalities, and osteoarthritis of the facet joint in asymptomatic volunteers. *Radiology* 209(3):661-666, 1998.

28. Jarvik JJ et al: The longitudinal assessment of imaging and disability of the back (LAID back) study. *Spine* 15; 26(10):1158-1166, 2001.

29. Kjaer P et al: An epidemiologic study of MRI and low back pain in 13-year-old children. *Spine* 30:798-806, 2005.

30. Salminen JJ et al: Recurrent low back pain and early disc degeneration in the young. *Spine* 24:1316-1321, 1999.

31. Takatalo J et al: Prevalence of degenerative imaging findings in lumbar magnetic resonance imaging among young adults. *Spine* 34:1716-1721, 2009.

32. Schmid MR et al: Changes in cross-sectional measurements of the spinal canal and intervertebral foramina as a function of body position: in vivo studies on an open-configuration MR system. *AJR Am J Roentgenol* 172(4):1095-1102, 1999.

33. Danielson B, Willen J: The diagnostic effect from axial loading of the lumbar spine during computed tomography and magnetic resonance imaging in patients with degenerative disorder. *Spine* 26(23):2607-2614, 2001.

34. Jinkins R, Dworkin J, Damadian R: Upright, weight-bearing, dynamic-kinetic MRI on the spine: initial results. *Eur Radiol* 15(9):1815-1825, 2005. Epub 2005 May 20.

35. Fardon DF, Milette PC: Nomenclature and classification of the lumbar disc pathology: recommendations of the combined task forces of the North American Spine Society, American Society of Spine Radiology, and American Society of Neuroradiology. *Spine* 26:E93-E113, 2001.

36. Nathan H: Osteophytes of the vertebral column: an anatomic study of their development according to age, race, and sex with consideration as to their etiology and significance. *J Bone Joint Surg* 44:243-268, 1962.

37. Hancock M et al: Systematic review of tests to identify the disc: SIJ, or facet joint as the source of low back pain. *Eur Spine J* 16:1539-1550, 2007.

38. Bogduk N: Point of view: Predictive signs of discogenic lumbar pain on magnetic resonance imaging with discography correlation. *Spine* 23(11):1259-1260, 1998.

39. Bogduk N, editor: *Practice guidelines for spinal diagnostic procedures*, San Francisco, 2004, International Spine Intervention Society.

40. Guyer R, Ohhnmeiss D: Lumbar discography. *Spine J* 3(3 suppl):11S-27S, 2003.

41. Manchikanti L et al: Systematic review of lumbar discography as a diagnostic test for chronic low back pain. *Pain Physician* 12(3):541-559, 2009.

42. Chou R et al: Interventional therapies, surgery, and interdisciplinary rehabilitation for low back pain: evidence-based clinical practice guidelines from the American Pain Society. *Spine* 1; 34(10):1066-1077, 2009.

43. Cohen S, Larkin T, Barna S: Lumbar discography: a comprehensive review of outcome studies, diagnostic accuracy, and principles. *Reg Anesth Pain Med* 30(2):163-183, 2005.

44. Walsh T et al: Lumbar discography in normal subjects: a controlled, prospective study. *J Bone Joint Surg Am* 72:1081-1088, 1990.

45. Ito M et al: Predictive signs of discogenic lumbar pain on magnetic resonance imaging with discography correlation. *Spine* 23:1252-1258, 1998.

46. O'Neill C et al: Accuracy of MRI for diagnosis of discogenic pain. *Pain Physician* 11:311-326, 2008.

47. Kang C et al: Can magnetic resonance imaging accurately predict concordant pain provocation during provocative disc injection? *Skeletal Radiol* 38: 877-885, 2009.

48. Osti O, Fraser R: MRI and discography of annular tears and intervertebral disc degeneration. *J Bone Joint Surg [Br]* 74-B(3):431-435, 1992.

49. Horton C, Daftari T: Which disc visualized by magnetic resonance imaging is actually a source of pain? *Spine* 17(suppl 6):S164-S171, 1992.

50. Weishaupt D et al: Painful Lumbar disc derangement: relevance of endplate abnormalities at MR imaging. *Radiology* 218:420-427, 2001.

51. Pearce R et al: Magnetic resonance imaging reflects the chemical changes of aging degeneration in human intervertebral disc. *J Rheumatol* 27(suppl):42-43, 1991.

52. Lim C et al: Discogenic lumbar pain: association with MRI imaging and CT discography. *Eur J Radiol* 54(3):431-437, 2005.

53. Lei D et al: Painful disc lesion: can modern biplanar magnetic resonance imaging replace discography. *J Spinal Disord Tech* 21:430-435, 2008.

54. Pfirrmann CW et al: Magnetic resonance classification of lumbar intervertebral disc degeneration. *Spine* 1; 26(17):1873-1878, 2001.

55. Modic M et al: Degenerative disc disease: assessment of changes in vertebral body marrow with MR imaging. *Radiology* 166(1 pt 1):193-199, 1988.

56. Ohtori S et al: Tumor necrosis factor-immunoreactive cells and PGP 9.5-immunoreactive nerve fibers in vertebral endplates of patients with discogenic low back pain and Modic type 1 or type 2 changes on MRI. *Spine* 31; 9:1026-1031, 2006.

57. Toyone T et al: Vertebral bone-marrow changes in degenerative lumbar disc disease: an MRI study of 74 patients with low back pain. *J Bone Joint Surg [Br]* 76:757-764, 1994.

58. Albert HB, Manniche C: Modic changes following lumbar disc herniation. *Eur Spine J* 16(7):977-982, 2007.

59. Buttermann GR et al: Vertebral body MRI related to lumbar fusion results. *Eur Spine J* 6:115-120, 1997.

60. Lang P et al: Lumbar spinal fusion: assessment of functional stability with magnetic resonance imaging. *Spine* 15:581-588, 1990.

61. Chataigner H, Onimus M, Polette A: Surgery for degenerative lumbar disc disease: should the black disc be grafted [in French]? *Rev Chir Orthop Reparatrice Appar Mot* 84:583-589, 1998.

62. Esposito P et al: Predictive value of MRI vertebral end-plate signal changes (Modic) on outcome of surgically treated degenerative disc disease: results of a cohort study including 60 patients. *Neurochirurgie* 52:315-322, 2006.

63. Braithwaite IJ et al: Vertebral end-plate (Modic) changes on lumbar spine MRI: correlation with pain reproduction at lumbar discography. *Eur Spine J* 7:363-368, 1998.

64. Kokkonen S et al: Endplate degeneration observed on magnetic resonance imaging of the lumbar spine. *Spine* 27(20):2274-2278, 2002.

65. Aprill C, Bogduk N: High-intensity zone: a diagnostic sign of painful lumbar disc on magnetic resonance imaging. *Br J Radiol* 65(773):361-369, 1992.

66. Schellhas K et al: Lumbar disc high-intensity zone: correlation of magnetic resonance imaging and discography. *Spine* 21(1):79-86, 1996.

67. Ricketson R, Simmons J, Hauser W: The prolapsed intervertebral disc: the high intensity zone with discography correlation. *Spine* 21(23):2758-2762, 1996.

68. Smith B et al: Interobserver reliability of detecting lumbar intervertebral disc high-intensity zone on magnetic resonance imaging and association of high-intensity zone with pain and annular disruption. *Spine* 23(19):2074-2080, 1998.

69. Saifuddin A et al: The value of magnetic resonance imaging in the demonstration of annular tears. *Spine* 23(4):453-457, 1998.

70. Carragee E, Paragioudakis S, Khurana S: Lumbar high-intensity zone and discography in subjects without low back problems. *Spine* 25(23):2987-2992, 2000.

71. Peng B, Hou S, Wu W: The pathogenesis and clinical significance of a high-intensity zone (HIZ) of lumbar intervertebral disc on MRI imaging in the patient with discogenic low back pain. *Eur Spine J* 15(5):583-587, 2006.

72. Korecki C, Costi J, Iatridis J: Needle puncture injury affects intervertebral disc mechanics and biology in an organ culture model. *Spine* 33(3):235-241, 2008.

73. Carragee E et al: Does Discography cause accelerated progression of degenerative changes in the lumbar disc: a ten-year matched cohort study. *Spine* 34(21):2338-2345, 2009.

74. Watanabe A et al: Classification of intervertebral disc degeneration with axial T2 mapping. *Am J Radiol* 189:936-942, 2007.

75. Johannessen W et al: Assessment of human disc degeneration and proteoglycan content using T1ρ-weighted magnetic resonance imaging. *Spine* 31(11):1253-1257, 2006.

76. Wang C et al: Validation of sodium magnetic resonance imaging of intervertebral disc. *Spine* 35(5):505-510, 2010.

4 Provocation Discography

Richard Derby, Milton H. Landers, Lee R. Wolfer, and Philip Kim

CHAPTER OVERVIEW

Chapter Synopsis: Chronic discogenic pain is a common problem. Its diagnosis presents significant challenges and should include multiple components. Perhaps no diagnostic tool has been as controversial as discography, a process in which contrast dye is injected into an intervertebral disc. However, discography can represent one useful component in the arsenal of diagnostic procedures under proper circumstances. This chapter provides a guide to the indications, technical considerations, and complications associated with discography. Although the primary concern with discography is the likelihood of a false positive finding, when current standards are utilized the validity of the procedure is sound. As an invasive procedure, discography carries significant risks to the patient and should not be used as an initial screening tool. Though initially used only for visualization of a disc's anatomical position, clinicians determined that the technique could be used for diagnosis when dye injection evoked discogenic pain familiar to patients. In its current state, discography can be used as a prelude to appropriate therapeutic interventions.

Important Points:

- Patient selection is of the utmost importance. This includes an appropriate history, physical examination, and interpretation of a recent MRI or CT scan by the physician performing the discography.
- Careful patient positioning allows for good fluoroscopic visualization and ease of disc access.
- The discographer must be experienced and skilled in needle placement, and understand the intricacies of the procedure.
- Informed consent is necessary to ensure that the patient understands and is comfortable with the provocative nature of the procedure and the need to provide appropriate information and dialogue with the physician.
- High quality fluoroscopic equipment and procedure table allow good visualization and safe disc access.
- Sedation should be used only to the extent as to provide adequate comfort for the patient without compromise of the pain responsiveness.
- Prophylactic antibiotic IV and intradiscal anesthetic help to prevent possible discitis.
- Sterile technique should be used.
- Use a true anterioposterior view with the endplate closest to the target parallel to the x-ray beam and appropriate obliquity, unique for each disc level accessed.
- Pain produced ipsilaterally to the needle insertion site must be evaluated carefully. The needle can be jiggled gently to distinguish needle pain from discogenic pain.
- Transient pain may be provoked. A true positive response is concordant pain, ≥7/10, sustained for greater than 30 to 60 seconds, at a pressure of ≤50 psi above opening, and volume of ≤3.5 mL.
- The injection into each disc should be slow.
- All positive responses should be confirmed with repressurization with a small volume of contrast.
- Discography performed at levels of prior discectomy have a higher false-positive response rate, and low pressure and volume criteria must be upheld.
- Pain reproduced at all levels tested should not be considered a positive discogram.

Clinical Pearls:

- If the patient has significant pain in a disc without a grade 3 tear, consider pain referred from a contiguous disc, overlap of innervations, or a fissure too small to discern by fluoroscopy.
- All positive responses should be confirmed with manual repressurization with a small volume. If repressurization does not provoke concordant ≥7/10 pain at <50 psi a.o., the response is considered indeterminate.
- If the patient provokes pain in a disc without a grade 3 tear, (adjacent to a positive response disc) one mL of 4% lidocaine (Xylocaine) should be injected into the painful adjacent disc and provocation testing repeated in about 5 minutes. One may find that the normal-appearing disc is no longer painful. If still painful, one should look for a small annular tear on the post-discogram CT scan.

Clinical Pitfalls:

- Pain provocation is difficult to interpret if one provokes excessive pain during needle insertions.
- Pain produced ipsilaterally to the needle insertion site must be evaluated carefully. Referred pain may be caused by the discogram needle adjacent to the dorsal root ganglion. The needle can be jiggled gently to distinguish needle pain from discogenic pain.
- Transient pain may be provoked if an asymptomatic fissure or previously healed annular tear with a fibrous cap is opened abruptly during pressurization. A true positive pain response is ≥7/10 and sustained for greater than 30 to 60 seconds; true discogenic pain is less likely to decrease rapidly. Pain that resolves within 10 seconds should be discounted. Clinically, patients with discogenic pain tend to have increased pain post procedure, and may note some exacerbation of symptoms for 3 to 7 days.
- False positive pain provocation will occur in a severely degenerated disc if excessive volume is injected. Injected volume should be limited to about 3.5 mL if the disc has an intact annulus or the disc is so degenerated that more volume is needed to fill the disc.
- The false-positive response rate is high in previously operated discs. Pain provocation should be reported as indeterminate unless the disc is painful at low volume and low pressure.

Introduction

Until the introduction of discography by Lindblom in the 1940s and 1950s,[1-3] oil-based contrast myelography was used to diagnose intervertebral disc herniations.[4] During the era of the "herniated disc" in the 1930s,[5] both axial and referred pain were thought to be caused by the disc-compressing neural elements. Myelography has always been limited in that it only visualized the thecal sac and dural root sleeves. Discography allowed visualization of the disc itself, including internal morphology and lateral protrusions, which were missed on myelography.

Discography was initially used to diagnose disc herniations before surgery in patients with radicular pain.[1,6,7] Interestingly, however, most of the discs examined by discography exhibited annular disruption but no frank herniation or protrusion. More important, on injection of contrast media into these internally disrupted discs, some patients experienced reproduction of their familiar pain.[8,9] These observations led surgeons to use provocation discography not only to reveal structural abnormalities but also to identify and treat painful internally disrupted discs. Discography became a sophisticated extension of the physical examination, a means of "palpating" the disc to elicit pain.[10]

Over the last decades histochemical and anatomical studies have provided evidence that the disc is an innervated structure capable of transmitting pain. There is no doubt that the disc can be a source of pain. Typically in a normal disc innervation is limited to the outer annulus; however, we know that pathologically painful discs (based on positive discogram pre-fusion) show neoinnervation to the inner annulus and nucleus pulposus.[11-13] It is believed that injection of contrast dye into the nucleus stimulates nerve endings[14] via two mechanisms: a chemical stimulus from contact between contrast dye and sensitized tissues and a mechanical stimulus resulting from fluid-distending stress. What is controversial is not whether the disc is a source of pain but whether disc pain can be reliably diagnosed. The validity and accuracy of discography has been challenged, particularly in the last 10 years, with reports of unacceptably high false-positive rates in asymptomatic subjects, particularly in patients with chronic pain or evidence of psychological pathology. However, these negative studies have been refuted after close review and a performance of a meta-analysis of false-positive rates of lumbar discography. Combining all the major studies on discography in asymptomatic subjects, a false-positive rate of less than 10% can be achieved if the discographer adheres to strict operational standards and interpretation criteria.[15]

Although magnetic resonance imaging (MRI) and computed tomography (CT) are the most commonly used advanced imaging modalities for low back pain, discography still occupies a critical place in the diagnostic algorithm. We know that abnormal disc morphology alone is not diagnostic of discogenic pain because many individuals with abnormal CT scans or MRIs are asymptomatic of low back pain.[16,17] However, MRI cannot distinguish between a painful and painless disc. In contemporary practice the criterion standard for diagnosis of a painful internally disrupted disc by provocation discography is pain ≥7/10, pressure <50 psi a.o. (pounds per square inch above opening), concordant pain, ≥grade 3 annular tear, volume ≤3.5 mL, and the presence of a negative control disc.[18]

In its proper context discography is not a stand-alone test but rather a diagnostic test used to confirm one's hypothesis that a particular disc is the source of the patient's pain.

In this chapter the indications for discography, both technical considerations and complications of lumbar discography, are discussed. Procedural descriptions have also been extensively described in our prior publications.[19-21] The technical section of the chapter is followed by a brief updated literature review regarding the role of discography as a diagnostic test (vs. MRI and CT), the false-positive controversy, and both predictive value and analgesic discography.

Indications and Contraindications

Discography is not an initial screening examination. Disc stimulation follows failed conservative treatment modalities and is only used when other less invasive diagnostic tests are inconclusive. Discography is invasive, and irreversible surgical procedures may be chosen based on the results. The principal indication for provocation discography is to determine whether or not a disc is pathologically painful and the extent of annular or endplate disruption. Pertinent clinical information is then used to establish a diagnosis of discogenic pain for targeted disc therapies. Only discography followed by CT scanning can define the internal anatomy of the disc.[22] Postdiscography CT scanning is also particularly useful in postdiscectomy patients with suspected residual or recurrent disc herniations. Discography is useful in problematic cases unresolved by MRI or myelography and in patients for whom surgery is contemplated.[23] It can offer a potential solution to the diagnostic dilemma concerning which patients to treat surgically and at what segmental level. When a single disc is found to be symptomatic in the presence of adjacent asymptomatic discs, focused intradiscal or surgical therapy can be entertained. A no less important application is to identify discs which are non-pristine by imaging studies, but are asymptomatic, and therefore require no treatment intervention.

Patients with symptomatic or abnormal discs at multiple levels (≥3) constitute a greater surgical challenge. If the patient is not a surgical candidate, discography is useful to provide a diagnosis to bring the workup to closure and direct the patient to non-interventional pain management care.

The position statement of the North American Spine Society on discography is as follows:[22] Discography is indicated in the evaluation of patients with unremitting spinal pain, with or without extremity pain, of greater than 4 months' duration, when the pain has been unresponsive to all appropriate methods of conservative therapy. Before discography the patients should have undergone investigation with other modalities that have failed to explain the source of pain; such modalities should include but not be limited to CT scanning, MRI scanning, and/or myelography.

Indication criteria include the following:

- Conservative treatment for low back pain of probable spinal origin has failed.
- Pain has been ongoing for greater than 3 months.
- Other pain generators have been ruled out (e.g., facets; sacroiliac joints).
- Symptoms are clinically consistent with disc pain.
- Symptoms are severe enough to consider surgery or percutaneous interventions.
- Surgery is planned, and the surgeon desires an assessment of the adjacent disc levels.
- The patient is capable of understanding the nature of the technique and can participate in the subjective interpretation.
- Both the patient and physician need to know of the source of pain to guide further treatments.

Contraindications include the following:

- Unable or unwilling to consent to the procedure
- Inability to assess patient response during the procedure

- Inability of patient to cooperate
- Known localized or systemic infection
- Pregnancy
- Anticoagulants or bleeding diathesis

Relative contraindications to discography follow:

- Allergy to contrast medium, antibiotics, or local anesthetics
- Significant psychological overlay
- Any other condition, medical, congenital, postsurgical, anatomical or psychological, that would increase the risk of performing the procedure to an acceptable level

Preprocedure Evaluation

Before discography, a complete history and physical examination should be obtained to reveal any procedural contraindications. The patient may have multiple symptoms that may be attributed to various spinal structures. It is important to identify the discogenic symptoms because these are the symptoms that will be provoked on discography. Red flags such as fever, night pain, history of malignancy, or unexplained weight loss should alert the physician to an alternate diagnosis. Before discography, informed consent should be obtained from the patient. The purpose and nature of the procedure; its risks, benefits, alternatives and complications; and what to expect after the procedure are explained. Patients are instructed in the use of a 0-to-10 pain scale.

Specifically the patient should understand that discography is commonly painful and that they will need to describe the location, intensity, and concordance of any provoked pain in respect to their ongoing complaints. A trained observer can independently monitor patient pain responses during the procedure. Some discographers have their patients fill out a brief psychometric test such as the Distress and Risk Assessment Method (DRAM) to assess if the patient has a normal, at risk, distressed depressive, or distressed somatic profile.[24]

In patients with a history of allergy to nonionic water-soluble contrast media (iohexol or iopamidol) or other drugs, the risks vs. benefits of the procedure must be weighed and discussed with the patient. Patients with suspect iodine allergies should be pretreated with corticosteroids and H_1 and H_2 blockers before the procedure. If the risk of allergic reaction to contrast is significant, saline can be substituted with the addition a very small volume of gadolinium considered. The addition of gadolinium allows assessment of the internal disc by MRI performed immediately post-procedure.[25,26]

In all cases of lumbar discography, an MRI or CT scan should be reviewed. The majority of discographers select test levels according to the appearance of the MRI T2 weighted images. Most test discs with decreased T2 weighted signal intensity; an adjacent, less degenerated disc is usually selected as a control. Rarely is it necessary to inject greater than four levels.

Patient Preparation

Antibiotic Prophylaxis

Intravenous (IV) access is standard. Discitis is the most common serious (although rare) complication. Prophylactic antibiotic (cefazolin 1 g, gentamicin 80 mg, clindamycin 900 mg, or ciprofloxacin 400 mg) is given within 30 minutes of needle insertion. Sheep studies confirmed optimal antibiotic levels in the annulus 30 minutes after IV administration; no antibiotics were present at 60 minutes.[27,28] Following the procedure aminoglycosides are not required for prophylaxis.[29] Along with IV antibiotics, many discographers mix antibiotics with the contrast dye (between 1 and 6 mg/mL of cefazolin or an equivalent dose of another antibiotic) for intradiscal administration.[30-33] Klessig, Showsh, and Sekorski[33] reported that cefazolin and gentamicin, 1 mg/mL; and clindamycin, 7.5 mg/mL, exceed the minimum inhibitory concentrations (MICs) for the three most common organisms causing discitis: *Escherichia coli, Staphylococcus aureus*, and *Staphylococcus epidermidis*. All procedures should be performed under sterile conditions with double gloves. Another concern is patients with histories of surgical infection who are methicillin-resistant *S. aureus* carriers. Preoperative nasal cultures have been used to identify carriers and treated with mupirocin topical to nares with reduction in surgical infection.

Sedation

As a provocative test, discography is at best uncomfortable and at worst very painful. How much and which drug to use for preoperative sedation varies according to the discographer's skill and training. IV sedation should be titrated to maintain patient comfort during needle insertion and minimize masking of the evoked pain response. The patient must be awake and conversant during disc stimulation. Doses of midazolam (Versed) between 2 and 5 mg provides effective sedation and anxiolytic effect during discography but may cause retrograde amnesia. Many spine interventionalists with an anesthesia background use propofol (Diprivan) (an ultrashort-acting hypnotic) in intermittent boluses of 10 to 30 mg. Propofol causes rapid sedation and amnesia during needle insertion; but, because of its short half-life, the patient will be awake during disc stimulation. Other anesthesia drugs such as ketamine, clonidine, and dexmedetomidine should be used with caution since they have analgesic properties.

Some discographers, including one of the authors (MHL), believe that opioids should not be used before or during discography.[21,34-36] They assert that discography is a provocational test; therefore pain intensity needs to be compared and quantified in relation to the patient's usual pain intensity, and opioid analgesics could decrease the pain response and increase the chance of a false-negative response. Alternatively, others[32] believe that a small dose of analgesics (meperidine [Demerol], 50 mg; fentanyl, 50 mcg; or morphine, 5 mg) before the procedure helps to decrease the rate of false positives in patients with clinically insignificant discogenic pain.

Most discographers agree that chronically opiate-tolerant patients (who have also been NPO) should be given a reasonable dose of IV opiate to avoid false-positive responses in the setting of early opiate withdrawal and possible heightening pain responses. One of the authors uses opioids and IV ketorolac at the end of the provocation discography. During discography, patients must be monitored appropriately. Although respiratory depression is uncommon with this protocol, subjects should have a pulse oximeter and blood pressure cuff.

Supplemental oxygen is supplied by nasal cannula. Personnel competent in airway management and resuscitation should be present during the procedure. General, epidural, or spinal anesthesia is inappropriate as it negates any diagnostic potential.

Sterile Technique

The skin and draping technique for discography is similar to the sterile technique used for surgery. Standard draping to provide a sterile field may include the use of sterile towels or fenestrated drapes per the injectionist's preference. Povidone-iodine 10% (Betadine solution), and/or DuraPrep (iodophor 0.7% and isopropyl alcohol 74%) are the preparations of choice.

Chlorhexidine and alcohol may be substituted if the patient has allergies to the aforementioned solutions. Recent studies[37] suggest that chlorhexidine and alcohol preparation are superior to povidone-iodine solution in reducing postoperative infection. Other suggested protocols may include a chlorhexidine shower the night before the procedure. Some authors scrub the area of the procedure before sterile preparation. This is done to remove the top layer of grime and material that may be hoarding skin bacteria. The procedure room staff should be dressed in clean clothes (scrub suits). Surgical caps and masks are mandatory for any personnel in close contact to the sterile field. Many injectionists scrub, gown, and glove as for an open surgical procedure. The C-arm image intensifier should also be draped to prevent detritus from falling onto the sterile field, and allows the injectionist to easily position the instrument for optimum visualization using safe, sterile technique.

Lumbar Discography: Technique

Discography can be performed in a procedure room appropriate for aseptic procedures. Fluoroscopy is required for safe visualization of spinal anatomy in anteroposterior (AP), lateral, and oblique projections. Biplanar fluoroscopy can be used, but most discographers use C-arm units, which allow excellent visualization without repositioning the patient. An adjustable, radiolucent procedure table is useful.

Patient Position

The patient lies in a prone position on a fluoroscopy table. Most discographers place a pillow or bolster under the patient's abdomen to slightly flex the spine and decrease the lumbar lordosis. Elevating the target side approximately 15 degrees allows the fluoroscopy tube to remain in a more AP projection and reduces radiation scatter. If needed, a folded towel or soft wedge can be placed under the patient's flank to prevent side bending of the lumbar spine. Monitoring and light sedation are initiated. On the side selected for puncture, a wide area of the skin of the back is prepared and draped from the costal margin to the mid buttock and from the midline to the flank.

Disc Puncture

Until the 1960s discography was performed with a posterior interpedicular or transdural approach; however, this technique is seldom used today because it requires two punctures of the dura. Currently a lateral, or extrapedicular, approach[38,39] is used, except in rare situations in which anatomical variation or postsurgical changes prevent disc access from a lateral approach. Before injection a fluoroscopic examination of the spine is performed to confirm segmentation and determine the appropriate level for needle placement. The target disc is identified on AP view. The image intensifier of the C-arm is tilted in a cephalad or caudad direction until the endplate of the vertebral body, caudad to the target disc, is parallel to the x-ray beam (**Fig. 4-1**). The endplate is visualized as a line rather than an oval. After selecting the target disc on AP view, the fluoroscopic beam is rotated obliquely until the superior articular process of the facet joint is at the midpoint of the upper vertebral endplate. On occasion at L5-S1, due to the wider dimension of the vertebral body, increased interfacetal distance, and the iliac crest, the fluoroscopy tube can only be rotated far enough to bring the SAP approximately 25% of the distance between the lateral margins of the inferior endplate of the level above. In this oblique view the insertion point is 1-3 mm lateral to the lateral margin of the superior articular process (SAP) (**Fig. 4-2**).

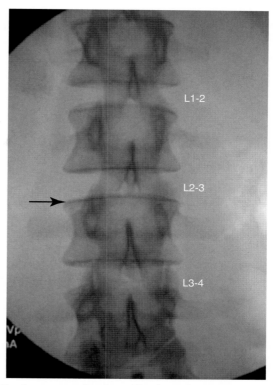

Fig. 4-1 Anteroposterior view of lumbar spine. Target disc is at L2-L3. Black arrow indicates superior endplate of L3 parallel to x-ray beam. Adapted from Derby R et al: Discography. In Pinheiro-Franco JL et al, editorss: *Advanced concepts in lumbar degenerative disc disease*, Brazil, 2010, Dilivros, p 86.

This positioning of the fluoroscope allows needles to be passed using tunnel vision (i.e., parallel to the beam when the skin puncture site is aligned with the target structure) just lateral to the SAP. The disc is preferentially approached from the side opposite the patient's usual pain to avoid the patient mistaking discomfort secondary to needle placement with provoked pain secondary by disc stimulation. If the patient has central pain or the pain is equal bilaterally or if there are other impeding technical factors, needle insertion from either side is fine.

The needle insertion point is marked on the skin. The distance between the two segmental superior articular processes increases at the lower lumbar levels. At T12-L1 the needle insertion point is about 3 to 4 cm lateral to the midline; at L5-S1 it is approximately 6 to 7 cm lateral. However, this lateral deviation is highly dependent on body habitus with a more lateral insertion required with obese patients.

Before needle placement a skin wheal is made with lidocaine 1% ($\approx$1 mL) using a 25-gauge, 1.5-inch needle. To anesthetize the needle track, one can use a 25-gauge, 3.5-inch needle advanced under tunnel vision (i.e., parallel to the x-ray beam to the level of the SAP). Exercise caution so as not to anesthetize the dorsal root ganglion within the foramen. Overenthusiastic anesthetization may obscure nerve root impalement and could potentially anesthetize the sinuvertebral and ramus communicans nerves, thus altering the evoked pain response during disc stimulation and creating a false-negative response. A one- or two-needle technique may be used; however, most discographers currently use a two-needle technique. Before the routine use of prophylactic antibiotics, Fraser, Osti, and Vernon-Roberts[40] reported a rate of discitis

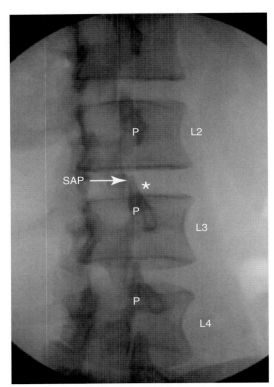

Fig. 4-2 Right oblique view. Tip of SAP of L3 is at approximate midpoint of the inferior endplate of the L2 vertebral body. *P*, pedicle; *SAP*, superior articular process; ***, target point. Adapted from Derby R et al: Discography. In Pinheiro-Franco JL et al, editors: *Advanced concepts in lumbar degenerative disc disease*, Brazil, 2010, Dilivros, p 86.

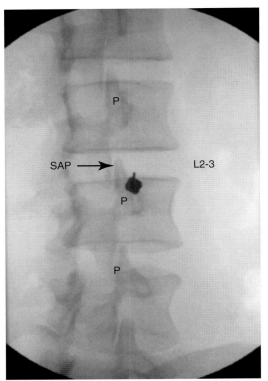

Fig. 4-3 Right oblique view. Introducer needle is lateral to SAP at L2-L3 target disc *(black arrow)*. *P*, Pedicle; *SAP*, superior articular process. Adapted from Derby R et al: Discography. In Pinheiro-Franco JL et al, editors: *Advanced concepts in lumbar degenerative disc disease*, Brazil, 2010, Dilivros, p 87.

with single nonstyleted vs. double needles of 2.7% vs. 0.7%. Both the North American Spine Society and the International Spinal Injection Society recommend a two-needle approach.[18,22] The two-needle technique uses a shorter, larger-gauge introducer needle through which a longer, smaller-gauge needle is advanced past the tip of the introducer needle into the targeted intervertebral disc, theoretically avoiding picking up any skin flora.. The trend is to use a 20-gauge, 3.5-inch introducer with the 25-gauge, 6-inch disc puncture needle. The 25-gauge needle theoretically minimizes any trauma to the disc. Less experienced operators may start with the 18/22-gauge needle combination, particularly because the curve of the disc puncture needle is easier to maintain. The body habitus of the patient will dictate if longer needles are necessary (i.e., a 5-inch introducer and an 8-10-inch disc puncture needle). A slight bend, opposite the bevel, is typically made at the tip of the disc puncture needle to allow the operator to "steer" the needle.[41-44] At times a larger curve, at the distal third of the disc puncture needle, must be used to compensate for less than ideal anatomy or postsurgical changes. The introducer needle is passed through the skin wheal at the skin puncture point, using a "down the beam" or tunnel-vision technique on the oblique fluoroscopic view (**Fig. 4-3**). To avoid potential neural injury, the needle should be directed into the region below the segmental nerve, just lateral to the superior articular process and above the endplate (**Figs. 4-3 and 4-4**). The disc puncture needle must travel under the segmental nerve coursing medial to lateral and dorsal to ventral to puncture the annulus fibrosus of the disc at the midpoint of the disc when seen in lateral and AP views. To minimize nerve trauma, a needle with a short, noncutting bevel or blunt pointed tip with a side port might be

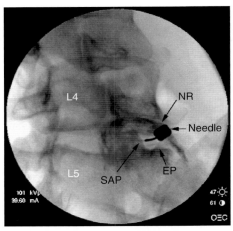

Fig. 4-4 Location for discogram needle insertion. *EP*, Endplate; *NR*, nerve root outlined by contrast media; *SAP*, superior articular process. Adapted from Slipman CW et al, editors: *Interventional spine: an algorithmic approach*, Philadelphia, 2008, Saunders Elsevier, p 292.

considered. Forward advancement is stopped at the approximate level of the SAP, although placement within the dorsal foramen is acceptable. A lateral fluoroscopic view should be used to check needle depth (**Fig. 4-5**).

The stylet is then removed from the introducer; and the longer, smaller-gauge disc puncture needle is advanced slowly under real-time lateral fluoroscopy. The needle is seen to transverse the intervertebral foramen; then firm but resilient resistance is noted as the needle touches and punctures the annulus fibrosus. On the lateral view the needle typically contacts the posterior disc margin 1 to 3 mm posterior to the vertebral margin. On AP projection the discogram needle ideally contacts the disc margin on a line drawn

between the midpoints of the pedicles above and below (**Fig.** 4-6). The patient may experience a brief sharp, pinching, or sudden aching sensation when the needle pierces the innervated outer annulus fibrosus. In no case should one advance the introducer or discogram needle medial to the inner pedicle margins before contacting the intervertebral disc. Using lateral fluoroscopy, the needle is then advanced to the center of the disc as seen on both lateral and AP projections (**Figs.** 4-7 and 4-8). Lateral and AP projections are used to ensure good needle placement, and spot films are saved

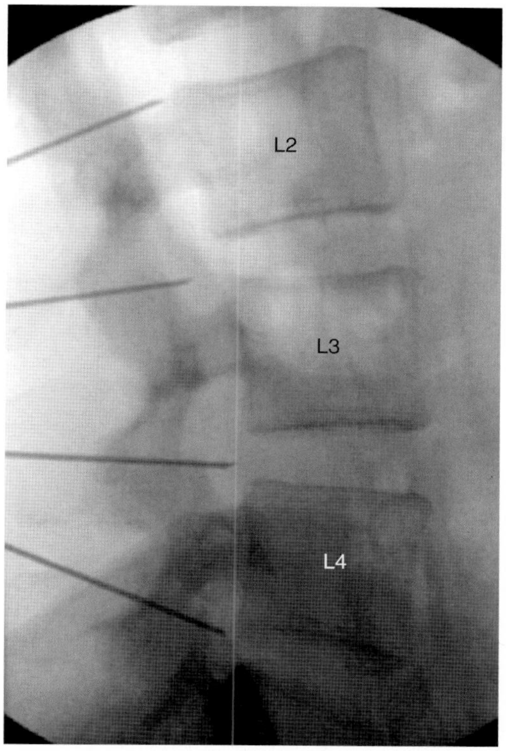

Fig. 4-5 Lateral fluoroscopic view of lumbar spine. All introducer needles are in place at or just ventral to the posterior elements for L1-2 through L5-S1 discs. Adapted from Derby R et al: Discography. In Pinheiro-Franco JL et al, editors: *Advanced concepts in lumbar degenerative disc disease*, Brazil, 2010, Dilivros, p 88.

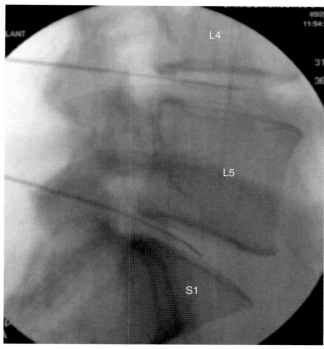

Fig. 4-7 Lateral fluoroscopic view. Discogram needles placed into center of intervertebral discs.

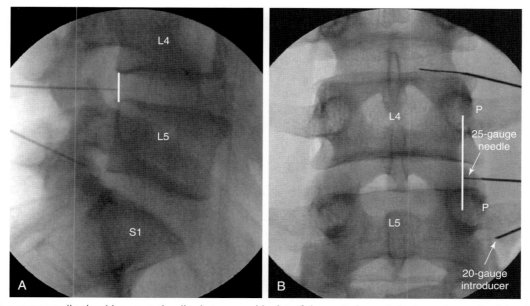

Fig. 4-6 The discogram needle should contact the disc between midpoint of the posterior vertebral margins on the lateral view (**A,** *white vertical line*) and at the line between the midpoint of the pedicles on the anteroposterior view (**B,** *white vertical line*). P, pedicle. Modified from Slipman CW et al, editors: *Interventional spine: an algorithmic approach*, Philadelphia, 2008, Saunders Elsevier, p 293.

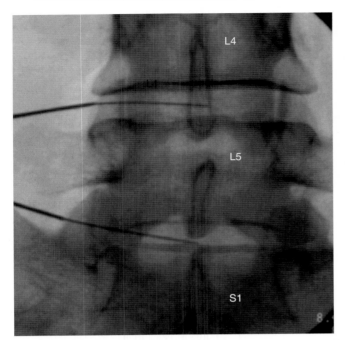

Fig. 4-8 Anteroposterior view. Disc puncture needles in center of nucleus pulposus of each intervertebral disc.

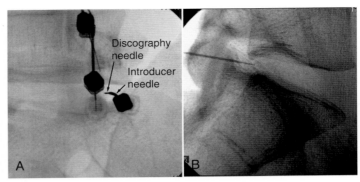

Fig. 4-9 A, Oblique view of L5-S1 needle position. The tip of the discogram needle can be seen just beyond the introducer just lateral to the S1 superior articular process and medial to the iliac crest. **B,** Lateral view. The needle is advanced slowly under direct fluoroscopic vision, and the guide needle is retracted simultaneously. The inner needle should contact the disc 2 to 3 mm posterior to the vertebral margin. Modified from Slipman CW et al, editors: *Interventional spine: an algorithmic approach*, Philadelphia, 2008, Saunders Elsevier, p 293.

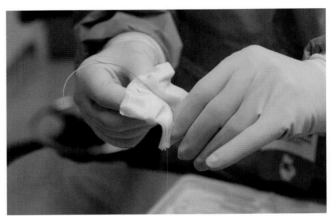

Fig. 4-10 Operator uses sterile gauze to bend distal tip of the discogram needle (bevel facing out). This technique is often used at the L5-S1 disc space. Photo courtesy Richard Derby, MD. Adapted from Derby R et al: Discography. In Pinheiro-Franco JL et al, editors: *Advanced concepts in lumbar degenerative disc disease*, Brazil, 2010, Dilivros, p 86.

for documentation before injection of contrast. If bony obstruction is encountered, the physician should utilize varying fluoroscopic views to determine whether the needle has contacted the superior articular process or the vertebral body. If the SAP is contacted, the introducer needle can be withdrawn slightly, and its trajectory modified. The introducer needle can be advanced to just over the lateral edge of the superior articular process or though the foramen to the margin of the disc where soft, "rubber-like" resistance to insertion will be noted. If the vertebral body is contacted, the introducer needle must be withdrawn towards the SAP and then re-advanced at a slightly different trajectory using active lateral fluoroscopy using to guide the needle positioning. If the patient experiences any radicular pain or dysesthesia during needle advancement, insertion of the needle must halt. The ventral ramus may be encountered because it crosses the posterior lateral aspect of the disc in close proximity to the disc entry site. In such a case, the needle is partially withdrawn to alter its course and redirected toward the disc. A slight bend in the needle tip facilitates small directional adjustments. Typically redirection of the needle more medially and caudally avoids the segmental nerve. If greater direction changes are needed, the introducer needle is also withdrawn and redirected. This technique can be used for disc puncture in more than 95% of lumbar disc levels; however, occasionally because of anatomical variations (i.e., overriding iliac crest, osteophytes) or postsurgical changes (i.e., posterior intertransverse fusion mass or fusion hardware), the procedure must be varied. A detailed description of the myriad modifications with which a discographer might be faced is beyond the scope of this chapter; however, most involve either a more lateral or medial needle insertion with the disc puncture needle bent or curved to varying degrees. Rarely the posterior interpedicular, transdural approach must be used for disc puncture. This technique increases the chance for morbidity since the dura is punctured twice. Risks and benefits of this technique must be weighed. At the L2-L3 level and above, the posterior approach should not be used because of the increased risk of impaling the

spinal cord. Disc puncture at L5-S1 is technically more challenging than the L1-L4 levels because of the increased interfacet distance and the proximity of the iliac crest. When identifying the L5-S1 target disc under fluoroscopy, the tube is rotated obliquely to bring the superior articular facet of S1 approximately 25% of the distance between lateral vertebral borders. Approximately 1 to 2 cm of the L5-S1 disc is visualized between the superior articular process of S1 and the sacral ala (**Fig. 4-9**). Unlike the direct lateral approach at the previous levels, a slight curve or "hockey-stick" bend is required for the discogram needle insertion at this level. Under the oblique fluoroscopic view, the introducer needle is advanced toward the bony notch between the S1 SAP and sacral ala. The needle tip should be immediately adjacent to the anterolateral aspect of the S1 SAP (see **Fig. 4-9**). Next, sterile gauze is used to curve the distal 2 to 3 cm of the discogram needle into a smooth arc in the direction opposite the bevel (**Fig. 4-10**). The degree of curve is operator-dependent, based on the amount of deflection required to reach the center of the disc. Under a live lateral fluoroscopic view, the curved discogram needle is advanced through the guide needle until the tip emerges. The needle is then directed in a medial and slightly posterior course around the SAP to stay within the safe region (see **Fig. 4-4**). For some discographers, the 18/22-gauge needle combination may be easier to direct vs. the 20/25-gauge needle combination used at upper levels. Obese or muscular patients may require longer needles. Once the discogram needle reaches the annulus fibrosus, its position is checked in both AP and lateral views. In the lateral view the needle should contact the disc 2 to 3 mm posterior to the vertebral margin (see **Fig. 4-9, B**), and in the AP view the needle ideally should be on a line bisecting the midpoint of the L5 and S1 pedicles. The needle course must be closely monitored; if the needle does not curve sufficiently in the medial direction, it will not reach the center of the disc; moreover, it may strike the ventral ramus. If the needle does not track medially and posteriorly, it must be removed, and its curvature accentuated. However, if an excessive curve is used the central spinal canal can be trespassed with dural or spinal cord puncture. As mentioned previously, if the needle contacts bone, it must be determined whether the superior articular process or the vertebral body has been encountered, and appropriate adjustments must be made. Ideally the final needle position is the center of the disc; however, there is leeway. In severely degenerated discs the needle position is not as crucial because the contrast spreads throughout the disc. Ideally the needle should be within 4 to 5 mm of the disc center on AP and lateral fluoroscopy.

Disc Provocation

Discography is a provocational test that attempts to mimic physiological disc loads and evoke the patient's pain by increasing intradiscal pressure with an injection of contrast medium. This concordance of pain reproduces that the index pain which the patient experiences in sitting and bending forward. Increased intradiscal pressure is thought to stimulate annular nerve endings, sensitized nociceptors, and/or pathologically innervated annular fissures. Until recently, pressure standards have been lacking, no doubt leading to erroneous conclusions. This approach is taxonomically unsound; emerging standards require unambiguous operational criteria that establish a threshold intensity for both pain response and stimulation intensity.

Both require a precise method to apply the stimulus and strict criteria for interpretation. The intensity of the provocation stimulus must be carefully controlled through the skilled operation of a manometer syringe or an automated manometer. A 3-mL syringe with manual thumb pressure is still used by some operators, but this does not reflect current standards.

Stimulus intensity can also be quantified with a controlled inflation syringe and digital pressure readout, permitting more precise comparisons between patient discs and between discographers. Most abnormal discs are painful between 15 and 50 psi[45] and are termed *mechanically sensitive* on the basis of a four-type classification introduced in the 1990s by Derby and associates in respect to annular sensitivity.[46] Discs that are painful at pressures <15 psi a.o. are termed *low-pressure positive* or *chemically sensitive* discs[46]; if painful between 15 and 50 psi a.o., they are termed *mechanically sensitive* discs. Indeterminate discs are painful between 51 and 90 psi a.o., and normal discs have no pain provocation. An important caveat is that a normal disc can hurt if pressurized too high with uncontrolled, manual thumb pressurization. Much of the recent research reporting a high false-positive rate for lumbar discography in asymptomatic subjects used uncontrolled, manual thumb pressurization to 100 psi.[47,48] If a disc is painful at >50 psi,

the response must be reported as indeterminate because it is difficult to distinguish between a pathologically painful disc and the pain evoked from simply mechanically stimulating a normal or subclinically symptomatic disc.[32] To limit false-positive responses, the most up-to-date discography standards set a pressure criteria of <50 psi to define a positive response.[18]

Injection speed is also a confounding factor and may account for interoperator variability in results and increased false-positive responses. At high injection speeds the true intradiscal pressure (dynamic pressure) is higher than the recorded static pressure.[49] The dynamic pressure, measured only in research settings, is the actual pressure that would be recorded with an intradiscal pressure sensor. Currently we measure pressure indirectly via a manometric syringe that records plateau static pressures after injection. The pain during activities of daily living (ADLs) is more closely correlated to dynamic peak pressure.[46] Static pressure is reflective of dynamic pressure when recorded by needle sensor and manometer only at slower injection speeds (<0.08 mL/sec).[49] Currently injection speed can be standardized with an automated manometer or manually by a skilled operator. When all needles are positioned in the nucleus pulposus of the target discs, injection can commence. The patient should be awake and able to describe sensations produced by disc stimulation. He or she should be blinded as to both the level and onset of injection. Nonionic contrast medium combined with antibiotic is injected into each disc at a slow velocity using a calibrated injection syringe or automated manometer with digital pressure readout. The total volume injected should probably be limited to ≤3.5 mL. A standardized procedure form is recommended. Opening pressure is reported first, with typical values from 5 to 25 psi, varying with the degree of disc degeneration. If the opening pressure is greater than 30 psi, it usually indicates that the needle tip is in the inner annulus and therefore must be repositioned. At each 0.5-mL aliquot the following data are collected: total volume, static and dynamic pressures, pain response (intensity and concordance), pain behaviors (vocal or physical), and contrast pattern. Injection continues until one of the following end points is reached: pain response ≥7/10, intradiscal pressure ≥50 psi above opening in a disc with a grade 3 or greater annular tear or 80 to 100 psi in a disc with a normal-appearing nucleogram, epidural or vascular pattern is evident, or a total of 3.5 mL of contrast medium has been injected. Some severely degenerated discs may accept greater volume; however, the incidence of false-positive pain responses may increase. If the disc cannot be pressurized >50 psi above opening pressure at ≤3.5-mL volume (because of an annular or endplate leak or severe disc degeneration), a rapid manual injection of a small volume can elicit a dynamic pressure of 50 psi above opening. However, the discographer should be aware that, in the setting of a leak, stimulation of structures adjacent to the disc (e.g., posterior longitudinal ligament, dorsal root ganglion [DRG], nerve roots) could provoke back or referred pain.

Imaging

Anteroposterior and lateral images of all injected discs are saved as part of the permanent record. A descriptive classification[50] is used for the fluoroscopic images: cotton ball, lobular, irregular, fissured, and ruptured (**Fig. 4-11**). A variety of patterns may occur in abnormal discs.[50] The appearance of the normal nucleus following the injection of contrast medium is classic: the contrast medium assumes either a lobular pattern or a bilobed "hamburger" pattern (see **Fig. 4-11**). Contrast medium may extend into radial fissures of various lengths but remain contained within the disc (see **Figs. 4-11** and **4-12**). Contrast may escape into the epidural

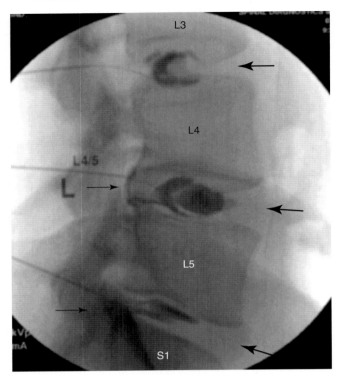

Fig. 4-11 Lateral fluoroscopic view after disc injection. Large, closed black arrows point to discs. L3-L4 disc: classic bilobed, "hamburger" pattern; L4-5 disc: posterior annular fissure with contrast dye outlining disc protrusion and a minimal leak *(thin black arrow)*; L5-S1: posterior annular tear extends to the outer posterior protrusion with leak into epidural space *(thin black arrow)*.

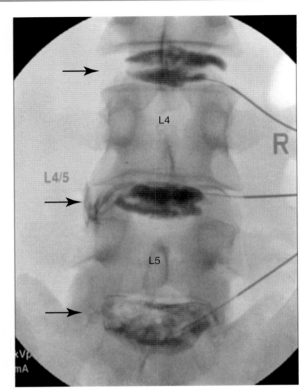

Fig. 4-12 Anteroposterior fluoroscopic view of patient in Fig. 4-11. Closed black arrows point to disc spaces. L3-L4 disc, bilobed dye pattern; L4-L5 disc, left-sided annular fissure extending into lateral protrusion; L5-S1 disc, marked annular disruption with small leak visible inferiorly. Adapted from Derby R et al: Discography. In Pinheiro-Franco JL et al, editors: *Advanced concepts in lumbar degenerative disc disease*, Brazil, 2010, Dilivros, p 93.

spaces through a torn annulus (see **Figs. 4-11** and **4-13**). In **Fig. 4-13** note how epidural contrast outlines the location of the left S1 nerve root as it passes under the right S1 pedicle.

This might explain how a patient could experience both axial and referred radicular type pain. In some cases the contrast medium may escape through a defect in the vertebral endplate.[51] In other cases the disc is completely fissured and disrupted (**Fig. 4-14**). However, none of these patterns alone indicates whether the disc is painful; that can be ascertained only by the patient's subjective response to disc injection. Postdiscography axial CT scanning provides the most accurate depiction of internal disc architecture. The degree of degeneration is described by dividing the disc into four quadrants.[52] If the contrast is confined to the nucleus, no quadrant disruption is present; if the contrast is dispersed, its location is described (e.g., single-quadrant disruption, right posterior; two-quadrant disruption, left anterolateral and right posterior). The degree of radial and annular disruption is most commonly described[52,53] using the modified Dallas discogram scale (**Fig. 4-15**)[18,54,55]: grade 0 describes contrast contained within the nucleus; grades 1 to 3 describe degree of fissuring extending to the inner, middle, and outer annulus, respectively; grade 4 describes a grade 3 annular fissure with a greater than 30-degree circumferential arc of contrast (**Figs. 4-16** to **4-20**); and a grade 5 annular tear indicates rupture or spread of contrast beyond the outer annulus (see **Fig. 4-13**).

Discography Standards

Both the techniques for performing discography and the criteria for interpreting the findings have been in a constant state of

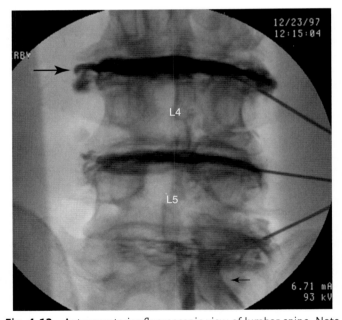

Fig. 4-13 Anteroposterior fluoroscopic view of lumbar spine. Note how contrast outlines the location of the S1 nerve root *(small black arrow)*. Large black arrow shows right lateral disc protrusion below L3 osteophyte and evidences an epidural leak at the right L5-S1 level. Adapted from Derby R et al: Discography. In Pinheiro-Franco JL et al, editors: *Advanced concepts in lumbar degenerative disc disease*, Brazil, 2010, Dilivros, p 94.

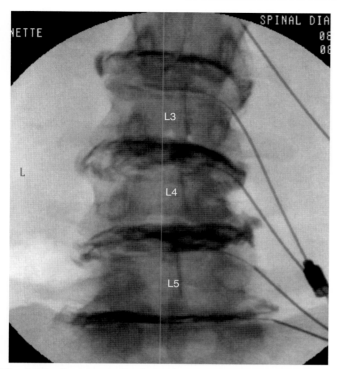

Fig. 4-14 Anteroposterior fluoroscopic view of lumbar spine. Multilevel severe degenerative disc disease from L2-L3 to L5-S1.

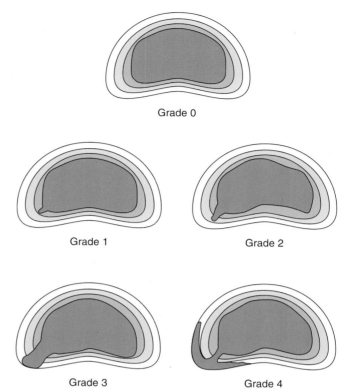

Fig. 4-15 Modified Dallas discogram scale. Grade 0, no annular disruption; grade 1, radial disruption into the inner third of the annulus; grade 2, contrast spread into the middle third of the annulus; grade 3, contrast into the innervated outer third of the annulus; grade 4, grade 3 with >30-degree circumferential tear; grade 5, spread of contrast into epidural space. Modified from Bogduk N: Lumbar disc stimulation. In Bogduk N, editor: *Practice guidelines for spinal diagnostic and treatment procedures, International Spine Intervention Society,* San Francisco, CA, 2004, p 23.

evolution since their introduction in the 1940s. Until recently,[32] discography has been performed without strict operational standards with respect to pressure limits, injection speed, volume, and validated clinical end points. The current standard for determining a positive response to discography with the use of pressure-controlled discography is: pain ≥7/10, pressure <50 psi a.o., concordant pain, grade 3 or greater annular tear, ≤3.5 mL volume, and at least one negative control disc.[18] One can refine the criteria by adding the Walsh criteria, which stipulate that a positive response includes ≥2/5 pain behaviors (guard/brace/withdraw, rubbing, signing, verbalizing, and grimacing).[56] Provocation discography is the best diagnostic test we have to diagnose discogenic pain. However, if performed without consistent operational and interpretation standards, discographers can obtain inaccurate results.

Caveats

The following are techniques used by experienced discographers to optimize performance of the test and limit false-positive and false-negative responses:

- The discographer must be skilled in needle placement; otherwise further pain provocation is hard to interpret. Inexperienced discographers often impale adjacent nerve roots or create significant tissue trauma from multiple needle insertion attempts.
- Pain produced ipsilaterally to the needle insertion site must be evaluated carefully. Referred pain may be caused by the discogram needle impinging on the dorsal root ganglion. The needle can be "jiggled" gently to distinguish needle pain from discogenic pain.
- Transient pain may be provoked if an asymptomatic fissure or previously healed annular tear with a fibrous cap is opened abruptly during pressurization. A true positive pain response is

≥7/10 and sustained for greater than 30 to 60 seconds; true discogenic pain is less likely to decrease rapidly. Pain that resolves within 10 seconds should be discounted. Clinically patients with discogenic pain tend to have increased pain postprocedure, and may note some exacerbation of symptoms for 3 to 7 days.

- All positive responses should be confirmed with manual repressurization with a small volume. If repressurization does not provoke concordant ≥7/10 pain at <50 psi a.o., the response is considered indeterminate.
- If the patient has significant pain in a disc without a grade 3 tear (adjacent to a positive response disc), consideration should be given to injecting 1 mL of 4% lidocaine (Xylocaine) into the painful adjacent disc and retesting the normal-appearing disc in 10 minutes. One may find that the disc is no longer painful. On rare occasion, a very small annular tear may be present that does not appear with fluoroscopy, but may be evidenced on a post-procedure CT scan. Another possibility involves segmental overlap of innervation.
- Injected volume should be limited to 3.5 mL. Painless, morphologically severely degenerated discs can be made painful if excessive volume is injected.
- When discography is performed on discs status post prior discectomy, the false-positive response is likely higher. The results should be reported as indeterminate unless the disc is painful at low volume and low pressure.

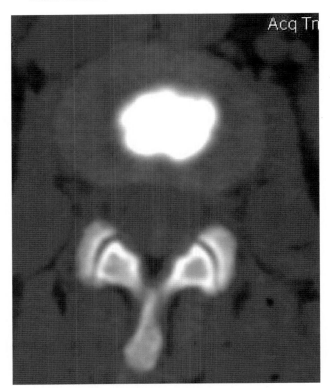

Fig. 4-16 Axial postdiscography computed tomography scan with grade 0 annular tear. Contrast is contained in the nucleus pulposus with an intact annulus.

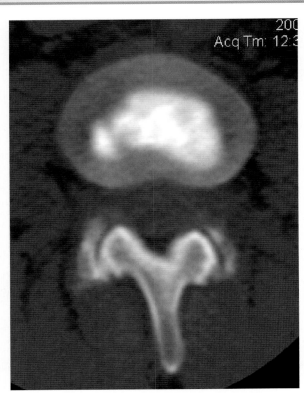

Fig. 4-18 Axial postdiscography computed tomography scan with grades 1 and 2 annular tears. Contrast extends slightly into the inner annulus in the right posterior quadrant and into the middle annulus iin the left posterior quadrant. Adapted from Derby R et al: Discography. In Pinheiro-Franco JL et al, editors: *Advanced concepts in lumbar degenerative disc disease*, Brazil, 2010, Dilivros, p 95.

Postprocedure Care

After the procedure patients are taken to the recovery room for monitoring of vital signs and clinical status by nurses trained in spine injection management. The patient is checked immediately following the transfer and 30 minutes after the procedure for any subcutaneous bleeding.

Analgesic medications (oral, IV or intramuscular [IM]) are provided as needed. The patient is advised that he or she may experience an exacerbation of their typical symptoms for 2 to 7 days. The patient is instructed to contact the office if fever, chills, or severe (or delayed) onset of pain develops. Patients are observed and discharged according to institutional protocol. Typically the patient is discharged to the care of a responsible adult and instructed not to drive for the remainder of the day. All patients should be contacted by phone 2 to 4 days after the procedure to screen for complications or adverse side effects.

Potential Risks and Complications

Postdiscography complications are well described.[28,57] Complications can occur secondary to the disc puncture itself or to misadventures during needle placement or related to medications used. Complications vary from minor (e.g., increased low back pain, nausea, headache) to major (discitis, seizure, permanent neurological injury, and death).[58] Concern over prolonged pain after discography has been overblown. In the 1960s Holt reported prolonged low back pain after discography[59]; however, serious criticisms were

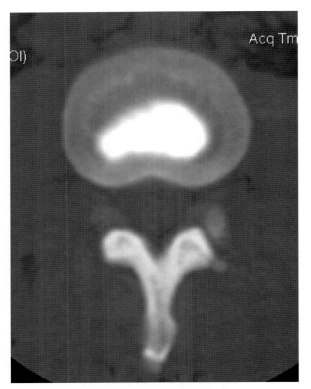

Fig. 4-17 Axial postdiscography computed tomography scan with grade 1 annular tear. Contrast extends slightly into the inner annulus in the right posterior quadrant. Adapted from Derby R et al: Discography. In Pinheiro-Franco JL et al, editors: *Advanced concepts in lumbar degenerative disc disease*, Brazil, 2010, Dilivros, p 95.

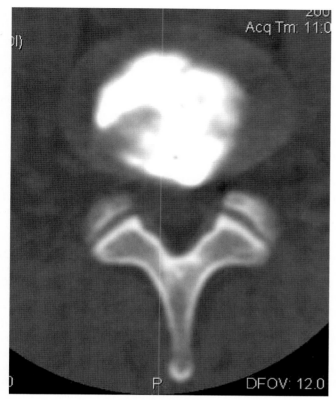

Fig. 4-19 Axial postdiscography computed tomography scan with grade 3 annular tear. Contrast extends posteriorly to the outer annulus within a contained protrusion.

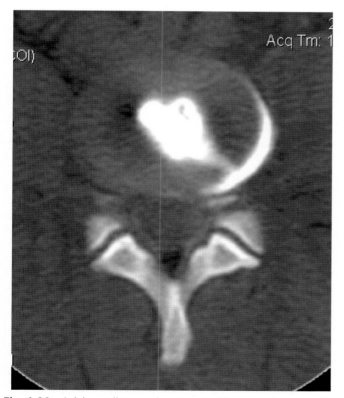

Fig. 4-20 Axial postdiscography computed tomography scan with grade 4 annular tear. Contrast extends into right posterior quadrant and into a circumferential tear of >30 degrees.

raised about this author's patient population (prisoners), technique, and use of noxious Hypaque dye. More recent studies also have serious shortcomings. The claim that discography causes prolonged pain at 1 year in subjects asymptomatic of low back pain who underwent discography is based on six patients.[60] Two of the six patients were chronic pain patients with postfailed cervical fusion status on opiate medications with active workers' compensation claims. The psychometric testing of these two patients also revealed that they were distressed somatics. The other four patients had a primary diagnosis of somatization disorder; two of the four were unable to tolerate the initial needle placement at more than one or two levels and discontinued their participation in the study.

Such a small sample size limits generalizability of the conclusions; moreover, it is well recognized that persons with somatization disorder commonly complain of recurrent pain and conversion phenomena (pseudoneurological symptoms) and are at risk for iatrogenic illness.[61] Furthermore, patients with somatization disorder are hospitalized or undergo surgery three times as often as depressed patients.[62]

Discitis is the most common serious complication of discography, reported to be less than 0.15% per patient and 0.08% per disc.[22] The incidence of discitis has been clearly diminished with the double- vs. single-needle technique.[27] In addition, with careful preprocedure screening for infection (e.g., urinary tract or skin), aseptic skin preparation, styleted needles, and IV and intradiscal antibiotics, discitis is now very rare. Over a 10-year period in the clinic of three of the authors (RD, LW, PK) only one case of discitis per over 2000 patients has been recorded. In the practice of the other author (ML), no cases of discitis have occurred in the same time period with injection into >6,000 individual discs. To prevent discitis, the authors recommend IV prophylaxis with antibiotics before the procedure and intradiscal antibiotics. However, even with prophylactic antibiotics, an epidural abscess after discography has been reported.[63,64] The most common causative organisms for discitis after lumbar discography are *S. aureus*, *S. epidermis*, and *E. coli*,[28,65,66] suggesting inoculation with surface flora or inadvertent bowel perforation. Clinically the patient with discitis presents with severe, unremitting, disabling pain in the days to weeks after the procedure. The patient may report a change in the quality of their pain and typical relieving factors. Some patients have a fever, although this is not a universal symptom. The workup should include physical examination, laboratory work, and imaging. Laboratory work includes complete blood count with differential (CBC), C-reactive protein (CRP), erythrocyte sedimentation rate (ESR), and blood cultures. The CRP usually increases within days of onset of infection; the ESR is not as sensitive and may not be elevated for a month. If the endplates have not been breached, the blood cultures and CBC are normal. MRI is the preferred imaging modality.[67-69] Technectium-99 bone scan is less sensitive and specific than MRI.[70] MRI within 3 to 4 days of symptoms shows increased T2 signal in the disc and endplate hyperemia. Biopsy in the acute phase before endplate breach is more likely to be positive. After endplate breach a sterile environment is created by activation of the immune system.[71] Treatment of discitis typically requires prolonged antibiotic therapy, although some mild self-limiting cases have been reported.[71]

Emphysema or abscess formation requires CT-guided drainage or surgical intervention.[72-74] Striking a ventral ramus is a potential hazard but may be avoided by careful attention to correct technique. The needle should be prevented from straying beyond its required and intended course. In a conscious patient contact with the ventral ramus is obviously indicated by a severe, sharp lancinating pain. Other complications include spinal cord or nerve root injury; cord compression or myelopathy; urticaria; retroperitoneal hemorrhage; nausea; convulsions; headache; and most commonly, increased pain.[22] Disc herniation following discography is very rare,[75] and there is little evidence that discography damages the disc.[76] Freeman and associates (2003)[77] recently reported no histological damage following needle insertion into sheep discs. Death after discography was reported in a patient who inadvertently received contrast dye mixed with cefazolin (12.5 mg/mL) intrathecally. She developed intractable seizures and coma and ultimately died.[78]

Discography Controversies: Brief Literature Review

Usefulness of Provocation Discography

While numerous papers have examined the usefulness of discography, some physicians still question its reliability.[60,79] Critics point toward mismatches between morphological features and clinical complaints and false-positive rates. Lumbar provocation discography for the diagnosis of abnormalities involving intervertebral discs has been used extensively as a diagnostic tool for evaluating low back pain since the 1950s. Almost from the beginning discography has been controversial, with both staunch proponents and opponents.

Discography is not meant to be a stand-alone test. Its proper use is in the diagnostic algorithm for chronic, intractable low back pain unresponsive to conservative care and when the patient is considering intradiscal or surgical treatments. Perhaps unappreciated is the value of discography in ruling out adjacent segment discogenic pain and limiting the number of levels treated surgically. Discography remains the criterion standard for visualizing internal disc architecture. As a provocation test, despite its liabilities and limitations, discography is also our best means of diagnosing discogenic pain. Provocation discography has 81% sensitivity and 64% specificity for pain.[80] It is commonly compared to CT or MRI imaging of the spine, yet it is distinctive in that it combines both an imaging and a provocation test. MRI is unable to discern a painless from a painful disc. We are well aware that morphological abnormalities of the disc are common in patients both with and without chronic low back pain. In one series 78% of patients with chronic low back pain had abnormal imaging findings on discography combined with post-CT-scanning (Grubb, Lipscomb, and Guilford, 1987[19,75]). Morphological abnormalities also increase with age.[81,82] Admittedly abnormal morphological structures revealed by discography without provocation are too nonspecific to be clinically useful; therefore positive results should be limited to those eliciting concordant pain.[79,83] In 1982 Millete and Melanson[84] reported retrospectively that concordant pain was evoked by injection in 37% of patients with a discographic morphological abnormality. Studies in the 1990s and 2000s on the prevalence of painful internal disc disruption in patients presenting to tertiary referral centers with chronic low back pain range from 26% to 39%.[85,86]

For most cases MRI is sufficient for advanced imaging; however, provocation discography adds additional useful diagnostic information to confirm or refute the hypothesis that a particular disc is the source of the patient's pain. Neither high-resolution CT scanning nor MRI demonstrates annular morphology with the same detail as discography.[87,88] CT discography was found to be more sensitive than MRI in detecting early annular disruption. In 18 of 177 discs with a normal T2 weighted MRI, annular and radial fissures were revealed on CT discography (Bernard).[89] When compared to surgical findings, in 94% of patients CT discography correctly diagnosed the type of disc herniation, including in the previously operated spine.[89] Discography has also been correlated to pain drawings.[90]

The high intensity zone (HIZ) has been proposed as a marker for a painful disc[91,92]; but, although highly specific, the sensitivity of this finding is only 26%, limiting the usefulness of the HIZ in selecting patients for surgery.[93] However, if an HIZ is contained within a protrusion, there is a correlation with a positive discogram response.[94] Discography remains a critical tool in surgical planning. Surgical decision making requires a high level of diagnostic confidence, and research has shown that MRI cannot always reliably predict which discs will be symptomatic with discography.[95,96]

False-Positive Rates

The greatest liability of discography at this time is the series of studies reporting high false-positive rates in asymptomatic subjects.[48,59] These recent negative studies also reported a correlation between the presence of chronic pain and abnormal psychometric scores with positive discogram responses. Early work by Holt in 1968[59] reported a 36% rate of positive discography in asymptomatic subjects, although this study contained serious methodological flaws. Reanalysis of the Holt data actually reveals a false-positive rate of 3.7%.[15]

Holt's findings were also refuted by Walsh and associates,[56] who demonstrated a 0% rate of positive discography in 10 asymptomatic volunteers and established reproducible criteria for positive discography (criteria: ≥3/5 pain [pain thermometer], concordant pain, ≥2/5 pain behaviors, pressure limited to approximately 60 to 70 psi a.o. [manual pressurization by a highly skilled discographer], and abnormal disc morphology). Using strict pressure criteria and pressure manometry, Derby and associates[97] studied 13 asymptomatic volunteers and also reported a 0% false-positive rate.

Carragee[47,48,60,98] performed discography on several subject populations asymptomatic of low back pain and reported the following false-positive rates: residual pain after iliac crest bone harvest, 50%; no low back pain, no chronic pain, 10%; chronic cervical pain, 40%; postdiscectomy, 35%; and somatization disorder, 75%. He also studied symptomatic subjects with "benign" or "mild persistent low back pain" and reported a false-positive rate of 36%.

Recent literature has reached a different conclusion. A critical examination of all the studies since the 1960s, including a systematic review and a meta-analyses of false-positive rates,[15] shows that an acceptably low false-positive rate can be achieved using provocation discography with the International Spine Intervention Society (ISIS)/ International Association for the Study of Pain (IASP) standards for a positive discogram: pain ≥7/10, concordant pain, pressure <50 psi a.o., ≥grade 3 annular tear, volume limit ≤3.5 mL, and presence of a negative control disc. Excluding the two studies from the 1960s, if all subject data from discography on asymptomatic subjects are analyzed together, a false-positive rate of 9.3% per patient and 6% per disc can be obtained. Among subjects asymptomatic of any confounding factors, one can obtain a false-positive rate of 3% per patient and 2.1% per disc; for subjects with chronic pain the rate is 5.6% per patient and 3.85% per disc. Taken alone as a group, postdiscectomy subjects appear to have a slightly higher false-positive rate of 15% per patient and 9.1% per disc. Given our limited knowledge of discography in postdiscectomy patients and the possibility that provocation may open previously healed granulation tissue along surgical planes, discographers may consider pressure and speed-controlled manometry and low pressure and volume limits for defining a positive value. Among subjects with somatization disorder, the false-positive rate is 50% per patient (95% confidence interval [CI] 0% to 100%) and 22% per disc. A recent meta-analysis of all studies of asymptomatic subjects undergoing discography (excluding 1960s studies; two patients with somatization disorder with an incomplete data set and subjects with chronic persistent low back pain) obtained a specificity of 0.94 (95% CI 0.89 to 0.98) or a false-positive rate of 6%.[15]

Concern has also been raised regarding chronic pain and psychological co-morbidity as significant confounding factors in patients undergoing discography. Is chronic pain a significant confounding factor? Evidence indicates that patients with chronic or chronic intermittent low back pain respond similarly to disc stimulation as do asymptomatic volunteers undergoing discography. Derby and associates[99] studied the effect of chronic low back pain on negative and positive discs vs. asymptomatic controls. For example, comparing asymptomatic volunteers vs. chronic low back pain patients (both with grade 3 discs) at 50 psi a.o. obtained pain scores of 1.6/10 pain and 1.1/10, respectively. Patients undergoing discography can readily distinguish between a negative and positive disc level.[99,100] Shin and associates[100] also recently reported that a majority of patients with grade 4 discs could distinguish between positive and negative discs by magnitude of pain response.[100] The argument that a majority of patients with chronic pain who undergo discography overreport pain is not supportable.

Are psychological co-morbidities confounding factors? Perhaps, but the data are conflicting.

Carragee[48] studied six subjects with somatization disorder. Only four of six subjects were able to complete their discogram because of pain (the cause of the pain is not reported—i.e., secondary to placement of discogram needles vs. disc stimulation). From this small sample size, a 75% false-positive rate with a 95% confidence interval from 0% to 100% was reported. Given the type of patients studied and the statistical shortcomings of the analysis, the generalizability of these findings is limited. Furthermore, contrary to these previous findings, larger, randomized controlled trial comparing discography results of 25 patients with and without somatization disorder found no significant difference in positive responses among groups.[101] There was also no difference in positive responses in patients with depression and/or general anxiety disorder. Derby and colleagues[24] reported DRAM scores of 81 patients undergoing discography: 15% (12 of 81) were normal; 52% (42 of 81) at risk, and 33% (27 of 81) were abnormal (distressed, depressive, or somatic). The positive rates of discography were not statistically significant by subgroup (p >0.05). In patients with chronic low back pain, no correlation was found between presenting DRAM score and discography result.

Concern has also been raised that discography is falsely positive in patients with "benign" or chronic persistent mild low back pain. To be considered a subject with "benign" low back pain, subjects reported that they did not restrict their activity or seek medical care for their back pain. They reported their pain as mild to moderate or 2 to 4 on a scale of 0 to 10. Provocation discography was reported as positive in 9 of 25 patients, obtaining a 36% false-positive rate. Of note, 72% (18 of 25) of the patients had chronic pain resulting from failed cervical surgeries and were on medications, including opiates for their pain, which may have masked their pain. Moreover, such subjects may have been understandably reluctant to seek medical care for their low back pain after a failed cervical surgery. The 36% reported false positives are arguably true positives. One could argue that these chronic low back pain volunteers are no different from patients undergoing discography who often have varying degrees and duration of pain flare-ups. Given the history of neck pain in these patients, the fact that some have painfully internally disrupted discs in their lumbar spine is not surprising. In fact, the reported prevalence of positive discograms in patients referred for chronic low back pain ranges from 26% to 39%.[86,102]

The argument that these positive responses represent false-positive responses is not supportable. Discography was not developed and should not be used to determine the clinical significance of a patient's perceived suffering and disability related to chronic low back pain.

In fact, one of the reasons Carragee[47,48,60,98] obtained so many false-positive responses may have been because of the high pretest probability of discogenic disease in most of his research subjects. All subjects, except for the somatization disorder and iliac crest pain patients, had a history of known discogenic pain severe enough to require surgery. Carragee's subjects may have had asymptomatic or minimally symptomatic disease provoked with high pressurization (up to 100 psi a.o.) or high dynamic pressures in the setting of manual discography. In addition, we know that the co-occurrence of cervical and lumbar discogenic disease is commonplace. MRI studies of twins showed 79% and 64% heritability for severe disease in the cervical and lumbar spine, respectively.[103] In one follow-up study of 200 patients who underwent cervical surgery, 100% had significant low back pain episodes (suggestive of disc herniation) and/or underwent back surgery.[104] Another reason for reported high false-positive rates may have been the use of uncontrolled manual pressurization (to 100 psi a.o.) with measurement of only static pressures.[49] Last, in some prior studies false-positive rates are reported per patient instead of per disc (iliac crest, somatization disorder, postdiscectomy), leading to a significantly higher absolute number. Provocation discography is a test designed to confirm or refute the hypothesis that a particular disc is the source of a patient's pain.

Analgesic Discography

The first reported use of analgesic discography (AD) was in 1948 by Hirsch.[105] He injected 0.5 mL of 1% procaine (Novocain) into the discs of patients who reported pain during disc puncture or needle movement. For the ensuing 2 to 4 hours, after local anesthetic injection these subjects were essentially free of back pain with normal mobility and negative straight–leg raise testing. Subsequently various surgeons have used the injection of local anesthetic to confirm the results of provocation discography.[13,105,106] In the 1970s Roth[106] studied AD in the cervical spine and reported that it was diagnostically superior to provocation discography. He had 93% good-to-excellent surgical outcomes in 71 patients undergoing cervical fusion.

Other descriptions of AD have largely been "embedded" in the methods sections of various discography studies. Coppes and associates[13] used 0.5 to 1 mL of bupivacaine as a confirmatory test and reported 1- to 4-hour pain relief. Theoretically AD makes sense. The disc has nociceptors that should be susceptible to anesthetization. Specifically, the pathological disc is innervated beyond the outer annulus, including the inner and middle annuli, the nucleus pulposus, and along annular fissures.[11-13]

Alamin[107] and Alamin, Arawal, and Carragee[108] recently co-developed a balloon-tipped catheter (functional analgesic discography [FAD], Discyphor Kyphon, Sunnyvale, Calif) that can be anchored in the disc for prefunctional and postfunctional positional testing. They reported that, using FAD immediately following provocation discography, the false-positive rate of PD could be significantly reduced. However, DePalma[109] found that provocation discography followed by FAD obtained similar results, with 80% of positive provocation discography discs demonstrating >50% pain reduction during FAD. Approximately 10% demonstrated partial pain reduction. Derby, Lee, and Wolfer[110] performed provocation discography with and without the addition of local anesthetic instead of following traditional provocation discography with FAD and found that the groups receiving local anesthetic reported a statistically significant decrease in visual analog scale (VAS) (≥2) in sitting at 15 and 45 minutes vs. the control group.

Two studies have reported on surgical outcomes using FAD or AD. Alamin[107] and Alamin, Arawal, and Carragee[108] have followed 16 patients out to 6 months: the mean Oswestry score decreased from 55 to 25; mean back pain VAS decreased from 6.9 to 2.6. Ohtori, Kinoshita, and Nakamura[111] performed a randomized clinical trial comparing surgical outcomes of 15 patients undergoing provocation discography vs. AD. At 3 years the VAS score, Japanese Orthopedic Association Score, Oswestry Disability Index, and patient satisfaction score were superior (p <0.05) in the AD group.

At this time the evidence is insufficient to recommend that AD or FAD replace provocation discography. However, these tests may be useful confirmatory tests. Further research is needed to compare provocation discography to AD, to refine technical performance of the test, to determine if AD has a lower false-positive rate than provocation discography, and to determine if surgical outcomes are superior with AD.

Predictive Value

Surgical fusion is the current standard treatment for discogenic low back pain unresponsive to conservative therapy. Several studies have reported on surgical outcomes in patients undergoing discography.[112] They studied 195 patients with axial pain and reported that, of 137 patients with discogram positive for disc disease and provoked concordant pain, 89% derived significant, sustained clinical benefit from operation. Twenty-five patients showed morphological disc abnormalities but no provocation of concordant pain on discography.

Among this group, only 52% had clinical success. Blumenthal and associates (1988)[113] reported that 74% of patients with internal disc disruption returned to work following anterior lumbar fusion performed on the basis of discography. In a multicenter surgical and nonsurgical outcome study after pressure-controlled discography, Derby and associates (1999)[46] stated that precise prospective categorization of positive discographic diagnoses may predict treatment outcomes, surgical or otherwise, thereby greatly facilitating therapeutic decision making. In addition, patients with highly sensitive discs at low pressure appear to achieve significantly better long-term outcomes with interbody/combined fusion than with intertransverse fusion.[34] Finally, although imperfect, discography is relatively safe, shows substantial sensitivity for identifying painful discs, and may predict surgery-related outcomes.

Recently Cooper, Kahn, and Lutz[114] studied the prognostic value of lumbar disc stimulation to validate the ability of disc stimulation to predict treatment response, using the ISIS guidelines for positive (>70 points), negative (40 to 60 points), and indeterminate (<40 points) responses[18] and physician determination of discography: positive, indeterminate and negative. They performed an opportunistic audit of patients who underwent discography and their surgical outcomes; the data were collected retrospectively; thus no interference occurred with respect to discographer or surgeon. Patients agreed to be followed up regarding response to treatment, pain scores, use of health care, and functional status. Eighty-nine patients were included in the study. The results demonstrated that discography was predictive of treatment response. A cutoff score of >50 and physician interpretation both showed statistical significance. A patient undergoing fusion with a score of >50 had the following results: five times more likely to return to >25% ADLs; 3.4 times more likely to return to >50% ADLs, and 3.3 times more likely to have less pain than patients who did not choose fusion.

With an ISIS score of >50, fusion outcome was superior to intradiscal electrothermal treatment. With a score of <50, conservative treatment was superior to fusion. Cooper, Kahn, and Lutz's final recommendation[114] was to use an ISIS score of 50 as a cutoff with clinical judgment to obtain the best patient outcome.[35]

Summary

For over 50 years lumbar discography has been widely used for evaluating discogenic low back pain. Since these earlier negative studies, discography techniques and diagnostic criteria have also advanced. Complications are minimal in skilled hands. Most important, pressure- and speed-controlled manometric discography has been introduced. Previous discogram studies assessing false-positive rates had limitations, including use of manual injections; uncontrolled injection rates; unrecorded and/or unreported opening; and dynamic pressures, volumes, and maximal volumes. In Walsh and colleague's study,[56] (performed by a skilled operator) with strict criteria, a 0% false-positive rate was reported. Derby and associates[97] used pressure-controlled manometry and precise criteria for positive discography and also obtained a 0% false-positive rate. We recommend positive criteria for lumbar pressure-controlled manometric discography as follows per ISIS/IASP standards: pain ≥7/10, concordant pain, <50 psi a.o., at least grade 3 annular tear, ≤3.5 mL total volume, and at least one negative control disc.[18] Based on the use of these standards, our best estimate of the false-positive rate for lumbar discography is acceptable. Our recent meta-analysis combining all the recent discography studies in asymptomatic subjects (including data from Carragee[47,48,60,98]) obtained a 6% false-positive rate per disc.[15] Discography remains the criterion standard for the diagnosis of discogenic pain.

References

1. Lindblom K: Diagnostic puncture of intervertebral discs in sciatica. *Acta Orthop Scand* 17(3-4):231-239, 1948.
2. Lindblom K: Technique and results in myelography and disc puncture. *Acta Radiol* 34(4-5):321-330, 1950.
3. Lindblom K: Technique and results of diagnostic disc puncture and injection (discography) in the lumbar region. *Acta Orthop Scand* 20(4):315-326, 1951.
4. Dandy WE: Loose cartilage from intervertebral disc simulating tumor of the spinal cord, by Walter E. Dandy, 1929. *Clin Orthop Relat Res* 238:4-8, 1989.
5. Mixter W, Barr J: Rupture of the intervertebral disc with involvement of the spinal canal. *N Engl J Med* 211:210, 1934.
6. Lindblom K: Technique and results in myelography and disc puncture. *Acta radiol* 34(4-5):321-330, 1950.
7. Lindblom K: Technique and results of diagnostic disc puncture and injection (discography) in the lumbar region. *Acta Orthop Scand* 20(4):315-326, 1951.
8. Gardner WJ et al: X-ray visualization of the intervertebral disc, with a consideration of the morbidity of disc puncture. *AMA Archive Surg* 64(3):355-364, 1952.
9. Wise RE, Gardner, WJ, Hosier RB: X-ray visualization of the intervertebral disc. *N Engl J Med* 257(1):6-10, 1957.
10. Bogduk N, Aprill C, Derby R: Discography. In White A, Schofferman J, editors: *Spine Care: Diagnosis and Conservative Treatment*, St. Louis, 1995, Mosby, pp 219-236.
11. Peng B et al: The pathogenesis of discogenic low back pain. *J Bone Joint Surg* 87(1):62-67, 2005.
12. Freemont AJ et al: Nerve ingrowth into diseased intervertebral disc in chronic back pain. *Lancet* 350(9072):178-181, 1997.
13. Coppes MH et al: Innervation of "painful" lumbar disc. *Spine* 22(20):2342-2349; discussion 2349-2350, 1997.

14. O'Neill C, Derby R: Percutaneous discectomy using nucleoplasty. Paper presented at International 21st course for percutaneous endoscopic spinal surgery and complementary techniques, Zurich, Switzerland, January 23, 2003.

15. Wolfer LR et al: Systematic review of lumbar provocation discography in asymptomatic subjects with a meta-analysis of false-positive rates. *Pain Physician* 11(4):513-538, 2008.

16. Boden SD et al: Abnormal magnetic-resonance scans of the cervical spine in asymptomatic subjects: a prospective investigation. *J Bone Joint Surg [Am]* 72(8):1178-1184, 1990.

17. Jensen MC et al: Magnetic resonance imaging of the lumbar spine in people without back pain. *N Engl J Med* 331(2):69-73, 1994.

18. Bogduk N, editor: *Practice guidelines for spinal diagnostic and treatment procedures: lumbar disc stimulation*, San Francisco, 2004, International Spine Intervention Society.

19. Derby R, Lee SH, Kim BJ: Discography. In Slipman CW et al, editors: *Interventional spine: an algorithmic approach*, Philadelphia, 2008, Saunders Elsevier, pp 291-302.

20. Landers MH et al: Lumbar spinal neuroaxial procedures. In Raj PP et al, editors: *Interventional pain management: image-guided procedures*, Philadelphia, 2008, Saunders Elsevier, pp 322-367.

21. Landers MH: Discography. In Waldman SD, editor: *Pain Management*, Philadelphia, 2007, WB Saunders, pp118-144.

22. Guyer RD, Ohnmeiss DD: Lumbar discography: Position statement from the North American Spine Society Diagnostic and Therapeutic Committee. *Spine* 20(18):2048-2059, 1995.

23. Greenspan A et al: Is there a role for discography in the era of magnetic resonance imaging? Prospective correlation and quantitative analysis of computed tomography-discography, magnetic resonance imaging, and surgical findings. *J Spinal Disord* 5(1):26-31, 1992.

24. Derby R et al: The influence of psychologic factors on discography in patients with chronic axial low back pain. *Arch Physical Med Rehabil* 89(7):1300-1304, 2008.

25. Huang TS et al: Gadopentetate dimeglumine as an intradiscal contrast agent. *Spine* 27(8):839-843, 2002.

26. Falco FJ, Moran JG: Lumbar discography using gadolinium in patients with iodine contrast allergy followed by postdiscography computed tomography scan. *Spine* 28(1):E1-4, 2003.

27. Fraser RD, Osti OL, Vernon-Roberts B: Discitis after discography. *J Bone Joint Surg [Br]* 69(1):26-35, 1987.

28. Fraser RD, Osti OL, Vernon-Roberts B: Iatrogenic discitis: the role of intravenous antibiotics in prevention and treatment: an experimental study. *Spine* 14(9):1025-1032, 1989.

29. Polk HC, Jr, Christmas AB: Prophylactic antibiotics in surgery and surgical wound infections. *Am Surg* 66(2):105-111, 2000.

30. Osti OL, Fraser RD, Vernon-Roberts B: Discitis after discography: the role of prophylactic antibiotics. *J Bone Joint Surg [Br]* 72(2):271-274, 1990.

31. Aprill C: Diagnostic disc injections. II. Diagnostic lumbar disc injection. In Frymoyer JW, Ducker TB, Hadler NM et al, editors: *In The adult spine: principles and practice*, ed 2, Philadelphia, 1997, Lippincott-Raven, pp 539-562.

32. Endres S, Bogduk N: International Spine Intervention Society Practice Guidelines and Protocols: lumbar disc stimulation. Presented at the ISIS 9th Annual Scientific Meeting, Boston, MA, 2001.

33. Klessig HT, Showsh SA, Sekorski A: The use of intradiscal antibiotics for discography: an in vitro study of gentamicin, cefazolin, and clindamycin. *Spine* 28(15):1735-1738, 2003.

34. Carrino JA, Morrison WB: Discography: current concepts and techniques. *Appl Radiol* 31:32-40, 2002.

35. Aprill C: Diagnostic disc injections. I. Cervical disc injection. In Frymoyer JW, Ducker TB, Hadler NM et al, editors: *In The Adult Spine:Principles and Practice*, ed 2, Philidelphia, 1997, Lippincott-Raven Publishers, pp 523-538.

36. Fenton DS, Czervionke LF: Discography. In Fenton DS, Czervionke LF, editors: *Image guided spine intervention*, Philadelphia, 2003, Saunders, pp 227-255.

37. Darouiche RO: Chlorhexidine-Alcohol versus Povidone-Iodine for Surgical-Site. Antisepsis *N Engl J Med* 362(1):18-26, 2010 Jan 7.

38. Day PL: Lateral approach for lumbar discogram and chemonucleolysis. *Clin Orthop Relat Res* 67:90-93, 1969.

39. Edholm P, Fernstrom I, Lindblom K: Extradural lumbar disc puncture. *Acta Radiol Diagn (Stockholm)* 6(4):322-328, 1967.

40. Fraser RD, Osti OL, Vernon-Roberts B: Discitis after discography. *J Bone Joint Surg [Br]* 69(1):26-35, 1987.

41. Drummond GB, Scott DH: Deflection of spinal needles by the bevel. *Anaesthesia* 35(9):854-857, 1980.

42. Sitzman BT, Uncles DR: The effects of needle type, gauge, and tip bend on spinal needle deflection. *Anesth Analg* 82(2):297-301, 1996.

43. Dreyfus P: The power of bevel control. *International Spinal Inject Soc Scientific Newsletter* 3(1):16, 1998.

44. Kumar N, Agorastides ID: The curved needle technique for accessing the L5/S1 disc space. *Br J Radiol* 73(870):655-657, 2000.

45. Derby R: Lumbar discometry. *International Spine Inject Soc Newsletter* 1:8-17, 1993.

46. Derby R et al: The ability of pressure-controlled discography to predict surgical and nonsurgical outcomes. *Spine* 24(4):364-371; discussion 371-372, 1999.

47. Carragee EJ et al: False-positive findings on lumbar discography: reliability of subjective concordance assessment during provocative disc injection. *Spine* 24(23):2542-2547, 1999.

48. Carragee EJ et al: The rates of false-positive lumbar discography in select patients without low back symptoms. *Spine* 25(11):1373-1380; discussion 1381, 2000.

49. Seo K-S et al: In vitro measurement of pressure differences using manometry at various injection speeds during discography. *Spine J* 7(1):68-73, 2007.

50. Adams MA, Dolan P, Hutton WC: The stages of disc degeneration as revealed by discograms. *J Bone Joint Surg [Br]* 68(1):36-41, 1986.

51. Bogduk NC, April C, Derby R: Discography. In White A, Schofferman A, editors: *Spine care: diagnosis and conservative treatment*, St Louis, 1995, Mosby, pp 219-236.

52. Vanharanta H et al: The relationship of pain provocation to lumbar disc deterioration as seen by CT/discography. *Spine* 12(3):295-298, 1987.

53. Derby R et al: The relation between annular disruption on computed tomography scan and pressure-controlled discography. *Arch Physical Med Rehabil* 86(8):1534-1538, 2005.

54. Aprill C, Bogduk N: High-intensity zone: a diagnostic sign of painful lumbar disc on magnetic resonance imaging. *Br J Radiol* 65(773):361-369, 1992.

55. Sachs BL et al: Dallas discogram description: a new classification of CT/discography in low-back disorders. *Spine* 12(3):287-294, 1987.

56. Walsh TR et al: Lumbar discography in normal subjects: a controlled, prospective study. *J Bone Joint Surg* 72(7):1081-1988, 1990.

57. Vanharanta H et al: Pain provocation and disc deterioration by age: a CT/discography study in a low-back pain population. *Spine* 14(4):420-423, 1989.

58. Thomas PS: *Image-guided pain management*, Philadelphia, 1997, Lippincott-Raven.

59. Holt EP: The question of lumbar discography. *J Bone Joint Surg [Am]* 50(4):720-726, 1968.

60. Carragee EJ et al: Provocative discography in patients after limited lumbar discectomy: a controlled, randomized study of pain response in symptomatic and asymptomatic subjects. *Spine* 25(23):3065-3071, 2000.

61. Ketterer MW, Buckholtz CD: Somatization disorder. *J Am Osteopath Assn* 89(4):489-490, 495, 1989.

62. Zoccolillo MS, Cloninger CR: Excess medical care of women with somatization disorder. *South Med J* 79(5):532-535, 1986.

63. Tsuji N, Igarashi S, Koyama T: Spinal epidural abscess—report of 5 cases. *No Shinkei Geka* 15(10):1079-1085, 1987.

64. Junila J, Niinimaki T, Tervonen O: Epidural abscess after lumbar discography: a case report. *Spine* 22(18):2191-2193, 1997.

65. Agre K et al: Chymodiactin postmarketing surveillance: demographic and adverse experience data in 29,075 patients. *Spine* 9(5):479-485, 1984.

66. Guyer RD et al: Discitis after discography. *Spine* 13(12):1352-1354, 1988.

67. Arrington JA et al: Magnetic resonance imaging of postdiscogram discitis and osteomyelitis in the lumbar spine: case report. *J Fla Med Assn* 73(3):192-194, 1986.

68. Modic MT et al: Vertebral osteomyelitis: assessment using MR. *Radiology* 157(1):157-166, 1985.

69. Ledermann HP et al: MR imaging findings in spinal infections: rules or myths? *Radiology* 228(2):506-514, 2003.

70. Szypryt EP et al: A comparison between magnetic resonance imaging and scintigraphic bone imaging in the diagnosis of disc space infection in an animal model. *Spine* 13(9):1042-1048, 1988.

71. Aprill C: Diagnostic disc injections. In Aprill C, editor: *The adult spine: principles and practice*, Philadelphia, 1997, Lippincott-Raven, pp 523-538.

72. Baker AS et al: Spinal epidural abscess. *N Engl J Med* 293(10):463-468, 1975.

73. Ravicovitch MA, Spallone A: Spinal epidural abscesses. surgical and parasurgical management. *Eur Neurol* 21(5):347-357, 1982.

74. Lownie SP, Ferguson GG: Spinal subdural empyema complicating cervical discography. *Spine* 14(12):1415-1417, 1989.

75. Grubb SA, Lipscomb HJ, Guilford WB: The relative value of lumbar roentgenograms, metrizamide myelography, and discography in the assessment of patients with chronic low-back syndrome. *Spine* 12(3):282-286, 1987.

76. Johnson RG: Does discography injure normal discs? An analysis of repeat discograms. *Spine* 14(4):424-426, 1989.

77. Freeman BJC et al: Does intradiscal electrothermal therapy denervate and repair experimentally induced posterolateral annular tears in an animal model? *Spine* 28(23):2602-2608, 2003.

78. Boswell MV, Wolfe JR: Intrathecal cefazolin-induced seizures following attempted discography. *Pain Physician* 7(1):103-106, 2004.

79. Resnick DK, Malone DG, Ryken TC: Guidelines for the use of discography for the diagnosis of painful degenerative lumbar disc disease. *Neurosurg Focus* 13(2):1-9, 2002.

80. Antti-Poika I et al: Clinical relevance of discography combined with CT scanning: a study of 100 patients. *J Bone Joint Surg [Br]* 72(3):480-485, 1990.

81. Smith SE et al: Outcome of unoperated discogram-positive low back pain. *Spine* 20(18):1997-2000; discussion 2000-2001, 1995.

82. Vanharanta H. et al: Pain provocation and disc deterioration by age: a CT/discography study in a low-back pain population. *Spine* 14(4):420-423, 1989.

83. Walsh TR et al: Lumbar discography in normal subject: a controlled, prospective study. *J Bone Joint Surg [Am]* 72(7):1081-1988, 1990.

84. Milette PC, Melanson D: A reappraisal of lumbar discography. *J Can Assn Radiol* 33(3):176-182, 1982.

85. Manchikanti L, et al: Influence of psychological factors on the ability to diagnose chronic low back pain of facet joint origin. *Pain Physician* 4(4):349-357, 2001.

86. Schwarzer AC et al: The prevalence and clinical features of internal disc disruption in patients with chronic low back pain. *Spine* 20(17):1878-1883, 1995.

87. Osti OL, Fraser RD: MRI and discography of annular tears and intervertebral disc degeneration: a prospective clinical comparison. *J Bone Joint Surg [Br]* 74(3):431-435, 1992.

88. Milette PC, Raymond J, Fontaine S: Comparison of high-resolution computed tomography with discography in the evaluation of lumbar disc herniations. *Spine* 15(6):525-533, 1990.

89. Bernard TN: Lumbar discography followed by computed tomography: refining the diagnosis of low-back pain. *Spine* 15(7):690-707, 1990.

90. Ohnmeiss DD, Vanharanta H, Guyer RD: The association between pain drawings and computed tomographic/discographic pain responses. *Spine* 20(6):729-733, 1995.

91. Aprill C, Bogduk N: High-intensity zone: a diagnostic sign of painful lumbar disc on magnetic resonance imaging. *Br J Radiol* 65(773):361-369, 1992.

92. Schellhas KP et al: Lumbar disc high-intensity zone: correlation of magnetic resonance imaging and discography. *Spine* 21(1):79-86, 1996.

93. Saifuddin A et al: The value of lumbar spine magnetic resonance imaging in the demonstration of anular tears. *Spine* 23(4):453-457, 1998.

94. Kang CH et al: A correlation of MR imaging and provocative discography in patients with discogenic low back pain: analysis of high intensity zone and disc contour. Can the MRI imaging accurately predict concordant pain? Unpublished work.

95. Simmons JW et al: Awake discography: a comparison study with magnetic resonance imaging. *Spine* 16(6 suppl):S216-S221, 1991.

96. Zucherman J et al: Normal magnetic resonance imaging with abnormal discography. *Spine* 13(12):1355-1359, 1988.

97. Derby R et al: Pressure-controlled lumbar discography in volunteers without low back symptoms. *Pain Med* 6(3):213-221, 2005.

98. Carragee EJ: Provocative discography in volunteer subjects with mild persistent low back pain, *The Spine Journal* 2:25-34, 2002.

99. Derby R et al: Comparison of discographic findings in asymptomatic subject discs and the negative discs of chronic LBP patients: can discography distinguish asymptomatic discs among morphologically abnormal discs? *Spine J* 5(4):389-394, 2005.

100. Shin D et al: Diagnostic relevance of pressure-controlled discography. *J Korean Med Sci* 21:911-916, 2006.

101. Manchikanti L et al: Provocative discography in low back pain patients with or without somatization disorder: a randomized prospective evaluation. *Pain Physician* 4(3):227-239, 2001.

102. Manchikanti L et al: Evaluation of the relative contributions of various structures in chronic low back pain. *Pain Physician* 4(4):308-316, 2001.

103. Sambrook PN, MacGregor AJ, Spector TD: Genetic influences on cervical and lumbar disc degeneration: a magnetic resonance imaging study in twins. *Arthr Rheum* 42(2):366-372, 1999.

104. Jacobs B, Ghelman B, Marchisello P: Coexistence of cervical and lumbar disc disease. *Spine* 15(12):1261-1264, 1990.

105. Hirsch C: An attempt to diagnose the level of a disc lesion clinically by disc puncture. *Acta Orthop Scand* 18:132-140, 1948.

106. Roth DA: Cervical analgesic discography: a new test for the definitive diagnosis of the painful-disc syndrome. *JAMA* 235(16):1713-1714, 1976.

107. Alamin T: Discography versus functional analgesic discography: comparative results and post-operative outcomes. In International Society for the Study of the Lumbar Spine. Bergen, Norway, pp 52-53, June 2006.

108. Alamin T, Arawal V, Carragee EJ: FAD versus provocative discography: comparative results and post-operative clinical outcomes, Proceedings of the NASS 22nd Annual Meeting. *Spine J* 7:39S-40S, 2007.

109. DePalma M: Functional analgesic discography: a retrospective chart review, unpublished manuscript, 2008.

110. Derby R, Lee JE, Wolfer LR: Analgesic discography: a comparison of provocation discography with and without local anesthetics, Unpublished work.

111. Ohtori S, Kinoshita T, Nakamura S: Surgical results for discogenic low back Pain: randomized study using discography versus discoblock, Proceedings of the International Society for Study of the Lumbar Spine. Geneva, Switzerland, 2008, pp 59.

112. Colhoun E et al: Provocation discography as a guide to planning operations on the spine. *J Bone Joint Surg [Br]* 70(2):267-271, 1988.

113. Blumenthal SL et al: The role of anterior lumbar fusion for internal disc disruption. *Spine* 13(5):566-569, 1988.

114. Cooper G, Kahn S, Lutz G: Predictive value of provocative lumbar disc stimulation. In International Spine Intervention Society, Las Vegas, NV, July 23-25 2008, pp 174-179.

5 Analgesic Discography

Richard Derby, Ray M. Baker, and Lee R. Wolfer

CHAPTER OVERVIEW

Chapter Synopsis: Although discography remains a controversial procedure, it represents a useful tool in diagnosis and even treatment of discogenic pain when certain guidelines are closely observed. Provocation discography (PD) can be used to confirm a disc as a suspected pain generator. Analgesic discography (AD) represents the correlate to this technique; analgesic drugs are injected into the disc in hope of relieving pain. Functional analgesic discography (FAD) uses input from the patient to gain a better understanding of the condition. This chapter provides a comparison of these techniques with a focus on AD, including technical considerations and risk avoidance. Although some recommendations are offered, they are subject to change as more data become available; strong evidence for or against the procedure remains scant.

Important Points:
- There is currently little data to support or refute the value of analgesic disc testing and there are no published standards for evaluation.
- Ideally, one would perform analgesic testing as a separate procedure on one disc at a time and probably no more than two discs per session.
- The test is perhaps best used to persuade a patient or surgeon that the disc is not the source of pain.
- A negative test does not rule out other segmental pain sources, including perhaps mechanical pain secondary to outer annular strain.
- Conceptually, pain relief of approximately 70% or more following local anesthetic injection would better predict outcome following intradiscal injection of a neurolytic solution.
- Requiring a positive response to local anesthetic infiltration to justify fusion or arthroplasty for internal disc disruption (IDD) would significantly reduce the number of authorized surgical cases.
- The predictive use of analgesic testing may be robust or at least better than provocative testing, but only two case series studies are published. Both studies injected local anesthetic after provocative testing.

Clinical Pearls:
- Relief of pain is conceptually more convincing than provocation.
- Analgesic testing should be considered in patients with low pain tolerance and abnormal psychological scores as the results of provocation testing are considerably less robust in this patient group.
- If pain originates from nociceptors within a torn annulus, one may expect relief of pain within 30 minutes after injection of local anesthetic. On the other hand, pain due to mechanical strain on the outer annulus or posterior longitudinal ligament may not be relieved.
- Convincing relief is a minimum of 50%, but a 70% cut-off should be considered.
- When a dark disc is the only pathology and one is considering percutaneous or open surgery, convincing relief of central axial pain following 1 cc of local anesthetic or less should be considered.
- Requiring 70% relief of pain will eliminate the disc as the primary source of pain in a majority of patients.

Clinical Pitfalls:
- Injected local anesthetic will slowly diffuse through the annulus and pain relief may be delayed. Test the patient for several hours after local anesthetic disc block.
- Whereas provocational testing is prone to false-positive responses, analgesic testing is likely prone to false-negative responses.
- With recent published data showing toxicity of bupivacaine to cultured disc cells, consider using Xylocaine or ropivacaine.
- Although injecting a small volume of local anesthetic following provocation discography is perhaps the most common and arguably the most logistically convenient protocol, relief of pain may be confounded by annular distention.

Introduction

Only 60 years ago discs were thought to be incapable of producing pain. Much has changed in the interim—scientifically, financially, and politically. As treatment options expand and health care costs spiral, governments, insurers, providers, and patients are demanding more definitive tests to diagnose discogenic pain or, at minimum, tests that clearly lead to improved treatment outcomes. Lacking standard proof, some are again disputing the existence of discogenic pain.[1-3] It is in this environment that analgesic discography (AD) and other methods for diagnosing painful disc degeneration are being actively pursued.

Absent definitive evidence, the diagnosis of discogenic pain evolved into judging a preponderance of the evidence. In some cases, history and physical examination combined with imaging findings were deemed sufficient. Unfortunately, features of the history and physical examination are unreliable,[4-6] and imaging modalities cannot differentiate disc, facet joint, or sacroiliac joint mediated low back pain (LBP) from similar imaging findings in asymptomatic adults.[7-12] In addition, magnetic resonance imaging (MRI) may show multiple potential pain sources or be normal.[13-15] Provocation discography (PD) was used in such cases as an aid in confirming or refuting one's hypothesis that a particular disc was a source of a patient's pain. The premise was simple: "If a particular disc is painful, instillation of contrast should reproduce the patient's pain. If the disc is not the source of a patient's pain, stressing it either should not be painful or should produce pain that is not the patient's familiar or accustomed pain."[16]

Indeed, recent analysis of all the published data on asymptomatic subjects undergoing PD shows that, if one limits pressure provocation, uses pressure-controlled manometry, and follows the standards of the International Spine Intervention Society (ISIS) and the International Association for the Study of Pain (IASP), the false-positive rate is less than 5% in asymptomatic volunteers without confounding factors. Even when volunteers with significant confounding factors (e.g., chronic pain, prior discectomy) are included, the false-positive rate is on average less than 10%.[17] However, if one does not adhere to these strict criteria, false-positive rates are undoubtedly higher. In addition, although such guidelines are increasingly accepted, most of those performing PD still rely on manual, unrestricted pressurization and provocation of concordant pain.

Thus, although useful as one of many data points in arriving at a diagnosis, PD is not a stand-alone test. It cannot rule out other sources of pain, determine whether the disc is the primary source of pain, or determine the significance of a patient's perceived suffering. PD can only determine if a patient's response is statistically different from an asymptomatic volunteer with similar annular disruption experiencing the same intradiscal distending pressure. As with any subjective test, PD results can also be altered, intentionally or unintentionally, by either the discographer or the patient. An inexperienced or biased operator can produce erroneous results.[1-3] Similarly, poor patient selection can increase the chance of erroneous results. Finally, the reliability of PD cannot be equated with outcome from treatment. Surgical treatment limitations do not necessarily negate the diagnostic value of discography or the diagnosis of painful internal disc disruption.

In many ways AD and PD are opposite sides of the same coin. Whereas PD attempts to confirm the disc as a source of pain by reproducing a patient's usual pain, AD attempts to relieve the patient's usual pain. AD can be used alone or in combination with PD. It can also be combined with functional testing, so-called *functional analgesic discography (FAD)*. In the following sections we explore our current understanding of the role of AD. However, we caution our readers that there are few current studies available that can either support or condemn its use and our conclusions and recommendations will likely change as new information becomes available.

History

The first reported use of AD was in 1948 by Hirsch.[18] He described diagnostic disc punctures in 16 patients with chronic LBP and negative myelograms. If disc puncture or needle movement

increased the patient's pain, he injected 0.5 mL of 1% procaine (Novocaine). "With addition of more volume into the disc, the patients experienced a temporary increase in pain, however, it resolved in 2 to 3 minutes. At 3 minutes the patient's straight–leg raise test was negative or markedly reduced, spine mobility normalized, and spasms resolved and "the patient considered himself quite free of his lumbago."

This effect lasted 2 to 4 hours. In contrast, other patients' pain was evoked by injection of normal saline, not by disc puncture or needle movement. These patients typically were worse for several hours and then returned to their baseline pain level.

Subsequently, injection of local anesthetic into a presumed painful disc following PD has been used sporadically over the decades to help surgeons confirm the diagnosis of discogenic pain.[4,19,20] In the late 1970s Roth[19] asserted that AD more precisely confirmed both the diagnosis of discogenic pain and the pathological level compared to PD. He reported a 93% good or excellent recovery rate in 71 patients over a 2-year follow-up period using cervical AD in patients undergoing fusion.

Until recently, descriptions of AD have largely been "embedded" in the methods sections of various studies based on the preference of the discographer in attempting to select the best surgical candidates. For example, in the study by Coppes and associates[14] local anesthetic was injected following PD as a confirmatory test before surgery. The authors reported that "additional injection of 0.5 to 1 mL of bupivacaine into the disc through the same needle relieved the pain for 1 to 4 hours."[4]

Alamin[21,22] was the first to place catheters in the disc as a part of the process of AD in 2006. This allowed for multilevel anesthetic and placebo testing of the disc and for functional testing in the recovery area using common provocative lumbar range-of-motion maneuvers. Working with Kyphon-Medtronic (Sunnyvale, Calif), Alamin co-developed a balloon-tipped catheter (Discyphor) to allow for anchoring of the device in the disc during functional testing and coined the term *functional analgesic discography* (**Fig. 5-1**).

Analgesic Discography: Construct Validity

Construct validity is considered the most important type of validity, referring to the degree to which a test assesses the underlying theoretical dimensions (constructs) that are trying to be measured.[23] Thus the question first arises: is the disc capable of being a pain generator? Anatomists demonstrated that the disc is indeed innervated. The normal, aging was first shown in 1981 to contain nociceptors in the outer one third of the posterior annulus and

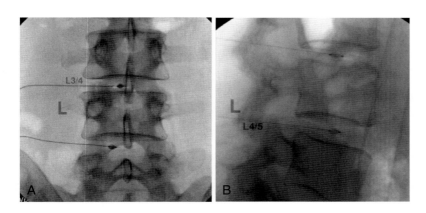

Fig. 5-1 Anteroposterior (*left*) and lateral (*right*) views. Case study: 51-year-old female reported no relief following L3-L4 injection of 1 mL 4% lidocaine (Xylocaine). Following injection of 1 mL 4% lidocaine in the L4-L5 disc, the patient reported 80% pain relief. (Note that the L4-L5 balloon is slightly in the anterior-lateral position in the disc nucleus.)

thus to be a potential pain generator.[24] More recently, pathologically painful discs demonstrated neoinnervation extending to the nucleus pulposus; these discs were positive at preoperative PD testing, and they were examined histologically after removal at fusion.[25] Compared to asymptomatic discs, painful internally disrupted lumbar intervertebral discs also have higher concentrations of sensory fibers in both their endplates and nucleus.[4,26] This high concentration of sensory fibers combined with increased levels of proinflammatory mediators such as interleukin (IL)-8 and prostaglandin E_2 (PGE_2) are theorized to cause hyperalgesia and pain on loading.[27,28] In fact, in this hyperalgesic state even normal mechanical loading, especially lateral shear and torsion, is painful.

Logically, if discogenic pain is caused by sensitized nociceptors within torn annular fissures or immediately adjacent to the endplates or outer annulus of the disc injection of local anesthetic into that disc should relieve pain to the extent that a sufficient concentration of local anesthetic reaches and blocks the offending nerve endings. However, despite the long-time occasional use of AD and the increasing use of FAD, the construct validity of AD has only been partially investigated. Questions remain related to the appropriate volume, type, and concentration of local anesthetic sufficient to fully anesthetize the disc and the onset and offset times of various anesthetics, particularly in the acidic, avascular environment of the disc. In addition, although it is assumed that the endplates are anesthetized along with the disc, the implications of this for treatment are unknown.

As with PD, AD is a procedure-based, subjective test; and the validity of the results depends on a variety of technical and nontechnical factors. Technically the placement of the catheter itself can be a source of pain, either through irritation of tissue during insertion or via a direct irritation of the adjacent nerve by the indwelling catheter. The quantity of local anesthetic injected may also be insufficient to affect an adequate block if pain is caused by abnormally high stress gradients within the endplates/vertebral bodies or the intact annulus, especially if anesthetic leaks from the disc.

Conversely, leakage of local anesthetic through an outer annular tear could block adjacent structures at the same or adjacent levels, including the sinuvertebral nerve that innervates the disc or the adjacent posterior longitudinal ligament, which is an integral part of the disc. Indeed, Bartynski and Rothfus[29] reported that pain relief during PD correlated with leak of local anesthetic through outer annular tears. However, their study was a retrospective review without controls. Patients "were continuously asked" whether their pain subsided after moderate-to-rapid manual injection contrast followed by 2% lidocaine (Xylocaine). The time after injection was not recorded; thus one might assume that the next level was injected within 5 minutes, an insufficient time for lidocaine to diffuse through the outer annulus. Regardless of whether or not local anesthetic is injected, experience shows that pain often subsides if it was provoked by the opening of an annular tear or if pressure on the outer annulus/endplates is not maintained as a result of a leak. Their finding that patients reported complete or partial relief in only 31% of the painful discs with intact outer annulus compared to 89% of leaking discs could also be caused by false-negative responses resulting from the activation of unblocked pain receptors within the annulus, posterior annular ligament, or endplates/vertebral bodies by persisting annular tension.

Nontechnical factors can also lead to erroneous AD results. Neurophysiological phenomenon with convergence of neurons from adjacent receptor fields might lead to false-positive results. On the other hand, central sensitization or uninvestigated alternative pain sources (e.g., multiple discs, secondary muscle spasms,

sacroiliac joint, zygapophyseal joint) may contribute to LBP and lead to a false-negative AD response. Even in patients in whom all other known sources of pain have been excluded, pain relief is rarely complete following AD. Although DePalma and associates[30] reported that 80% of patients achieved ≥50% reduction in visual analog scale (VAS), Alamin's,[21] Alamin, Arawal, and Carragee's,[22] Derby and Lee's,[31] and Derby and associates[32] patients reported considerably less pain relief. Indeed, in all of the studies of AD to date, most patients did not obtain pain relief approaching 75% to 100%. Where is the origin of the unrelieved pain? Does this pain originate from a source outside the disc or is it caused by the inherent limitations of AD? These questions remain unanswered.

Finally, as is documented well in the literature, psychosocial factors can be problematic in the LBP population. Currently analgesic testing is more often used to confirm provocation testing in patients in whom, for a variety of reasons, the surgeon is wary to offer a surgical procedure. These patients might be expected to often not report pain relief following AD since many are on significant doses of narcotics, have had no treatment that has provided any significant pain relief, and often claim that various interventional treatments made them worse. Equally one could argue that this is the appeal of AD. A patient may be counseled that he or she is unlikely to have more pain relief following a fusion or artificial disc replacement than that experienced following AD. Failure to have significant relief is a persuasive way to convince the patient to stop pursing a surgical treatment.

Comparisons of Analgesic Discography with Provocation Discography

Although the evidence largely supports the face validity (the extent to which a test superficially appears to measure what it is supposed to measure)[23] of AD, questions remain. First and foremost, without knowing the sensitivity or specificity or either AD or PD, we cannot know whether disagreement between them is caused by false-positive or false-negative results in one or the other test; that limitation notwithstanding, comparison studies of PD and AD have been published.

Alamin[21,22] compared the ability of FAD and PD to predict surgical outcome in 41 patients. All patients underwent preprocedure functional testing to determine which activities were painful and rated the pain that each activity elicited. Standard PD was then performed on all patients. Before leaving the operating suite, a balloon-tipped catheter was inserted into the PD-positive discs. In the recovery room he sequentially injected the catheter(s) with normal saline followed by testing with 0.75 mL of local anesthetic (4% lidocaine or 0.75% bupivacaine). The patients then underwent repeat functional testing within 20 minutes in positions that typically provoked their pain. Alamin, Arawal, and Carragee's 2007 NASS abstract[22] reports the following: "7 of the 41 (17%) patients had two-level findings on PD that were reduced to one-level findings on the FAD test. 11 patients (27%) had positive provocation discograms that were negative on FAD testing. Two patients (5%) had a negative provocation discogram and yet pain relief on the FAD. 21 patients (51%) had confirmatory findings on the FAD test. Distress and Risk Assessment Method (DRAM) profile of distressed depressive or distressed somatic was a significant predictor of negative findings on the FAD test."

Alamin reported a 44% false-positive PD rate per patient (27% of patients with single-level positive PD had a negative FAD, plus 17% with two-level positive PD reduced to one level with FAD), but it was not substantiated by DePalma and associates.[30] Using a similar protocol, DePalma and colleagues performed PD followed by insertion of Discyphor FAD catheters into each positive disc. Data were collected on all patients but, as per ISIS criteria, he excluded patients with more than two positive levels. After a post-PD computed tomography (CT) scan, patients graded provoked pain in sitting, lumbar flexion, flexion/axial rotation, and supine positions. The disc(s) were then sequentially injected with 0.8 mL of 4% lidocaine. Confirmation of successful disc anesthetization was performed using an intradiscal saline challenge to ensure that distention did not produce pain. The patients then underwent postprocedure functional retesting over the following 5- to 10-minute period. He found a strong correlation between PD and AD, with 80% of positive PD discs demonstrating ≥50% pain reduction during FAD and an additional 8% demonstrating a 25% to 50% or partial reduction. Patients with confounding psychological factors showed the same correlation; contrary to Alamin's findings,[21] co-morbid depression or somatization was a significant predictor of results. The predictive value for surgical outcomes was not studied.

Derby, Lee, and Lee[32] used a different approach to study the validity of AD. Using the ISIS standard (pain ≥7 on a scale of 1 to 10, pressure <50 psi a.o.[pounds per square inch above opening], concordant pain, ≥grade 3 annular tear, negative control disc, and maximum volume of 3.5 mL), they evaluated 70 patients with chronic LBP referred for PD. The control group underwent routine PD (n = 23 patients). The experimental group received 2.5 mL of an equal mixture of local anesthetic (either 4% lidocaine or 0.75% bupivacaine) and nonionic contrast media during PD. Among the control group, 18 of 23 patients (78 %) had positive discograms for a total of 63 positive discs. Among the experimental group, 30 of 47 patients (70%) had positive discograms, for a total of 107 positive discs. Among the positive discs, they compared pain relief in patients whose discs were injected with contrast alone vs. those discs receiving local anesthetic and contrast. He used functional testing, including range of motion (lumbar flexion and extension), static loading positions (sitting and standing), and walking. Testing was done before PD and at 15 and 45 minutes after PD. Among control patients, 6% (1 of 18) reported ≥50% subjective relief. Among local anesthetic subjects, 8% (2 of 25) reported ≥50% relief. There was no significant difference between groups. Moreover, neither the type of local anesthetic used nor the time tested made a significant difference, although there appeared to be a trend for greater pain relief at 45 vs. 15 minutes. Sitting and forward flexion did reveal significant difference vs. other testing positions. However, using Alamin's criteria for a positive response (≥2 point decrease in VAS), they found a statistically significant difference between groups. Of the local anesthetic group, 29% reported a 2/10 or greater decrease in VASs at 15 minutes and 39% at 45 minutes (in sitting position). In the control group, 8.3% of patients reported relief at 15 minutes, and 0% reported relief at 45 minutes. Contrary to Bartynski and Rothfus,[29] patients having one or more discs that leaked did not correlate with reported pain relief. Alamin[21] reported 51% of patients with a positive confirmatory FAD after PD, whereas Derby, Lee, and Lee[32] found approximately 30% to 40% of patients reporting relief after local anesthetic injection.

Suspecting a high false-negative rate using the former method, Derby and Lee[31] switched to stand-alone analgesic testing using 0.8 to 1 mL of bupivacaine. Their preliminary results show that 38% of patients report 50% or greater subjective pain relief, which is lower than the DePalma and associates' study,[30] but almost the same 39% prevalence of discogenic pain determined by provocation discography.[6] If percent improvement in VAS in flexion and sitting is used, 50% of patients report 50% or greater relief in both positions. Even so, 54% of patients reporting concordant pain

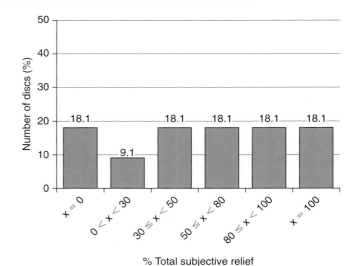

Fig. 5-2 Percentage total subjective relief in subgroup with concordant pain provocation (pain—visual analog scale ≥8) during analgesic injection.

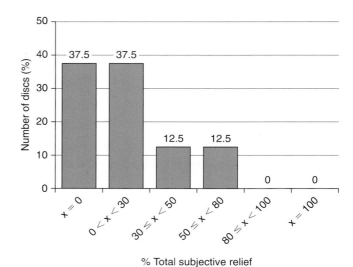

Fig. 5-3 Percentage of total subjective relief in subgroup with no pain provocation during analgesic injection.

provocation at 0.5 mL or less during injection reported 50% or greater relief, suggesting a probable high false-negative rate (**Fig. 5-2**). On the other hand, there was a statistically significant correlation (p <0.01, coefficient = 0.67) between no pain provocation during local anesthetic injection and the report of less than 50% pain relief consistent with a robust specificity (**Fig. 5-3**).

Predictive Value Comparisons between Provocation Discography and Analgesic Discography

The renewed interest in analgesic testing is the result of a perceived poor predictive value of PD. It is hoped that AD will provide a more reliable or at least a complementary method of selecting patients for surgical or interventional procedures. We have a few studies evaluating surgical outcomes after PD alone and AD alone and comparing PD to AD. Using PD to identify surgical levels, Derby and associates[33] showed that surgeons achieved good-to-excellent outcomes following single level interbody fusion supplemented with pedicle screw fixation and posterior lateral fusion in ≈62% of patients having a Short Form Health Survey (SF-36) mental component summary score (MCS) of >40. Using much stricter criteria for success, Carragee and associates[34] reported surgical outcome following single-level fusions for internal disc disruption (IDD) with positive discograms ranging from ≈33% for highly effective results to ≈75% meeting minimum Food and Drug Administration standards of a ≥2/10 decrease in VAS score and ≥10 decrease in Oswestry Disability Index (ODI).[34] More recently, Cooper, Kahn, and Lutz[35] showed that discography was a useful predictive tool for response to fusion. Discograms were assigned scores based on the ISIS scoring system. Both positive (score >70) and indeterminate discograms (score >50) predicted a favorable result with fusion surgery. The breakpoint was 50; with an ISIS discogram score of greater than 50, patients who underwent fusion surgery were 5 times more likely to return to ≥25% of normal daily activities, 3.4 times more likely to return to ≥50% daily activities, and 3.3 times more likely to have less pain compared with patients with a similar ISIS score who elected not to have surgery.

Using AD to identify surgical fusion candidates, several studies document pain relief following interbody fusion surgeries based on pain relief following AD. Alamin, Arawal, and Carragee[22] reported outcomes at a mean follow-up of 6 months (range 6 to 24 months) in 16 patients who underwent fusion after a positive FAD. ODI and VAS scores at 6 months after surgery decreased ≥50%. The mean ODI score decreased from 55 to 25 at follow-up. Mean back pain VAS decreased from 6.9 to 2.6. Ohtor, Kinoshita, and Nakamura[36] recently published a randomized controlled trial comparing surgical outcomes of patients with positive PD (1.5 mL contrast) vs. "discoblock" (AD with 0.75 mL 0.5% bupivacaine). Forty-two patients with severe LBP with L4-L5 or L5-S1 disc degeneration on MRI underwent either PD or AD. Twelve patients were excluded because of negative PD or AD testing. Surgical outcomes in 15 patients with positive PD vs. 15 patients with positive AD were compared following interbody fusion or disc replacement. Improvement in the VAS, Japanese Orthopedic Association Score (JOAS), ODI, and patient satisfaction score at 3 years' follow-up were statistically significant in the discoblock group vs. the PD group (p <0.05). Three patients were dissatisfied with surgical outcome after PD vs. one patient with AD. Unfortunately, the authors gave no details on the degree of pain relief required and the timing or testing after local anesthetic injection, which was performed immediately following provocative testing.

Indications/Contraindications

Analgesic testing of the disc shares the same indications as provocative disc testing. Since the specificity and sensitivity of the test has not been well studied, analgesic testing is a complementary test to provocative testing. However, the provocation of pain is monitored during the injection of local anesthetic; thus analgesic testing as a stand-alone test provides low-volume provocative testing in addition to analgesic testing.

Discography is not an initial screening test. PD is pursued only after failed conservative care. Discography is only used when less invasive diagnostic tests are inconclusive. Discography is an invasive procedure, and irreversible surgical procedures may be considered based on the testing outcome. The primary indication for discography is to ascertain whether or not a disc is pathologically painful and the extent of annular or endplate disruption. Minimally invasive percutaneous, intradiscal, or surgical therapies can be pursued if the diagnosis of discogenic pain is presumed. In spite of the attempts of some insurers to "unbundle" CT scanning from discography, it is well known that *only* CT scanning can definitively detail internal disc anatomy.[37] Postdiscography CT scanning is particularly invaluable in postdiscectomy patients with suspected residual or recurrent disc herniations. When using stand-alone AD without contrast, contrast should be injected into the disc at a separate session either on a different day or on the same day after AD testing. Discography is used in challenging cases unresolved by MRI or myelography and in general for patients in whom surgery is contemplated.[38] It can offer a resolution to the diagnostic dilemma regarding whom to treat surgically and at what segmental level. When a single disc is painful among neighboring asymptomatic discs, focused intradiscal or surgical therapy can be considered. A critically important application is to identify asymptomatic discs that do not need intervention; moreover, patients with multiple-level (≥3) positive discs pose much greater surgical challenge and risk to the patient.

If the patient is not a surgical candidate, discography is useful to provide a diagnosis to bring the workup to closure and direct the patient to pain management.

The position statement of the North American Spine Society on discography is as follows:[37]

Discography is indicated in the evaluation of patients with unremitting spinal pain, with or without extremity pain, of greater than 4 months' duration, when the pain has been unresponsive to all appropriate methods of conservative therapy. Before discography, the patients should have undergone investigation with other modalities that have failed to explain the source of pain; such modalities should include but not be limited to CT scanning, MRI scanning, and/or myelography.

Indications include the following:

1. Failed conservative treatment for LBP of probable spinal origin.
2. Pain has been ongoing for greater than 3 months.
3. Other pain generators have been ruled out (e.g., facets, sacroiliac joints).
4. Symptoms are clinically consistent with disc pain.
5. Symptoms are severe enough to consider surgery or percutaneous interventions.
6. Surgery is planned, and the surgeon desires an assessment of the adjacent disc levels.
7. The patient is capable of understanding the nature of the technique and can participate in the subjective interpretation.
8. Both the patient and physician need to know of the source of pain to guide further treatments.

Contraindications include the following:

1. Unable or unwilling to consent to the procedure
2. Inability to assess patient response during the procedure
3. Inability of patient to cooperate
4. Known localized or systemic infection
5. Pregnancy
6. Anticoagulants or bleeding diathesis

Relative contraindications to discography:

1. Allergy to contrast medium, antibiotics, or local anesthetics
2. Significant psychological overlay
3. Any other condition (i.e., medical, congenital, postsurgical, anatomical, or psychological) that would increase the risk of the performance of the procedure to an acceptable level

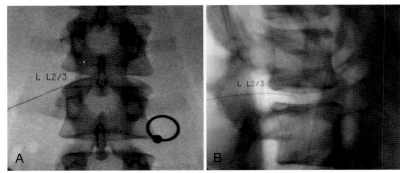

Fig. 5-4 Anteroposterior (*left*) and lateral (*right*) views. Case study: 27-year-old female 40% low back pain and 60% leg pain following a motor vehicle accident 2 years before evaluation. Workup negative for facet pain and temporary relief of leg pain following diagnostic TFE L2 block with 1 mL bupivacaine. Provocation discography was positive at L2-L3 and negative at three control levels. Analgesic testing was performed on a separate day. Following injection of 1 mL of 0.75% bupivacaine into the L2-L3 disc, the patient reported 60% pain relief of both back and leg pain. She continues to improve after 9 months' follow-up. L2-L3 biacuplasty reporting 50% back pain relief and 70% relief of her leg pain.

Technique

Before the procedure the patient typically undergoes standard functional testing in which the VAS on a 0 to 10 scale is recorded following various provocation maneuvers. At a minimum, testing should include the activities that typically increase a patient's pain.

Two methods are used to perform analgesic testing. We name the first *stand-alone analgesic disc testing*; the second, as named by its inventor, is *FAD*. The former method places a narrow-gauge needle (typically 25 gauge) into the intervertebral disc using standard disc access techniques (**Fig. 5-4**). For example, in the lumbar spine using a single-needle technique, an ≈3.5-inch, 25-gauge needle with a slight distal bend is corkscrewed into the disc using a down-the-beam approach beginning ≈8 cm from the midline. Before advancing the needle or needles, the endplate of the caudad vertebrae is aligned parallel to the beam, and the C-arm is rotated ipsilaterally until the oblique view projects the superior articular process of the caudad level halfway across the disc space. If one uses two needles, as is often done in the lumbar spine, typically a 20-gauge needle is passed using the same projection just over the medial aspect of the superior articular process; and a 6-inch, 25-gauge needle with or without a slight distal bend or curve is passed into the disc.

Once the needle is in the center of the disc, the disc is injected with 0.8 to 1 mL of local anesthetic. The injection should be done slowly, and the patient asked to report the intensity from 0 to 10 and concordance of pain as reflected by similar location and character. Most discographers either pretreat with 1 to 2 g of an intravenous cephalosporin antibiotic 30 to 60 minutes before the procedure and/or add antibiotics (e.g., 2 to 6 mg/mL cephalosporin) to the injected local anesthetic. The current consensus is to inject 0.8 to 1 mL of either 4% lidocaine or 0.75% bupivacaine into the disc(s), although an equivalent dose of ropivacaine (Naropin) may also be used instead of bupivacaine. Following intradiscal injection, the patient is transferred to the recovery area and is retested 10 to 15 minutes following injection of lidocaine or 45 minutes following injection of bupivacaine. Before discharge the patient should be given a pain diary to record the pain level for at least 6 to 12 hours.

If one chooses to use the FAD technique (Kyphon-Medtronic), an introducer is passed into the disk using the same standard access techniques, or a provocative discogram can be performed first (see **Fig. 5-1**). The original design included advancing a catheter over a guidewire. The new-generation device does not require a guidewire and uses a smaller-gauge needle (20 gauge, 7.5 or 8 inches) with a bullet point tip to reduce annular disruption. The new catheter is also softer and more flexible to reduce catheter-related pain. The smaller-gauge introducer is advanced in a standard fashion toward the dorsolateral disc annulus. If PD is to be performed, a 25-gauge discography needle is inserted through the introducer into the mid nucleus pulposus. Following PD, the 25-gauge needle is removed, and the Discyphor catheter is inserted through the introducer and directly into the annulus. If PD is not performed, the catheter is inserted directly through the introducer. The catheter has a port for injection, and a port to inflate a small balloon designed to prevent the catheter from being dislodged during provocation testing. The catheter is then secured at its skin exit point, and the patient is taken to the recovery area. Preblock testing or a placebo injection with the FAD technique can be performed after insertion of the catheter or repeated after anesthetization to confirm disc anesthesia. In the setting of sequential disc testing, the patient is tested 15 minutes after the injection of the first disc, and then the next level is injected and similarly tested. If a catheter is not used, the patient needs to either return on another day or be returned to the operating suite, and another level investigated.

The percentage or absolute amount of pain reduction required for a test to be deemed positive has not been validated, but Alamin's surgical outcomes provide a starting point. Alamin[21,22] and Derby[32] defined a positive response with disc analgesia as a decrease in VAS pain scale of ≥2/10. DePalma and associates[30] defined a positive response as ≥50% reduction in VAS before and after FAD. However, one could strongly argue that a decrease in only two VAS points is noise and that patients should report near 100% relief. Likewise, whether to perform AD as a stand-alone test or in the same session as PD is undecided. Although we recommend collecting the provocative information during injection of local anesthetic, our data show a probable unacceptable high false-negative rate if analgesic testing is performed following standard pressure-controlled discography. Currently FAD catheters are more often inserted directly following provocation testing into the positive or indeterminate discs. Alamin's[21,22] and DePalma's[30] studies both used this protocol. DePalma waited approximately 45 to 60 minutes following PD, during which time a CT scan was performed. Alternatively, one could inject contrast into all positive disc(s) at the end of AD and then send the patient for CT scanning.

The order of injection is an individual choice and may depend on what information is important. Typically PD is performed from the least to most clinically suspected level to mitigate the effect of lingering provoked pain. In the case of AD, lingering pain is not a concern. When surgery at a particular segment is inevitable because of undisputed indications, the primary question is the status of adjacent segments. Since the presence or absence of pain at a planned surgical level is less important, one might consider injecting the adjacent level first. No pain relief would indicate that this segment (or the disc at this segment) is not a significant source of pain. On the other hand, if used to validate a source of discogenic pain, consideration can be given to injecting the most clinically suspected disc first.

Postprocedure Care

After the procedure, patients are taken to the recovery room for vital sign and clinical status monitoring by nurses trained in spine injection management. The patient is checked immediately after transfer and 30 minutes after the procedure for any subcutaneous bleeding. Analgesic medications are withheld until after postprocedural testing and preferably omitted altogether so the patient can test the duration of pain relief.

If pain relief does not occur, analgesic medications (oral, intravenous, or intramuscular) are provided as needed. The patient is advised that they may experience an exacerbation of their typical symptoms for 2 to 7 days. The patient is instructed to contact the office if fever, chills, or severe (or delayed) onset of pain develop. Patients are observed and discharged according to institutional protocol. After testing at 45 minutes, the patients can be discharged and typically given a diary to record their pain over the next 12 to 48 hours. Typically the patient is discharged to the care of a responsible adult and instructed not to drive for the remainder of the day. All patients should be contacted by phone 2 to 4 days after the procedure to screen for complications or adverse side effects.

Test Selection

A variety of testing options exist, including PD only, AD only, PD immediately followed by confirmatory AD, or PD followed by confirmatory AD on another session (see **Figs. 5-1** and **5-4**). Performing AD as a stand-alone procedure or combining it with PD as a confirmatory test is an individual choice and often depends on the circumstances, including cost and authorization issues.

The senior author of this chapter is skeptical that same day PD-AD testing is reliable in all but the most obvious cases and especially when the structural pathology is minimal or when the capacity of the patient to get better or admit to getting better from any procedure is dubious. Potential confounding factors include acute pain sensitization, lingering adjacent level pain, and continued radial annular stress caused by injecting 1 to 3 mL of contrast into a disc. In addition, the local anesthetic effect might be reduced by dilution or by an unknown effect from the combination with contrast. DePalma's,[30] but not necessarily Alamin's, study[21,22] suggests that same-day discography followed by local anesthetic testing does not diminish the test sensitivity. On the other hand, Derby's data suggest that it may be difficult to evaluate patients after PD, which could theoretically increase the false-negative results. In any case, testing without the potential confounding effects of lingering pain, acute pain sensitization, or contrast pressurization from PD should be more reliable.

If one wants to globally rule in or out discogenic pain using AD, one can simply inject every disc with local anesthetic. If only one disc is in question, injection into that single disc is sufficient. Furthermore, if one or more segments will have to be surgically addressed for undisputed structural reasons, one may elect to only inject a questionable adjacent level to make sure pain that is not relieved.

The FAD technique is appealing and attractive when multiple levels need testing, retesting is necessary, or placebo testing is warranted. In fact, one could make the case that, if improved surgical results can be substantiated by disinterested investigators, FAD or AD could become the criterion standard to one's diagnosis that a particular disc is the source of the patient's pain.

Risk and Complication Avoidance

AD shares the same possible complications as PD and, for that matter, any procedure that requires disc puncture.[39,40] Complications can occur secondary to disc puncture itself or to misadventures during needle placement or related to medications used. Complications vary from minor (e.g., increased LBP, nausea, headache) to major (discitis, seizure, permanent neurological injury, and death).[41] Concern over prolonged pain after discography is overstated. Since analgesic testing requires lower volumes and pressures than provocative testing, the chance of permanently increasing pain is unlikely. In the 1960s Holt reported prolonged LBP after discography[42]; however, serious criticisms were raised about this author's patient population (prisoners), technique, and use of noxious Hypaque dye. More recent studies also have serious shortcomings. The claim that discography causes prolonged pain at 1 year in subjects asymptomatic of LBP who underwent discography is based on only six patients.[1] The claim of prolonged pain after PD has been perpetuated in the literature[43] and quoted as a significant negative effect in leading workers' compensation occupational health guidelines for the diagnosis of chronic LBP.[44] In the original study by Carragee and associates,[2] two of the six patients were chronic pain patients status post failed cervical fusions and on opiate medications with active workers' compensation claims. The psychometric testing of these two patients also revealed that they were distressed somatics. The other four patients had a primary diagnosis of somatization disorder; two of these four patients were unable to tolerate the initial disc access needle placement at more than one or two levels and discontinued their participation in the initial study from which these later data were harvested. A sample size of four patients with such a wide confidence interval grossly limits the precision and thereby generalizability of the conclusions. Moreover, all four subjects had somatization disorders, and it is well recognized that persons with somatization disorder commonly complain of recurrent pain and conversion phenomena (pseudoneurological symptoms) and are at risk for iatrogenic illness.[45] Furthermore, somatization disorder patients are hospitalized or undergo surgery three times as often as depressed patients.[46]

Potentially injecting any volume of solution into a disc could precipitate or enlarge an existing herniation. Disc herniation following discography is very rare.[47] There is a case series of five acute disc herniations following provocative testing.[48] Puncturing an intervertebral disc with a needle may potentially lead to progressive disc disruption. In fact, when disruption is purposefully initiated in rabbits weighing approximately 3.5 kg by puncturing the disc with 16-, 18-, or 21-gauge needles, the degree and rapidity of disruption directly correlates to the size of the needle.[49] However, in comparing animal with human studies in this situation, common sense is advised. A 16-gauge needle in a 3.5-kg rabbit disc may be comparable to putting a fire hose into a 70-kg human disc. Therefore as such these needles are huge compared to a 25-gauge needle typically used to puncture a human disc. It is generally accepted that discography does not accelerate disc degeneration, and a prior study using repeat discograms showed no change at an average of 17 months.[50] Freeman and associates[51] recently reported no histological damage following needle insertion into sheep discs. On the other hand, one opportunistic surgical audit found increased evidence of degeneration of cervical discs where a locator needle was initially passed into the wrong level.[52] In addition, a recent study by Carragee[43] followed 52 control and 50 lumbar discogram patients over 10 years. Using the Pfirrmann grading system[53] (grades 1 to 5), he reported greater progression of degenerative findings in postdiscography discs (n = 54 or 35%) vs. control discs (n = 21 or 14%) (p = 0.03). In addition, there was an increased likelihood of new "herniations" of unstated size in the discography group with more herniations on the same side as the needle insertion. Criticisms of this study have been raised.[54] The control group and postdiscography group may have subjects with differing severity of cervical disc disease. Subjects with multilevel cervical spondylosis vs. single-level disc herniations have a higher incidence of lumbar disc abnormalities.[55]

The most common serious complication of discography is discitis, reported to be less than 0.15% per patient and 0.08% per disc.[37] The incidence of discitis has been reduced with the double- vs. single-needle technique.[56] With the advent of careful preprocedure screening for infection (e.g., urinary tract or skin), aseptic skin preparation, styletted needles, and intravenous and intradiscal antibiotics, discitis is now very rare. In our clinic over a 10-year period we have reported one case of discitis per over 2000 patients. Intravenous prophylaxis with antibiotics before the procedure and intradiscal antibiotics are the standard for discitis prevention. However, even with prophylactic antibiotics, an epidural abscess after discography has been reported.[57,58]

The most common causative organisms for discitis after lumbar discography are *Staphylococcus aureus*, *Staphylococcus epidermis*, and *Escherichia coli*.[39,59,60] The presence of these organisms suggests inoculation with surface flora or inadvertent bowel perforation. After discography, a patient with discitis presents with severe, unremitting, disabling pain, usually within days to weeks after discharge. The pain may be unremitting and unlike the patient's preprocedure pain in intensity and quality. Fever may or may not be present and is a reliable, universal symptom. The workup for discitis should include physical examination, laboratory tests, and imaging. Specific laboratory work includes complete blood count with differential (CBC), C-reactive protein (CRP), sedimentation rate (ESR), and blood cultures. The CRP usually increases within days of onset of infection; the ESR is not as sensitive and may not be elevated for a month. If the endplates have not been breached, the blood cultures and CBC are normal. MRI is the preferred imaging modality.[61-63] Technectium-99 bone scan is less sensitive and specific than MRI.[64] MRI within 3 to 4 days of symptoms shows increased T2 signal in the disc and endplate hyperemia. Biopsy in the acute phase, before endplate breach, is more likely to be positive. After endplate breach, a sterile environment is created by activation of the immune system.[65] Treatment of discitis typically requires prolonged antibiotic therapy, although some mild self-limiting cases have been reported.[65] Empyema or abscess formation require CT-guided drainage or surgical intervention.[66-68]

Striking a ventral ramus is a potential hazard but may be avoided by careful attention to correct technique and the level of patient sedation. The needle should be prevented from straying beyond its required and intended course. In a conscious patient, contact with the ventral ramus is obviously indicated by a severe, sharp lancinating pain. Other complications include spinal cord or nerve root injury, cord compression or myelopathy, urticaria, retroperitoneal hemorrhage, nausea, convulsions, headache, and most commonly, increased pain.[69]

Death after discography was reported in a patient who inadvertently received contrast dye mixed with cefazolin (12.5 mg/mL) intrathecally. She developed intractable seizures and coma and ultimately died.[70]

Summary Recommendations

Because there is no gold standard test to identify discogenic pain, AD must, by necessity, be compared against the current criterion standard, PD. This circular testing logic means that disagreement between PD and AD cannot automatically be attributed to false-positive or false-negative results in one or the other test. However, it is likely that, in contrast to PD, AD has a low sensitivity. However, the value of AD is a probable robust specificity.

We recommend agreement of both PD and AD tests when IDD is the primary indication for an operation or interventional treatment. For example, confirmation by AD may be considered when one is planning surgical disc heating or fusion for disc pain in which the only structural abnormalities are one or more grade 3 annular tears.

For AD testing, we recommend that a positive response require both a 50% or greater overall subjective pain relief and preferably 70% or greater pain relief in one or more activities or positions that aggravate the patient's pain. An indeterminate response is 25% to 49% relief, and a negative response is <25% pain relief. Stricter criteria could be used if one wants to increase specificity. Recommendations on criteria for a positive response should be updated on the basis of further research. Because there is some concern that needle puncture may accelerate degeneration in ≈20% of cases, using the larger-bore FAD introducer needle is of some concern. Therefore we recommend stand-alone analgesic disc testing with a narrow-gauge needle that might potentially include even a smaller gauge than the standard 25 and perhaps using a bullet-point tip rather than a cutting tip needle.

Until more data are available, AD is a complement to provocative testing (although the provocation response during local anesthetic injection is indeed a provocative test). If therapy is directed specifically at the disc innervation (e.g., methylene blue, hypertonic dextrose injection, or disc heating), relief of pain following local anesthetic injection is conceptually the best test to predict outcome. Finally, if predictive value is confirmed, AD may become the criterion standard to surgical or interventional treatment for IDD using procedures such as fusion, arthroplasty, or various interventional procedures. Unlike PD, the worth of which is often challenged because many believe that provocative testing is prone to high false positives, we predict that analgesic testing will have a robust specificity, although most likely a low sensitivity.

Caveats

Injecting the contrast is a low-volume provocative test; therefore many of the same caveats that apply to PD apply to analgesic testing,

The following are techniques used by experienced discographers to optimize performance of the test and limit false-positive and false-negative responses:

1. The discographer must be skilled in needle placement; otherwise further pain provocation will be hard to interpret. Inexperienced discographers often impale adjacent nerve

roots or create significant tissue trauma from multiple needle insertion attempts.

2. Carefully evaluate pain produced ipsilaterally to the needle insertion site. Referred pain may be caused by the discogram needle impinging on the dorsal root ganglion. Gently jiggle the needle to distinguish needle pain from discogenic pain.

3. Transient pain may be provoked if an asymptomatic fissure or previously healed annular tear with a fibrous cap is opened abruptly during pressurization. A true positive pain response is ≥7 on a level of 0 to 10 and sustained for greater than 30 to 60 seconds; true discogenic pain is less likely to decrease rapidly. Pain that resolves within 10 seconds should be discounted. Clinically patients with discogenic pain tend to have increased pain after surgery and an exacerbation of symptoms for 3 to 7 days.

4. Confirm all positive responses with manual repressurization with a small volume. If repressurization does not provoke concordant ≥7/10 pain at <50 psi a.o., the response is considered indeterminate.

5. Limit the volume to 1 mL or less since larger volumes may increase the tensional forces of the outer annulus that may not be adequately anesthetized by the injected local anesthetic. Remember that one is only testing the hypothesis that the pain is caused by nociceptors within radial and communicating concentric annular tears.

6. Be sure to test the patient before the procedure in a variety of active and passive loading positions; one or more of those positions should clearly provoke the intensity of pain to at least a 5 on a level of 0 to 10. Use the same testing procedure at ≈15 to 45 minutes after the procedure.

7. If the patient clearly has 7 or greater on a level of 0 to 10 and concordant pain provocation at incremental ≈0.2- to 0.5-mL injection of local anesthetic and reports no significant relief in pain after the procedure, one cannot necessarily assume that the provocative testing is false positive. More likely the source of the patient's pain is not caused by sensitized annular tears, one did not fully anesthetize the tears, or the patient pain is mostly related to other structures. One is ideally looking for both provocation and relief to minimize the chance of false-positive provocative responses.

References

1. Carragee EJ et al: Provocative discography in patients after limited lumbar discectomy: controlled, randomized study of pain response in symptomatic and asymptomatic subjects. *Spine* 25:3065-3071, 2000.

2. Carragee EJ et al: The rates of false-positive lumbar discography in select patients without low back symptoms. *Spine* 25:1373-1380; discussion 1381, 2000.

3. Carragee EJ et al: False-positive findings on lumbar discography: reliability of subjective concordance assessment during provocative disc injection. *Spine* 24:2542-2547, 1999.

4. Coppes MH et al: Innervation of "painful" lumbar discs. *Spine* 22:2342-2349, discussion 2349-2350, 1997.

5. Kuslich SD, Ahern JW, Garner MD: *An in-vivo, prospective analysis of tissue sensitivity of lumbar spinal tissue*, Proceedings of the 12th Annual North American Spine Society, New York, 1997.

6. Schwarzer AC et al: The prevalence and clinical features of internal disc disruption in patients with chronic low back pain. *Spine* 20:1878-1883, 1995.

7. Gilbert FJ et al: Low back pain: influence of early MR imaging or CT on treatment and outcome–multicenter randomized trial. *Radiology* 231:343-351, 2004.

8. Ito M et al: Predictive signs of discogenic lumbar pain on magnetic resonance imaging with discography correlation. *Spine* 23:1252-1258; discussion 1259-1260, 1998.

9. Jarvik JG et al: Rapid magnetic resonance imaging vs radiographs for patients with low back pain: a randomized controlled trial. *JAMA* 289:2810-2818, 2003.

10. Jensen MC et al: Magnetic resonance imaging of the lumbar spine in people without back pain. *N Engl J Med* 331:69-73, 1994.

11. Sandhu HS et al: Association between findings of provocative discography and vertebral endplate signal changes as seen on MRI. *J Spinal Disord* 13:438-443, 2000.

12. Boden SD et al: Abnormal magnetic-resonance scans of the cervical spine in asymptomatic subjects: a prospective investigation. *J Bone Joint Surg [Am]* 72:1178-1184, 1990.

13. Bernard TN, Jr: Lumbar discography followed by computed tomography: refining the diagnosis of low-back pain. *Spine* 15:690-707, 1990.

14. Horton WC, Daftari TK: Which disc as visualized by magnetic resonance imaging is actually a source of pain? A correlation between magnetic resonance imaging and discography. *Spine* 17(suppl):S164-S171, 1992.

15. Zucherman J et al: Normal magnetic resonance imaging with abnormal discography. *Spine* 13:1355-1359, 1988.

16. Bogduk N: *Practice guidelines for spinal diagnostic and treatment procedures*, San Francisco, 2004, International Spine Intervention Society.

17. Wolfer LR et al: Systematic review of lumbar provocation discography in asymptomatic subjects with a meta-analysis of false-positive rates. *Pain Physician* 11:513-538, 2008.

18. Hirsch C: An attempt to diagnose the level of a disc lesion clinically by disc puncture. *Acta Orthop Scand* 18:132-140, 1948.

19. Roth DA: Cervical analgesic discography: a new test for the definitive diagnosis of the painful-disk syndrome. *JAMA* 235:1713-1714, 1976.

20. Osler GE: Cervical analgesic discography: a test for diagnosis of the painful disc syndrome. *South Afr Med J* 71:363, 1987.

21. Alamin T: *Discography versus functional analgesic discography: comparative results and post-operative outcomes*, Bergen, Norway, 2006, International Society for the Study of the Lumbar Spine, pp 52-53.

22. Alamin T, Arawal V, Carragee EJ: Fad versus provocative discography: comparative results and post-operative clinical outcomes, Proceedings of the NASS 22nd annual meeting. *Spine J* 7:39S-40S, 2007.

23. Lang TA, Secic M: *How to report statistics in medicine*, ed 2, Philadelphia, 2006, American College of Physicians.

24. Bogduk N, Tynan W, Wilson AS: The nerve supply to the human lumbar intervertebral discs. *J Anat* 132:39-56, 1981.

25. Freemont AJ et al: Nerve ingrowth into diseased intervertebral disc in chronic back pain. *Lancet* 350:178-181, 1997.

26. Brown MF et al: Sensory and sympathetic innervation of the vertebral endplate in patients with degenerative disc disease. *J Bone Joint Surg [Br]* 79:147-153, 1997.

27. Burke JG et al: Intervertebral discs which cause low back pain secrete high levels of proinflammatory mediators. *J Bone Joint Surg [Br]* 84:196-201, 2002.

28. Cunha JM et al: Cytokine-mediated inflammatory hyperalgesia limited by interleukin-1 receptor antagonist. *Br J Pharmacol* 130:1418-1424, 2000.

29. Bartynski WS, Rothfus WE: Pain improvement after intradiskal lidocaine administration in provocation lumbar diskography: association with diskographic contrast leakage. *Am J Neuroradiol* 28:1259-1265, 2007.

30. DePalma MJ et al: Are outer annular fissures stimulated during diskography the source of diskogenic low-back pain? An analysis of analgesic diskography data. *Pain Med* 10:488-494, 2009.

31. Derby R, Lee JE: Preliminary results for stand-alone analgesic discography (unpublished work), 2010.

32. Derby R, Lee JE, Lee SH: Analgesic discography: effect of adding a local anesthetic to routine lumbar provocation discography. *Pain Med* 11(9):1335-1342, 2010.

33. Derby R et al: Single-level lumbar fusion in chronic discogenic low-back pain psychological and emotional status as a predictor of

outcome measured using the 36-item short form. *J Neurosurg Spine* 3:255-261, 2005.

34. Carragee EJ et al: A gold standard evaluation of the discogenic pain diagnosis as determined by provocative discography. *Spine* 31:2115-2123, 2006.

35. Cooper G, Kahn S, Lutz G: *Predictive value of provocative lumbar disc stimulation*, Las Vegas, Nevada, 2008, International Spine Intervention Society, pp 174-179.

36. Ohtori S, Kinoshita T, Nakamura S: Surgical results for discogenic low back pain randomized study using discography versus discoblock: Proceedings of International Society for Study of the Lumbar Spine, Geneva, Switzerland, 2008, p 59.

37. Guyer RD, Ohnmeiss DD: Lumbar discography: position statement from the North American Spine Society diagnostic and therapeutic committee. *Spine* 20:2048-2059, 1995.

38. Greenspan A et al: Is there a role for diskography in the era of magnetic resonance imaging? Prospective correlation and quantitative analysis of computed tomography-diskography, magnetic resonance imaging, and surgical findings. *J Spinal Disord* 5:26-31, 1992.

39. Fraser RD, Osti OL, Vernon-Roberts B: Iatrogenic discitis: the role of intravenous antibiotics in prevention and treatment: an experimental study. *Spine* 14:1025-1032, 1989.

40. Vanharanta H et al: Pain provocation and disc deterioration by age: a CT/discography study in a low-back pain population. *Spine* 14:420-423, 1989.

41. Thomas PS: *Image-guided pain management*, Philadelphia, PA, 1997, Lippincott-Raven.

42. Holt EP: The question of lumbar discography. *J Bone Joint Surg [Am]* 50:720-726, 1968.

43. Carragee EJ et al: Does discography cause accelerated progression of degeneration changes in the lumbar disc: a ten-year matched cohort study. *Spine* 13(21):2338-2345, 2009.

44. Hegmann, Talmage: American College Of Occupational And Environmental Medicine (ACOEM). 2008.

45. Ketterer MW, Buckholtz CD: Somatization disorder, *J Am Osteopath Assn* 89:489-490, 495, 1989.

46. Zoccolillo MS, Cloninger CR: Excess medical care of women with somatization disorder. *South Med J* 79:532-535, 1986.

47. Grubb SA, Lipscomb HJ, Guilford WB: The relative value of lumbar roentgenograms, metrizamide myelography, and discography in the assessment of patients with chronic low-back syndrome. *Spine* 12:282-286, 1987.

48. Poynton AR et al: Discography-induced acute lumbar disc herniation: a report of five cases. *J Spinal Disord Tech* 18:188-192, 2005.

49. Masuda K et al: A novel rabbit model of mild, reproducible disc degeneration by an anulus needle puncture: correlation between the degree of disc injury and radiological and histological appearances of disc degeneration. *Spine* 30:5-14, 2005.

50. Johnson RG, Does discography injure normal discs? An analysis of repeat discograms. *Spine* 14(4):424-426, 1989.

51. Freeman BJC et al: Does intradiscal electrothermal therapy denervate and repair experimentally induced posterolateral annular tears in an animal model? *Spine* 28:2602-2608, 2003.

52. Nassr A et al: Does incorrect level needle localization during anterior cervical discectomy and fusion lead to accelerated disc degeneration? *Spine* 34:189-192, 2009.

53. Pfirrmann CW et al: Magnetic resonance classification of lumbar intervertebral disc degeneration. *Spine* 26:1873-1878, 2001.

54. Derby R, Wolfer L, Summers J: Does discography cause accelerated progression of degeneration changes in the lumbar disc? *Spine Line* Mar/April:26-30, 2010.

55. Jacobs B, Ghelman B, Marchisello P: Coexistence of cervical and lumbar disc disease. *Spine* 15:1261-1264, 1990.

56. Fraser RD, Osti OL, Vernon-Roberts B: Discitis after discography. *J Bone Joint Surg [Br]* 69:26-35, 1987.

57. Tsuji N, Igarashi S, Koyama T: Spinal epidural abscess—report of 5 cases. *No Shinkei Geka* 15:1079-1085, 1987.

58. Junila J, Niinimaki T, Tervonen O: Epidural abscess after lumbar discography: a case report. *Spine* 22:2191-2193, 1997.

59. Agre K et al: Chymodiactin postmarketing surveillance. demographic and adverse experience data in 29,075 patients. *Spine* 9:479-485, 1984.

60. Guyer RD et al: Discitis after discography. *Spine* 13:1352-1354, 1988.

61. Arrington JA et al: Magnetic resonance imaging of postdiscogram discitis and osteomyelitis in the lumbar spine: case report. *J Fla Med Assn* 73:192-194, 1986.

62. Modic MT et al: Vertebral osteomyelitis: Assessment using MRI. *Radiology* 157:157-166, 1985.

63. Ledermann HP et al: MR imaging findings in spinal infections: rules or myths? *Radiology* 228:506-514, 2003.

64. Szypryt EP et al: A comparison between magnetic resonance imaging and scintigraphic bone imaging in the diagnosis of disc space infection in an animal model. *Spine* 13:1042-1048, 1988.

65. Aprill C: Diagnostic disc injections. In Aprill C, editor: *The adult spine: principles and practice*, Philadelphia, 1997, Lippincott-Raven, pp 523-538.

66. Baker AS et al: Spinal epidural abscess. *New Engl J Med* 293:463-468, 1975.

67. Ravicovitch MA, Spallone A: Spinal epidural abscesses: surgical and parasurgical management. *Eur Neurol* 21:347-357, 1982.

68. Lownie SP, Ferguson GG: Spinal subdural empyema complicating cervical discography. *Spine* 14:1415-1417, 1989.

69. Guyer RD, Ohnmeiss DD: Lumbar discography: position statement from the North American Spine Society diagnostic and therapeutic committee [see comments]. *Spine* 20:2048-2059, 1995.

70. Boswell MV, Wolfe JR: Intrathecal cefazolin-induced seizures following attempted discography. *Pain Physician* 7:103-106, 2004.

6 Discogenic Pain: Intradiscal Therapeutic Injections and Use of Intradiscal Biologic Agents

Jeffrey D. Petersohn

CHAPTER OVERVIEW

Chapter Synopsis: Discogenic pain is a complex process with multiple components. After an annular tear of the intervertebral disc, nociceptors and blood vessels invade new areas of the disc that are normally noninnervated and avascular. Cytokine alterations promote nociception, both directly and indirectly, while altered anabolic-catabolic balance compromises the disc's hydraulic load-bearing function, also effecting changes in the intervertebral joints. This chapter assesses the nonsurgical therapies available to combat each of these components of lumbar discogenic pain. Growth factors in the bone morphogenetic protein family show promise in repairing metabolic and even structural disc abnormalities, but nonspecific anabolic effects of any growth factor must be considered. Although this treatment has potential, it is still in development. Intradiscal injection of fibrin sealants has been shown to improve cell proliferation and matrix production. Although still in an early stage, this therapy seems to address all the components of discogenic pain and disease. Many in the field are excited about the potential for stem cell therapy for discogenic disease. Mesenchymal stem cells transform into chondrocytes, which produce collagen and aggrecan to maintain the disc's structural integrity. Several currently available therapies are also considered, including pharmaceutical interventions and therapies to ablate nociceptive structures.

Important Points:
- Intradiscal ablative agents ethanol and methylene blue seem to be effective treatments for discogenic pain, requiring careful use to avoid potential epidural spread, but are readily available for use today.
- Intradiscal fibrin sealants may represent a useful interim step for addressing discogenic pain; studies are underway.
- Use of mesenchymal stem cells could be an emerging restorative agent but requires further research.

Clinical Pearls: Understanding the anatomy and pathophysiology of discogenic pain allows thoughtful consideration of emerging paradigms and techniques for treatment. The specific mechanism of delivery and confinement of any drug or biological modality to an anatomic disc target is critical to the success and safety of any of these techniques.

Clinical Pitfalls: Many published studies report on treatments for degenerated discs, radicular pain, or sciatica and overbroadly refer to these conditions as "discogenic pain." Many techniques applicable for radicular pain have not proven useful for discogenic pain originating from a painful posterior annular tear. Imprecision in nomenclature is frequent, even in contemporary surgical literature. Novel techniques require confirmation of safety and efficacy in human trials before widespread use.

In lumbar discogenic pain the injured intervertebral disc produces pain not only as a primary nociceptive structure but also as a result of reduced disco-vertebral mechanical load-bearing capacity and subsequently altered spinal biomechanics, including increased zygapophyseal joint loading. As a consequence, therapeutic strategies for discogenic pain are directed toward three general objectives: (1) resolution of primary nociception resulting from post-injury neoinnervation and neovascularization of the posterior annular tear; (2) restoring or mitigating the pro-nociceptive anabolic-catabolic imbalance, including restoration of normalized cytokine immunochemistry within the nucleoannular biochemical and cellular milieu; and (3) restoring lost mechanical and hydraulic function, including the loss of intervertebral hydrostatic pressure, intervertebral disc height, and annular integrity. Therapeutic approaches may rely on direct molecular effects, gene induction or suppression, or cellular replacement. This chapter discusses present and emerging clinical intradiscal therapies for discogenic pain within this triad of therapeutic objectives.

The adult lower lumbar intervertebral discs are the largest structures within the human body that have no dedicated primary arteriovenous vascular supply, except a small marginal circulation to the outermost annulus, since the vascular buds in the vertebral endplates have typically regressed by 10 years of age. As a consequence, delivery of oxygen and glucose, as well as removal of metabolic waste products, is dependent on diffusion of these substances through the vertebral body endplates, producing a nuclear milieu marked by low oxygen tension, low pH, and a predominance of lactate over glucose as a metabolic substrate. Age- and injury-related changes to the vertebral endplate region may further compromise diffusion transport of nutrients and waste, creating an increasingly challenging milieu for the survival and proliferation of nuclear chondrocytes. The possibility of improving diffusion transport across the vertebral endplates by 7% to 11% as measured by magnetic resonance imaging (MRI) with use of nimodipine has been reported by Rajasekaran and associates.[1] The minimal reparative capacity of nuclear chondrocytes following injury to the intervertebral disc is compounded by the absence of the typical macromolecular humoral and cellular responses to injury seen elsewhere in the human body. The spectrum of discal response to injury, including the immunobiochemistry of the intervertebral disc, has been recently reviewed by Freemont.[2]

The posterior annulus of the lumbar intervertebral disc is normally innervated only in its outermost third, with innervation of the middle or inner thirds or of the nucleus limited to pathologically painful states. Mechanical injury to the posterior annulus may tear the posterior annular lamellae, with the result that multiple torn lamellar defects overlap one another in order to combine as radial fissures. The fissure can be confined to the middle or outer annulus, but in painful states, more commonly extends from the nucleoannular junction into or through the posterior annulus. Small tears in the outer annulus appear to accompany neovascularization and neoinnervation of the normally avascular and non-innervated middle and inner third of the annulus. Annular tears and nuclear degeneration may result in compromise of the native broad distribution of loading forces across the intervertebral disc, leading ultimately to a preponderance of load bearing along the annular rim or limbus region, further exacerbating annular wall stress during mechanical loading.

Normal nuclear chondrocytes maintain the hygroscopic nuclear matrix by producing collagen II, aggrecan, and a regulatory protein, SOX-9, with resultant hydrostatic pressure that allows optimal load bearing by distribution of that load across the annulus and vertebral endplates by the intact disco-vertebral unit. While the loss of annular integrity is usually cited as the initiating event in discogenic pain, there is evidence that repetitive mechanical loading stress produces pro-nociceptive changes in the function of nuclear cells.[3] Interestingly, it appears that some moderate degree of dynamic cyclical mechanical stress is associated with improved production of collagen and glycosaminoglycan by cells in the annulus fibrosus and nucleus pulposus as compared to cells undergoing either no cyclic loading or those undergoing high compressive stress.[4] Homeostatic functioning of the nuclear cells also depends upon a delicate balance between cytokine interleukin-1 (IL-1) and its associated receptors and receptor antagonists. Disruption of the IL-1 system can initiate biochemical changes, including a transition from nuclear collagen II to collagen I production, induction of matrix metalloproteinases, and cellular apoptosis. Although tumor necrosis factor (TNF)-α initiates inflammation and pain when applied to a somatic nerve root or to a sciatic nerve, antagonists of TNF-α (such as etanercept) have not proven useful in the treatment of discogenic pain.[5,6] TNF-α may also play a role in promoting sensory neoinnervation of the injured disc.[7] Members of the transforming growth factor

(TGF)-β superfamily, which includes the bone morphogenetic protein (BMP) family and SOX-9, have been experimentally demonstrated to result in stimulation of collagen and proteoglycan production as well as the proliferation of nuclear cells; however, the relative stimulatory potency of the different BMPs varies.[8] BMP-7 (also called OP-1) has been shown to produce restoration of disc height and water content after initiation of degenerative changes using a rabbit stab injury model.[9] BMP-2 has been used experimentally to achieve intradiscal fusion. Concerns common to most BMPs include avoiding the formation of locally unwanted new bone or blood vessels and maintaining a specific locus of action with predictable termination or modulation of effect so unopposed anabolism does not produce distant or anatomically widespread adverse effects such as proliferative hyperostosis or neoplasm.

The cost of BMPs and injectable growth factors remains a concern. One alternative strategy is to seek inexpensive drugs that stimulate BMP production. Zhang and associates[10] have demonstrated that injection of intradiscal simvastatin (Zocor) in a PEG-PLGA-PEG gel stimulates BMP-2 and produces improvement in nuclear morphology and anabolic changes in a rat model. Although these growth factors and modulators represent an exciting and potentially transformative treatment for human discogenic pain, research using nonbipedal animal models may not translate to effective human treatments; and much additional research will be required to define optimal combinations of pharmacologic moiety and carrier. Human clinical trials with sufficiently lengthy follow-up to answer concerns regarding long-term potential for efficacy or harm will also be necessary.

Modulation of discogenic pain by a series of three intradiscal injections given at 2-month intervals using a solution of chondroitin sulfate, glucosamine, carboxycellulose, dextrose, and a cephalosporin antibiotic has been pioneered by Eek. Derby and Eek[11] published results of a prospective trial of chondroitin sulfate and glucosamine (35 patients) vs. intradiscal electrothermal treatment (IDET) (74 patients) in 2004. Some of the patients in each group had prior surgery or IDET treatment, and others had more than one level of identified discogenic pain generation on discography. As a treatment, they mixed 0.5% chondroitin sulfate and 20% glucosamine in 12% dimethylsulfoxide (DMSO) and 2% bupivacaine and then diluted this with equal quantities of contrast agent and 50% dextrose prior to injection. Postoperative flare of pain was seen in the majority of both treatment groups, with much briefer flare (9 days) seen in the mixture-treated group. Average visual analog scale (VAS) decrease of 2.2/10 for the mixture and 1.7/10 for IDET was reported. The results of this research are difficult to analyze due to the confounding factors of prior IDET or surgery as well as to the inclusion of patients with multilevel disc disease. The possible modest efficacy of this approach does not recommend further use at this time in light of superior results demonstrated with other modalities described later in this chapter.

In the field of orthopedic regenerative medicine, there is little that surpasses the excitement surrounding the use of stem cells, typically of mesenchymal origin, for repair of injured joint structures, including the intervertebral disc.[12] Mesenchymal stem cells (MSCs) can be induced to proliferate a chondrocyte phenotype by TGF-β.[13] Type II collagen can also induce and maintain chondrocytic lineage in a bovine model.[14] Interestingly, adult MSCs spontaneously differentiate into a chondrocytic lineage when inserted into disc nuclear tissue in vitro; so it is unclear whether any additional step is truly necessary to induce desired cellular differentiation.[15]

It has been demonstrated that MSCs can be harvested from the intervertebral disc, bone marrow, or the knee. These cells can be grown in culture before implantation, but viability of transplanted MSCs has been demonstrated only in animal models. Wuertz and associates[16] reported enhancement of matrix biosynthesis and nuclear cell proliferation in low-glucose environments; but low pH environments, similar to that of the degenerated disc, reduced both biosynthetic activity and the proliferation of MSCs. Sobajima and colleagues[17] demonstrated stem cell survival and engraftment in a rabbit model. In the knee the use of scaffolding may be superior to monolayer tissue culture for harvesting, but substantial challenges are related to specific details of culture technique, which are beyond the scope of this chapter. Particular note is made of the frequent use of animal models such as rabbit spine, ox tail, or ovine models, in which there is little or none of the repetitive axial loading that has been demonstrated to alter the production of collagen and aggrecan in chondrocyte tissue culture. Differences in epiphyseal and growth plate architecture and the effect of animal age on observed responses have been discussed in a comprehensive review of the limitations of animal models for study of discogenic pain.[18] Issues relevant to successful human therapeutic application include identification of optimal tissue source, ease of cellular harvesting, choice of implantation carrier, and assurance of clinically significant long-term viability of cellular transplants in the harsh disc nuclear environment. Research must also quantify the potential for malignant transformation of transplanted MSCs.

Platelet-rich plasma contains multiple cytokines and has been used for treatment of a variety of musculoskeletal pain processes by administration as prolotherapy. It has been postulated that intradiscal administration of platelet-rich plasma (PRP) may be beneficial in the treatment of discogenic pain, although the specific cytokines or factors contained in PRP that may effect this benefit remain unstudied.[19] Nonetheless, a randomized clinical trial of intradiscal PRP has been initiated by Lutz in 2009. No further information is available on this modality at the time of this writing.

Chymopapain (Chymodiactin) chemonucleolysis had been reported for many years and was popular in the United States in the 1970s when, due to frequent allergic reactions and reports of rare fatal anaphylactic reactions, it was withdrawn from clinical practice. Since that time, various investigators have considered a variety of substances for intradiscal injections that lyse or denature protein, including collagenase, ethanol, osmic acid, phenol, and 50% dextrose. Unfortunately, the chymopapain literature addresses efficacy in the context of lumbar disc herniation and radicular pain, but no reports address use of this modality specifically for axial discogenic pain. Furthermore, there is no evidence that chymopapain restores nuclear homeostasis or annular integrity.

As of this writing, several direct pharmaceutical modalities are presently available or in clinical trials for direct treatment of human discogenic pain. The following paragraphs review the available evidence supporting or questioning efficacy and safety.

Intradiscal steroids, theoretically effecting improvement in discogenic pain by suppression of inflammation, have been used for almost a half century for treatment of discogenic pain with varying success. Retrospective analyses dominated the literature until a rigorous double-blinded randomized controlled trial by Khot and associates failed to show efficacy.[20] Fayad and colleagues[21] reported improved efficacy of intradiscal steroids in patients with Modic I changes at 1 month. At 3 and 6 months, pain scores were not significantly different from baseline in any group, regardless of Modic categorization. If readers wish to consider this class of medications, avoidance of use of methylprednisolone (Depo-Medrol) is recommended because of its potential for intradiscal calcification.[22] At this time there is no evidence for improved long-term outcome with intradiscal steroid use and only weak evidence for a short-term effect.

One of the simplest pathways for treatment of discogenic pain involves chemical oxidation or denaturation of putative algogenic structures, which includes neurolysis. This class of treatments addresses neither restoration of nuclear homeostasis nor restoration of annular integrity. Discussion of intradiscal ozone, ethanol, methylene blue, and intradiscal 50% dextrose follows.

Intradiscal ozone is commercially available although not used in the United States. Therapeutic effectiveness is putatively associated with peroxide formation and oxidative injury. While free radical formation is possible, this mechanism appears less likely to be the predominant source of reputed efficacy. Administration must be carefully controlled to avoid gaseous emboli formation and adjacent structure injury caused by overwhelming of local tissue superoxide dismutase and catalase defenses. While the technique appears popular in Italy and India, no published literature addresses discogenic pain in the sense of internal disc disruption, addressing only applications in the treatment of radicular pain. Whereas original clinical series were reported for herniated nucleus pulposus and radicular pain[23,24] using concentrations of 27 mcg/mL, better outcomes were observed by concomitant infiltration of the nerve root with local anesthetic and steroids, with a reported 78% successful outcome at 6 months. Curiously, Gautam and colleagues[24] reported improved results with concomitant percutaneous intradiscal radiofrequency lesioning, a technique that, performed alone, has been shown to be entirely unhelpful for treatment of discogenic pain.[25] Unfortunately, serious complications, including basilar stroke,[26] epidural abscess,[27] and fulminating sepsis resulting in death[28] have been reported with this intradiscal ozone. As of this writing, no evidence supports the use of intradiscal ozone as being efficacious in the treatment of discogenic pain due to painful posterior annular tears.

Ethanol has been a traditional choice for regional anesthetic neurolytic block for many years. Intradiscal ethanol has been used by Riquelme and associates.[29] They reported a series of 118 patients in which discography was performed to identify the nucleoannular junction with subsequent injection of 0.4 mL of absolute ethanol at the junction of the middle and lateral thirds of the disc resulting in 98% of patients improved at 6 months. They did not inject full-thickness posterior annular tears (Dallas grade 5) because of concerns for potential epidural and dural structural injury, and no complications were noted in the series. These procedures were performed under propofol general anesthesia. It is unclear whether the patients had a diagnosis of discogenic pain since most of the patients treated had sciatica and no data on the proportion of patients with predominantly axial pain were included. Avoidance of spread into the epidural space or onto the dural surface by confinement of the drug to the target tissue has spurred use of a gel carrier using ethylcellulose, which has shown preliminary success in 91% of 221 patients studied by Theron and associates.[30] After injection of 0.4 to 0.8 mL of the gelled ethanol intradiscally with gentamicin for antibiotic prophylaxis, patients also underwent mandatory facet joint injection with triamcinolone, unilaterally or bilaterally, in this reported series. Successful use of gelified ethanol for treatment of 90% of cervical disc herniations without adverse effect has also been reported by Theron and associates.[31] They used tungsten or tantalum dust to opacify the gel, but both ethylcellulose and ethanol are relatively inexpensive and commercially available. These results are encouraging, but additional clinical studies will be necessary to determine the proper place of this moiety in treatment of discogenic pain.

Methylene blue is often thought to be a reducing agent, but at physiologic pH is more likely to function as an oxidizing agent. Intradiscal use has been studied by Peng and associates in a pilot study and then in a formal randomized controlled trial.[32,33] They report use of a simple and inexpensive technique, mixing 1 mL of methylene blue in 2 mL of lidocaine (Xylocaine) 1% and injecting this mix into the putatively painful lumbar intervertebral disc nucleus immediately after completion of (positive) discography. Use of methylene blue raises concern since direct neurotoxicity of this drug has been reported in both intrathecal and epidural applications.[34] However, their results bear thoughtful consideration since there were neither reported complications nor patient injuries. Their randomized controlled trial of 72 patients showed that 91% of the patients studied were satisfied by this treatment at 2 years, with an average pain reduction of 52 on a 101-point numerical rating scale and mean reduction in Oswestry scores of 36 compared with placebo. Reduction in the use of medications was also demonstrated. These outcomes have been envied by researchers worldwide, but wide adoption of this technique must await duplication of these results by other researchers.

Miller, Mathews, and Reeves[35] reported using 50% dextrose, a preparation known to be neurotoxic, on patients with positive concordant discography and transient response to two epidural steroid injections. Forty-three percent of patients improved by 71/100 on VAS. Single injections were insufficient, and the average patient required 3.5 injections. Since many patients with discogenic pain have exclusively axial symptoms and most do not respond to epidural steroid injection, the highly selected nature of Miller's population limits inferences that may be drawn.

One technique that appears to meet all three goals for treatment of discogenic pain involves use of an injectable fibrin sealant. Fibrinogen and thrombin are delivered in a dual syringe and mixed at a Y connector to form an elastic coagulum that is injected into the disc. Fibrin has been shown to improve cell proliferation and matrix production in vitro by Sha'ban and colleagues.[36] Human use of injectable fibrin sealants has been reported following nucleoplasty or IDET by Derby and Kim[37] and as a stand-alone treatment by Yin and associates.[38] Proposed mechanisms for efficacy include (1) fibrin glue sealing a mechanically defective posterior annular rent; (2) improving annular integrity to promote improved mechanical load sharing and reduction of annular wall shear forces; (3) preventing algogenic substances from reaching the sensitized or neoinnervated annular defect; and (4) improving nuclear cell function, including improved aggrecan and collagen production. U.S. Food and Drug Administration phase III clinical trials have demonstrated clinical efficacy of the patented clinical product. Greater than 50% reduction in both back and leg pain was demonstrated at 12 weeks. A single case of discitis was the only reported complication in the clinical series reported by Yin and Pauza. A multicenter randomized controlled phase III trial began in 2009 and is underway in the United States.

In summary, multiple biological and pharmaceutical modalities for intradiscal treatment of discogenic pain are available and under development. Treatments using ethanol and methylene blue appear to be simple, presently available, and promising. These approaches only address pain and do not address restoration of hydrostatic forces and annular integrity. Intradiscal fibrin sealants may represent a useful interim step for addressing discogenic pain in comprehensive fashion. Use of BMPs, simvastatin, and mesenchymal stem cells appear to be emerging as agents capable of addressing the entire triad of goals for resolving discogenic pain, but their use will require much further research and development before incorporation in routine clinical practice.

References

1. Rajasekaran S et al: Pharmacological enhancement of disc diffusion and differentiation of healthy, aging and degenerated discs: results from in-vivo serial post-contrast MRI studies in 365 human lumbar discs. *Eur Spine J* 17(5):626-643, 2008.
2. Freemont AJ: The cellular pathobiology of the degenerate intervertebral disc and discogenic back pain. *Rheumatology* 48:5-10, 2009.
3. Adams MA et al: Mechanical initiation of intervertebral disc degeneration. *Spine* 25:1625-1636, 2000.
4. Hee HT et al: An in vitro study of dynamic cyclic compressive stress on compared human inner annulus fibrosus and nucleus pulposus cells. *Spine J* 10:795-801, 2010.
5. Korhonen T et al: The treatment of disc-herniation-induced sciatica with infliximab: one-year follow-up results of FIRST II, a randomized changes controlled trial. *Spine* 31:2759-2766, 2006.
6. Cohen SP et al: A double-blind, placebo-controlled, dose-response pilot study evaluating intradiscal etanercept in patients with chronic discogenic low back pain or lumbosacral radiculopathy. *Anesthesiology* 107(1):99-105, 2007.
7. Igarashi T et al: 2000 Volvo Award winner in basic science studies: exogenous tumor necrosis factor-alpha mimics nucleus pulposus induced neuropathology: molecular, histologic, and behavioral comparisons in rats. *Spine* 25:2975-2980, 2000.
8. Zhang Y et al: Comparative effects of bone morphogenetic proteins and sox 9 overexpression on extracellular matrix metabolism of bovine nucleus pulposus cells. *Spine* 31:2173-2179, 2006.
9. Masuda K et al: Osteogenic protein-1 injection into a degenerated disc induces the restoration of disc height and structural in the rabbit annular puncture model. *Spine* 31(7):742-754, 2006.
10. Zhang H et al: Intradiscal injection of simvastatin retards progression of intervertebral disc degeneration induced by stab injury. *Arthritis Res Ther* 11(6):R172, 2009. Epub Nov 13, 2009.
11. Derby R et al: Comparison of intradiscal restorative injections to intradiscal electrothermal treatment (IDET) in the treatment of low back pain. *Pain Physician* 7:63-66, 2004.
12. Crevensten G et al: Intervertebral disc cell therapy for regeneration: mesenchymal stem cell implantation in rat intervertebral discs. *Ann Biomed Eng* 32(3):430-434, 2004.
13. Steck E et al: Induction of intervertebral disc-like cells from adult mesenchymal stem cells. *Stem Cells* 23:403-411, 2005.
14. Bosnakovski D et al: Chondrogenic differentiation of bovine bone marrow mesenchymal stem cells in different hydrogels: influence of collagen type II extracellular matrix on MSC chondrogenesis. *Biotechnol Bioeng* 93:1152-1163, 2006.
15. LeMaitre CL et al: An in vitro study investigating the survival and phenotype of mesenchymal stem cells following injection into nucleus pulposus tissue. *Arthritis Res Ther* 11(1):R20, 2009.
16. Wuertz K et al: Behavior of mesenchymal stem cells in the chemical microenvironment of the intervertebral disc. *Spine* 33:1843-1849, 2008.
17. Sobajima S et al: Feasibility of a stem cell therapy for intervertebral disc degeneration. *Spine J* 8:888-896, 2008.
18. Alini M et al: Are animal models useful for studying disc disorders/degeneration. *Eur Spine J* 17(1):2-19, 2008.
19. Chen WH, et al: Intervertebral disc regeneration in an ex vivo culture system using mesenchymal stem cells and platelet-rich plasma. *Biomaterials* 30(29):5523-5533, 2009.
20. Khot A et al: The use of intradiscal steroid therapy for lumbar spinal discogenic pain: a randomized controlled trial. *Spine* 29(8):833-837, 2004.
21. Fayad F et al: Relation of inflammatory Modic changes to intradiscal steroid injection outcome in chronic low back pain. *Eur Spine J* 6:925-931, 2007.
22. Aoki M et al: Histologic changes in the intervertebral disc after intradiscal injections of methylprednisolone acetate in rabbits. *Spine* 22(2):127-131, 1997.
23. Andreula CF et al: Minimally invasive oxygen-ozone therapy for lumbar disk herniation. *Am J Neuroradiol* 24:996-1000, 2003.

24. Gautam S et al: Comparative evaluation of oxygen-ozone therapy and combined use of oxygen-ozone therapy with percutaneous intradiscal radiofrequency thermocoagulation for the treatment of lumbar disc herniation. *Pain Pract* Epub 19 July 2010.

25. Barendse GA et al: Randomized controlled trial of percutaneous intradiscal radiofrequency thermocoagulation for chronic discogenic back pain: lack of effect from a 90-second 70 C lesion. *Spine* 26(3):287-292, 2001.

26. Francesco C et al: A case of vertebrobasilar stroke during oxygen-ozone therapy. *J Stroke Cerebrovasc Dis* 13(6):259-261, 2004.

27. Bo W, Longyi C, Jian T: A pyogenic discitis at C3-C4 with associated ventral epidural abscess involving C1-C4 after intradiscal oxygen-ozone chemonucleolysis: a case report. *Spine* 34(8):E298-E304, 2009.

28. Gazzeri R et al: Fulminating septicemia secondary to oxygen-ozone therapy for lumbar disc herniation: case report. *Spine* 32(3):E121-E123, 2007.

29. Riquelme C et al: Chemonucleolysis of lumbar disc herniation with ethanol. *J Neuroradiol* 28(4): 219-229, 2001.

30. Theron J et al: Percutaneous treatment of lumbar intervertebral disk hernias with radiopaque gelified ethanol. *J Spinal Disord Tech* 20(7):526-532, 2007.

31. Theron J et al: Percutaneous treatment of cervical disk hernias using gelified ethanol. *Am J Neuroradiol* 31:1454-1456, 2010.

32. Peng B et al: Intradiscal methylene blue injection for the treatment of chronic discogenic low back pain. *Eur Spine J* 16:33-38, 2007.

33. Peng B et al: A randomized placebo-controlled trial of intradiscal methylene blue injection for the treatment of chronic discogenic low back pain. *Pain* 149(1):124-129, 2010.

34. Popper PJ et al: The effect of methylene blue on neural tissue. *Anesthesiology* 33(3):335-340, 1970.

35. Miller MR, Mathews RS, Reeves KD: Treatment of painful advanced internal disc derangement with intradiscal injection of hypertonic dextrose. *Pain Physician* 9:115-121, 2006.

36. Sha'ban M et al: Fibrin promotes proliferation and matrix production of intervertebral disc cells cultured in three-dimensional poly(lactic-co-glycolic acid) scaffold. *J Biomater Sci Polym Ed* 19(9):1219-1237, 2008.

37. Derby R, et al: Injection of fibrin sealant into discs following IDET and nucleoplasty: Early outcome in six cases, International Spine Intervention Society. *Interventional Spine* 5(2):12-19, 2005.

38. Yin W et al: Intradiscal injection of fibrin sealant for the treatment of symptomatic internal disc disruption: results of a prospective multicenter IDE pilot study with 6-month follow-up. *Pain Med* 10(5):955 (abstract), 2009.

7 Radiofrequency and Other Heat Applications for the Treatment of Discogenic Pain

Leonardo Kapural and Timothy R. Deer

CHAPTER OVERVIEW

Chapter Synopsis: In addition to surgical treatments for discogenic pain, some minimally invasive and nonsurgical options are available. Intradiscal electrothermal therapy (IDET) delivers heat via a resistive coil, whereas with biacuplasty a radiofrequency (RF) catheter is applied to the posterior annulus of the disc to create a lesion within the disc. The procedures are thought to denervate ingrown nociceptors and to coagulate the connective tissues within the disc, but there is little evidence that these outcomes provide the pain relief seen with the treatments. With biacuplasty, alternating current is delivered in the RF range by a cooled electrode, providing greater control over the size and extent of the lesion. Because the indications for IDET and biacuplasty are so specific to discogenic pain, patient selection is particularly important. Provocation discography is recommended as one of many diagnostic procedures to confirm that the treatment is indeed indicated. Chronic, nonspecific low back pain is not indicated for IDET or biacuplasty.

Important Points:
- Strict selection criteria improve results of annuloplasty procedures for lower back discogenic pain.
- Patients with evidence of one or two levels of disc degeneration on magnetic resonance imaging (MRI) and one or two levels positive on provocation discography are desired candidates for annuloplasty.
- Disc biacuplasty and IDET are both effective minimally invasive annuloplasty procedures. Biacuplasty may provide a procedural advantage over IDET in regard to the degree of disc disruption and changes to disc architecture. It is also easier to place the electrode in biacuplasty.

Clinical Pearls:
- Initially the biacuplasty introducer is positioned from the oblique view by rotating the fluoroscopy C-arm to position where the superior articular process of the vertebral level below is somewhere between one third and one half the width of the vertebral column. This view allows optimal placement of two electrodes to form a bipolar configuration with approximate distances of 2.5 to 3 cm or less.
- Postprocedurally an optimal rehabilitation step-by-step program is required to ascertain a good outcome.

Clinical Pitfalls:
- Patients with increased body mass index, a smoking habit, and multilevel degenerative disc disease have less chance to improve long term.
- Heavy sedation and general anesthesia may predispose patients to various neurological injuries.

Introduction

There are multiple potential sources of lower back pain. In approximately 45% of the cases, such pain appears to be discogenic in origin.[1,2] In clinical practice, often more than one cause can be found simultaneously that might be held responsible for the patients' pain. The development of various minimally invasive treatments for discogenic pain prompts the development of new diagnostic procedures producing better specificity and sensitivity to confirm or refute clinical suspicion that the patient's pain is of discogenic origin.

Establishing Diagnosis

The diagnosis of discogenic pain frequently remains unclear secondary to its nonspecific clinical features, including persistent, nociceptive low back and groin and/or leg pain that worsens with axial loading and improves with recumbency. These signs and symptoms are insufficient to establish the diagnosis of discogenic pain and to begin a comprehensive treatment plan for the patients with such complaints. To provide definite diagnosis many practitioners use provocation, functional, and analgesic lumbar discography (see Chapters 4 and 5) in conjunction with magnetic resonance imaging (MRI). Although MRI images may assist in visualizing pathological disc changes such as high intensity zones and loss of disc height, the results correlate poorly with clinical findings, leaving open the question of the clear source of the back pain. Currently provocation discography is the only method that may link pathological abnormalities recognized on MRI with the patient's pain. Relatively high false-positive rates of provocation discography reported in clinical studies have led to lack of clarity in its predictive value.[3-5]

Anatomy and Pathophysiology

The etiology of discogenic pain is not well understood. However, newer evidence has suggested that various pathophysiological changes may be associated with disc degeneration and in some cases discogenic pain.[6,7] Delamination or tearing of the posterior annulus and diffuse dehydration and progressive loss of nuclear material with increasing age are associated with disc degeneration. Physical changes observed in the degenerative disc are also closely associated with biochemical and cellular changes. The degenerating disc continues to produce inflammatory cytokines, including tumor necrosis factor-α (TNF-α), nitric oxide, and matrix metalloprotineases (MMPs).[8] Frequently nerve growth restricted to the outer third of the annulus in a normal disc extends farther into the degenerated disc along the fissures and is supported by extent of the vasculature.[9-13] Immunohistochemical studies have confirmed that these aberrantly ingrown nerves are of nociceptive origin (C- and A-beta fibers) and are responsible for transmitting pain responses.[6,12] The role of inflammatory cytokines is theorized to increase the sensitization of these ingrowth nerves. Elimination of the previously described nociceptive fibers may stop transmission of the pain signal. Therefore a potentially effective measure to reduce discogenic pain is to denervate the posterior annulus or neural supply to the disc.[14]

Mechanism of Therapeutic Efficacy

Thermal annular procedures were developed in an effort to provide a minimally invasive alternative to spinal surgeries. Thermal energy is delivered to the affected disc via a resistive heating coil (intradiscal electrothermal therapy [IDET], Smith and Nephew, London, UK) or a radiofrequency (RF) catheter (biacuplasty (Kimberly Clark, Atlanta, Ga; discTRODE; ValleyLab, Boulder, Col) in an attempt to denervate nociceptive fibers and coagulate collagenous tissues in the annulus. Scientific evidence to support such mechanisms of action in the literature is lacking.[15]

The rationale of disc thermal treatment for discogenic pain was largely influenced by the shoulder capsule studies, in which modifying and shrinking the same type of collagen is clearly documented.[16,17] Because the annulus is comprised of collagen, heating may cause collagen shrinkage, limit the leakage of inflammatory disc materials, and cause denervation of nociceptive fibers. Collagen shrinkage and denaturation require a temperature of at least

60° to 65° C.[16,17] However, at least when it comes to IDET, it seems that temperatures generated during the procedure are insufficient to alter the collagen architecture.[18] Tissue modulation, including shrinkage, denaturation, and structural changes to collagen fibers in the annulus to increase annular stability, is one hypotheses proposed to explain the mechanism of action for the thermal treatment of discogenic pain.[16,17]

Perhaps a more likely mechanism of action for intradiscal thermal minimally invasive procedures is denervation of ingrown nociceptors by neuroablation. Temperatures reached in the disc using biacuplasty or IDET are sufficient to produce denervation, which occurs at 42° to 45° C.[19,20] Still, lack of any evidence to confirm that neuroablation is the mechanisms of action for discogenic pain relief continues to be stumbling block to further clinical research in that area.

One means of delivering thermal energy to biological tissues is to use alternating current (AC). It is superior to direct current (DC) electricity since it can be delivered with less resistance and more control. A direct relationship exists between increased frequency of AC electricity and conductance through tissue.[21-23] The frequency used to create thermal lesions in modern RF generators is in the order of 400 to 600 kHz. This corresponds to the frequency of radio waves. At RFs, the flow of electrons does not interfere with physiological functions such as depolarization of muscle cells or neurons. During application of RF, the alternating flow of electrical current causes ions in the tissue to move back and forth. This alternating movement by the ions causes molecular vibration within the tissue and results in frictional heating.[22,23] This effect is called ionic heating and can lead to thermal injury to the cells when tissue temperature reaches 42° C.[24] The extent of cellular damage is a function of temperature and duration of heating. As the temperature increases, there is an exponential decrease in time needed to cause cellular destruction.[25] Increase in tissue temperature, produced by ionic heating, is a function of current density, or the amount of current-per-unit area. Current density is greatest at the proximity of the electrode and decreases with increasing distance from the electrode. However, by increasing the power output, current density around the electrode is increased; thus the lesion size produced by ionic heating is limited by the current density.

One method of increasing lesion size or volume is by cooling the RF electrode internally (**Fig. 7-1**). This technique was initially developed for tumor and cardiac ablation[26-28] and is currently used in the intradiscal biacuplasty procedure.[29-31] Cooled RF probes have hollow lumens that extend to the tip of the electrode. The cooling fluid circulates in a closed loop through the hollow lumens to the tip of the electrode and back to a pump. The coolant acts as a heat sink that removes heat from the tissue adjacent to the electrode. Consequently larger lesion volumes can be produced by increasing power deposition and the duration at which current is delivered without causing tissue charring around the electrode (see **Fig. 7-1**).[26] A larger lesion volume can be produced by using two internally cooled RF electrodes in a bipolar arrangement. **Fig. 7-1** compares a bipolar lesion formed

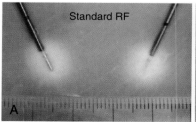
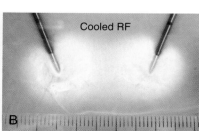

Fig. 7-1 Bipolar lesion in chicken breast (37° C) formed using standard (**A**) and cooled (**B**) radiofrequency electrodes for 25 minutes. The lesion temperatures for the standard and cooled radio frequencies were 80° C and 55° C, respectively.

with and without cooling. A large confluent lesion can be formed using cooled electrodes at a lower temperature than the small and nonconfluent lesion formed using noncooled electrodes at a higher temperature.

Guidelines

The current body of evidence in peer-reviewed literature does not provide clear support for using intradiscal heat treatments such as IDET and intradiscal biacuplasty for chronic, nonspecific low back pain originating from the intervertebral disc.[15] To improve results of minimally invasive intradiscal treatments, it is imperative to use a strict patient selection criteria and provocation discography with manometry appropriately.[14] Multiple studies on minimally invasive intradiscal therapies performed in recent years either were pilot trials, or they enrolled patients in a prospective manner but lacked randomization and blinding. This had adverse influence on the interpretation of clinical efficacy by the third-party payers and critics.

Indications

When considering indications for two commonly used annuloplasties, IDET and intradiscal biacuplasty, commonly used patient selection criteria include persistent discogenic lower back pain, which remains despite comprehensive conservative treatment, including physical therapy and a directed exercise program.[32-36] Furthermore, no neural compressive lesions should be seen on MRI, and provocation discography should reproduce concordant pain at low pressurization at one or two intervertebral disc levels.[33,36] When comparing published IDET studies, differences in outcomes are thought to be related to variability in patient selection.[33-36]

Strict selection criteria should also include Beck's depression inventory score of <20, less than 20% disc height narrowing on lateral radiograph,[37] and any signs of disc degeneration on MRI at more than two lumbar levels.[33] Patients with multilevel degenerative disc disease as shown on the MRI study are unlikely to benefit from the annuloplasty (**Fig. 7-2**). In their randomized, prospective trial Pauza and colleagues[37] used provocation discography as a selection criterion rather than a combination of MRI and discography criteria for the enrollment. That may have contributed to somewhat poorer outcomes in this IDET study.[37] Overweight patients[34] and patients receiving workers' compensation benefits[32,35] represent additional patient subsets that are less likely to improve following any annuloplasty.

A good example of the impact of poor patient selection influencing results of annuloplasty is seen in the randomized, double-blinded, controlled IDET study by Freeman and colleagues.[36] They reported no significant improvement between treatment and placebo groups of patients with discogenic pain. It should be noted that this study did not include critical factors in the selection criteria such a body mass index, depression scores, and the number of disc levels degenerated on MRI. It should also be noted that a large group of their enrolled patients were receiving workers' compensation benefits at the time of their participation in the study.[36]

Techniques and Equipment

Intradiscal Electrothermal Therapy

The current direction and proper use of IDET in the interventional pain medicine physician community is uncertain, but it is still available on the market, and the procedural technique is described here. IDET is performed under local anesthesia and mild

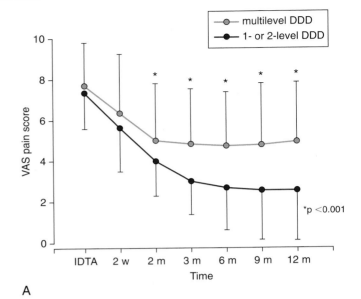

A

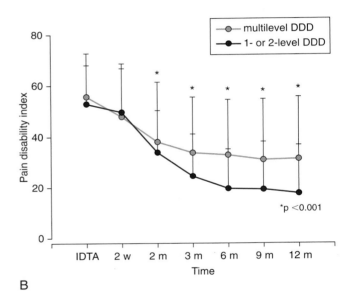

B

Fig. 7-2 Improvements in the VAS pain scores and Pain Disability Index over time in patients with discogenic pain following IDET (*IDTA*). Compared are three-or-more–level DDD (multilevel DDD) patients (*filled circles*) with one or two DDD (1- or 2-level DDD) patients (*open circles*). Note only modest improvements in multilevel-DDD group and robust, sustained low pain scoring and functional capacity improvements at 12 months after IDET in 1- or 2-level DDD patients. *DDD,* Degenerative disc disease; *IDET,* intradiscal electrothermal treatment; *IDTA,* intradiscal thermal annuloplasty; *VAS,* visual analog scale. Modified from Kapural L et al: Intradiscal thermal annuloplasty for discogenic pain in patients with multilevel degenerative disc disease, *Anesth Analg* 99:472-476, 2004.

intravenous sedation in sterile conditions. Intravenous antibiotics should be timed 30 to 60 minutes before the procedure. Patients are placed in the prone position, and midabdomen support rolls or cushions are used to correct for lumbar lordosis. After a 17-gauge needle is inserted under fluoroscopic guidance into the targeted disc, a thermal resistive coil (**Fig. 7-3**) is navigated through the same needle until it is positioned appropriately within the disc (**Fig. 7-4, C**).[38] It should be positioned across the posterior interphase between the annulus and nucleus. The thermal resistive coil generates gradual rising temperature inside the disc up to 90° C. Temperature is then maintained for 4 minutes according to manufacturer protocol (Smith and Nephews, London, UK).

Intradiscal Biacuplasty

The disc biacuplasty procedure using the TransDiscal system is a minimally invasive technique for RF delivery to the posterior annulus of the disc. The procedure is completed under fluoroscopy and minimal sedation. Heating itself usually is not painful, and it normally produces only mild transient back discomfort without significant leg pain. Two 17-gauge TransDiscal introducers are placed in the posterior annulus of the intervertebral disc bilaterally.[38] The C-arm of the fluoroscope is rotated by approximately 30 degrees oblique view such that one third to one half of the disc appears lateral to the superior articular process (SAP). The introducer should be directed in the "tunnel view" next to

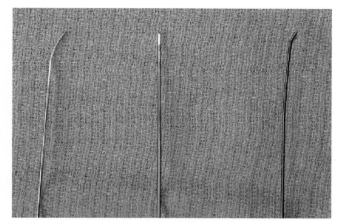

Fig. 7-3   Three annuloplasty electrode tips that are currently available for clinical use. *Far left,* DiscTRODE with elongated flexible tip designed to lie within the posterior annulus. *Middle,* Electrode tip is one of two bipolar electrodes used for biacuplasty. The electrode is cooled as high as the active tip. *Far right,* IDET resistive coil with slightly curved tip, facilitating placement of the coil in the circular fashion between the annulus and nucleus.

the SAP and enter the disc at approximately the center of the disc height. This ensures that the electrodes are away from the endplates to increase the safety of the procedure. The introducers are advanced into the disc until the tips appear to be within the medial edge of the pedicles in an anteroposterior (AP) view. Two 18-gauge TransDiscal probes (see **Fig. 7-3**) are then positioned inside the disc through the introducers. Appropriate positioning and depth of probe are assessed by checking AP and lateral views of the lumbar spine (**Fig. 7-5**). The generator controls the delivery of RF energy by monitoring the temperature measured by a thermocouple at the tip of the probe. The temperature increases gradually over a period of 7 to 8 minutes to 50° C, with final heating at 50° C for another 7 minutes. It should be noted that, although the temperature is set to 45° C on the RF generator, tissue temperature reaches 65° to 70° C because of ionic heating. During this time the patient should be awake and communicate with the physician. Following completion of the procedure, the patient should go through a specific physical therapy program over a rehabilitation period.

Outcomes Evidence

Intradiscal Electrothermal Therapy

A recent review article by Appleby and associates[39] compared 13 available studies on IDET and concluded that variation in patient selection and heating techniques may account for differences seen in clinical results of IDET.[39] Overall the average pain score improvements were between 1.5 to 5 visual analog scale (VAS) points. SF-36 physical function (PF) scores for evaluation of functional capacity improved from approximately 15 to 30 in four separate studies.[39] A commonly cited IDET study is carefully designed Pauza and colleagues' sham-controlled, prospective study.[37] Clinical improvements were seen in both sham and treatment groups, but greater improvements in mean pain and functionality scores were reported in patients who underwent IDET. Pauza and colleagues used provocation discography rather than combined MRI/discography criteria for enrollment, which may have contributed to the high number needed to treat (i.e., five) to achieve >75% improvement in one patient.[37] Again, as detailed in the patient selection section of this chapter, strict patient selection influenced most outcomes of the IDET studies (see **Fig. 7-2**).

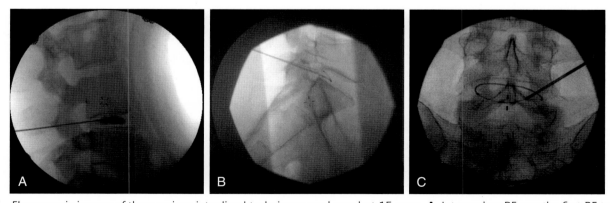

Fig. 7-4   Fluoroscopic images of three various intradiscal techniques used over last 15 years. **A,** Intranuclear RF was the first RF technique intended for the treatment of lumbar discogenic back pain. Electrode is positioned within the nucleus of the disc. It was shown to be largely ineffective. **B,** Lateral fluoroscopic view of properly positioned discTRODE. Idea was to cover most of the posterior annulus with an elongated RF electrode, but it was shown to be ineffective (see text). **C,** Cranial tilt view of the final position of an IDET resistive coil. The coil is within the disc borders of an L4-L5 intervertebral disc. *IDET,* Intradiscal electrothermal treatment; *RF,* radiofrequency.

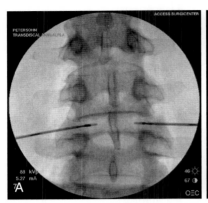
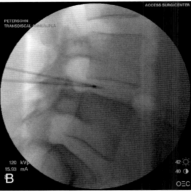

Fig. 7-5   **A,** Anteroposterior view of the lumbar spine with the tip of the probe inserted to the medial edge of the pedicles. **B,** Lateral view of the lumbar spine with the depth of the probe about 1 cm deep into the posterior annulus of the disc.

Biacuplasty

Before the initiation of clinical trials, temperature profile of the disc biacuplasty procedure had been investigated in both porcine and human cadaveric lumbar discs.[29-31] Acute histological effects were investigated initially using an in vivo porcine model by Petersohn to assess safety of the procedure.[31] Histological examination showed no evidence of injury to the surrounding neural structures or tissue charring in sections adjacent to the position of the probes. Temperature profiles in the porcine discs demonstrated increase in tissue temperature to 45° to 65° C, sufficient to cause neuroablation; temperatures around the nerve root and in the epidural space remained below 45° C. A temperature mapping study performed in human cadaveric specimens demonstrated that the disc biacuplasty procedure increases intradiscal tissue temperature to a neuroablative level. Temperature profiles similar to those in the porcine disc model were obtained. Temperatures in the inner two thirds of the posterior annulus reached 46° to 67° C and above 45° C in the outer third while maintaining temperature in the epidural space below 42° C.[29,30] When histological changes and temperature distribution were compared between degenerated and nondegenerated cadaveric lumbar discs, bipolar lesions formed in the posterior annulus maintained a consistent size and an effective temperature distribution. It is important to note that there was no heating at the epidural space and segmental nerve root.[29]

The clinical results of disc biacuplasty in two case series involving 8 and 15 patients showed significant pain relief 3 and 12 months after the procedure.[40-42] One case series involving eight patients demonstrated approximately 50% improvements in pain scores at 3 months after the procedure without postprocedural pain and/or any other complications.[42] Another pilot study reported patient improvements in several functional capacity and pain assessment measures after undergoing disc biacuplasty procedure for discogenic pain; again there were no procedure-related complications.[40,41] Significant reduction in the median VAS pain score from about 7 cm to 4 cm at 3 months was maintained at 12 months' follow-up. In addition, improvement in the Oswestry index from 23.3 to 16.5 points at 1 and 6 months was maintained at 12 months, with similar increases in the SF-36 subscales scores.[40,41]

Other subsets of patients with discogenic pain who have been treated using disc biacuplasty are those with previously discectomized discs and thoracic discogenic pain.[43,44]

Persistent lower back pain after discectomy in most of the patients could be of discogenic origin.[45] As many as 75% of the patients would require treatment of back pain following the discectomy; the back pain replaced the leg pain that preceded

discectomy.[45] It is reasonable to assume that discectomy produces permanent anatomical, biochemical, and functional changes to the treated intervertebral disc, potentially leading to the development of low back pain. We described successful treatment of discogenic pain using the disc biacuplasty procedure in a previously discectomized disc.[43]

Discogenic pain in the thoracic region is a challenging condition characterized by refractoriness to conservative treatments; unlike lumbar discogenic pain, there is a lack of effective surgical options. Improvements in functional capacity and pain scores were noted in two of three patients in the first published case series. The Oswestry index improved from 24 to 8 and 10 points in two responding patients, and similarly SF-36-PF score changed from 55 to 80 and 45 to 82. One patient showed no improvement.[44]

Possible advantages of disc biacuplasty when compared to other RF lesioning procedures within the disc are minimal disruption to the native tissue architecture and relative ease of electrode placement (**Fig. 7-5**), which eliminates the need to thread a long heating catheter (e.g., IDET).

Other Radiofrequency Lesioning Procedures for Discogenic Pain

Two additional techniques were described to treat discogenic lower back pain using RF lesioning.[46-48] Both were shown to be clinically ineffective. No appreciable differences in pain or functional capacity scores could be demonstrated between the sham and the treated patient groups during the randomized controlled trial with the original Sluijter RF technique (see **Fig. 7-3, A**) in which the nucleus (and not the annulus) was heated to 70° C for 90 seconds.[46] In addition, different annular RF probe (i.e., discTRODE) (see **Fig. 7-3, B**) studies confirmed what was suspected clinically (i.e., that only modest or no improvements in pain scores and functional capacity could be achieved).[47,48] Some clinicians have attributed this to poor electrode design in which proper heat distribution across the posterior annulus could not be achieved.

Avoiding Risks and Complications

The location of the intervertebral discs and structures that form the spine and the proximity of vascular and neural tissue may predispose patients to complications during any annuloplasty procedure. The onset of the clinical presentations of different complications varies according to their pathological mechanisms and/or presence of other co-morbidities. The incidence of various complications related to intradiscal procedures has been reported to range from 0% to as high as 10%.[49,50]

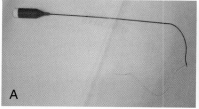

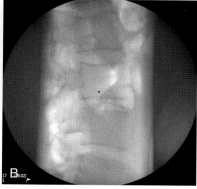

Fig. 7-6 **A,** Uncoiled IDET catheter that was carefully removed from the intervertebral disc after completion of the heating interval. **B,** Intradiscally retained uncoiled piece of the same IDET catheter visible on fluoroscopic lateral view. *IDET,* Intradiscal electrothermal treatment.

The most serious, dangerous, and difficult-to-treat complication of any intradiscal procedure is discitis. The prevalence is very low and may range from 0% to 1.3% per disc during provocation discography and is caused by contamination with skin flora.[51,52] The most common causative microorganisms are *Staphylococcus aureus* and *Staphylococcus epidermidis*.[52-54] Clinically, if worsening back pain days to weeks after the provocation discography is accompanied by laboratory findings of leukocytosis and elevated erythrocyte sedimentation rate, MRI is indicated.[55]

To prevent discitis preprocedural intravenous antibiotics are used more frequently than intradiscal antibiotics. Use of gentamicin (Garamycin), vancomycin, or cefazolin may be preferred since they penetrate into the intervertebral disc to a greater degree than other cephalosporins or oxacilli.[56,57] The best interval for intravenous administration of cefazolin or vancomycin is 15 to 81 minutes before disc penetration with needle.[58] The occurrence of infectious discitis may also be decreased when antibiotics are mixed with intradiscal, water-soluble contrast.[59] The antibiotics are frequently mixed with the contrast agent into a stable nonprecipitating solution before injecting them into the disc. Multiple studies reported absence of discitis in thousands of patients when these suggested protocols were followed.[60] The incidence of discitis after intradiscal annuloplasty procedures is not certain based on a literature review, but it seems to be rare. Only one published report described discitis after the IDET in a patient with increased low back pain, lethargy, night sweats, and spasm.[61] One of the suggested prophylactic approaches is to inject 1 g of cephalosporins mixed with local anesthetics on withdrawal of the RF electrode.[62] There is no prospective analysis to support or refute this recommendation.

Epidural abscess[63] and acute lumbar disc herniation[64] are other potential but very rare complications of intradiscal procedures, as is catheter breakage (**Fig. 7-6**),[60,62] vertebral osteonecrosis,[65] or cauda equina syndrome.[66] Overall, disc herniation is rare after IDET, with an incidence of 0.3%; it was speculated to be caused by thermally mediated loss of tensile strength of the collagen fibers.[67] One study reported four patients with transient radiculopathy that resolved in less than 6 weeks following the IDET procedure.[36] Similar transient radicular signs and symptoms were reported in several patients who underwent IDET; one patient had a foot drop.[62] Cauda equina syndrome was reported in a 56-year-old woman after the IDET who unfortunately did not improve even 5 months after the injury.[68] It seems that biacuplasty procedure may be somewhat safer since no such complications have been reported up to this date (personal communication with Kimberly Clark Inc, Atlanta, Ga, representatives). More outcome data on complications will become available as these procedures become more clinically common.

Conclusions

Discogenic pain is a debilitating condition that represents a major source of chronic low back pain. There are few minimally invasive effective treatment options available. The disc biacuplasty procedure uses an internally cooled electrode to deliver an effective heat distribution to the annulus for ablating ingrown nociceptive fibers that are a likely source of the pain generation. Although the current peer-reviewed literature suggests largely positive clinical effects in long-term improvement of function and lower back pain, it still does not provide enough evidence for use of intradiscal heat treatments for chronic, nonspecific low back pain originating from the intervertebral disc. Serious complications following percutaneous interventional procedures for back or leg pain are infrequent.

References

1. Kuslich SD, Ulstrom CL, Michael CJ: The tissue origin of low back pain and sciatica: a report of pain response to tissue stimulation during operations on the lumbar spine using local anesthesia. *Orthop Clin North Am* 22:181-187, 1991.
2. Schwarzer AC et al: The relative contributions of the disc and zygapophyseal joint in chronic low back pain. *Spine* 19:801-806, 1994.
3. Cohen SP et al: Lumbar discography: a comprehensive review of outcome studies, diagnostic accuracy, and principles. *Reg Anesth Pain Med* 30(2):163-183, 2005.
4. Carragee EJ, Alamin TF, Carragee JM: Low-pressure positive discography in subjects asymptomatic of significant low back pain illness. *Spine* 31(5):505-509, 2006.
5. Derby R et al: The ability of pressure-controlled discography to predict surgical and nonsurgical outcomes. *Spine* 24:364-371, 1999.
6. Peng B et al: The pathogenesis of discogenic low back pain. *J Bone Joint Surg* 87(B):62-67, 2005.
7. Peng B, Hao J, Hou S: Possible pathogenesis of painful intervertebral disc degeneration. *Spine* 31:560-566, 2006.
8. Podichetty VK: The aging spine: the role of inflammatory mediators in intervertebral disc degeneration. *Cell Mol Biol (Noisy-le-grand)* 53(5):4-18, 2007.
9. Ashton, IK et al: Neuropeptides in the human intervertebral disc. *J Orthop Res* 12(2):186-192, 1994.
10. Johnson WE et al: Immunohistochemical detection of Schwann cells in innervated and vascularized human intervertebral discs. *Spine* 26(23):2550-2557, 2001.

11. Melrose J et al: Increased nerve and blood vessel ingrowth associated with proteoglycan depletion in an ovine anular lesion model of experimental disc degeneration. *Spine* 27(12):1278-1285, 2002.

12. Palmgren T et al: An immunohistochemical study of nerve structures in the anulus fibrosus of human normal lumbar intervertebral discs. *Spine* 24(20):2075-2079, 1999.

13. Jackson HC, II, Winkelmann RK, Bickel WH: Nerve endings in the human lumbar spinal column and related structures. *J Bone Joint Surg Am* 48(7):1272-1281, 1966.

14. Kapural L: Indications for minimally invasive disc and vertebral procedures. *Pain Med* 9(S1):S65-S72, 2008.

15. Helm S et al: Systematic review of the effectiveness of thermal annular procedures in treating discogenic low back pain. *Pain Physician* 12(1):207-232, 2009.

16. Naseef GS, III et al: The thermal properties of bovine joint capsule: the basic science of laser- and radiofrequency-induced capsular shrinkage. *Am J Sports Med* 25(5):670-674, 1997.

17. Wall MS et al: Thermal modification of collagen. *J Shoulder Elbow Surg* 8(4):339-344, 1999.

18. Kleinstueck FS et al: Acute biomechanical and histological effects of intradiscal electrothermal therapy on human lumbar discs. *Spine* 26(20): 2198-2207, 2001.

19. Troussier B, Lebas JF, Chirossel JP et al., Percutaneous intradiscal radio-frequency thermocoagulation: a cadaveric study. *Spine* 20(15): 1713-1718, 1995.

20. Smith HP, McWhorter JM, Challa VR: Radiofrequency neurolysis in a clinical model: neuropathological correlation. *J Neurosurg* 55(2):246-253, 1981.

21. Kline M, Yin W: Radiofrequency techniques in clinical practice. In Waldman S, editor: *Interventional pain management*, Philadelphia, 2001, Saunders, pp 243-293.

22. Noe CE, Racz GB: Radiofrequency. In Raj P, editor: *Pain medicine: a comprehensive review*, St. Louis, 1996, Mosby, pp 305-308.

23. Organ LW: Electrophysiologic principles of radiofrequency lesion making. *Appl Neurophysiol* 39(2):69-76, 1976.

24. Dickson JA, CS: Temperature range and selective sensitivity of tumors to hyperthermia: a critical review. *Ann NY Acad Sci* 335:180-205, 1980.

25. Curley SA: Radiofrequency ablation of malignant liver tumors. *Ann Surg Oncol* 10(4):338-347, 2003.

26. Lorentze T: A cooled needle electrode for radiofrequency tissue ablation: thermodynamic aspects of improved performance compared with conventional needle design. *Acad Radiol* 3(7):556-563, 1996.

27. Wittkamp FHM, Hauer RN, Robles de Medina EO: Radiofrequency ablation with a cooled porus electrode catheter. *J Am Coll Cardiol* 11(17) (abstract): 102, 1988.

28. Goldberg SN et al: Radiofrequency tissue ablation: increased lesion diameter with a perfusion electrode. *Acad Radiol* 3(8):636-644, 1996.

29. Kapural L et al: Histological and temperature distribution studies in the lumbar degenerated and non-degenerated human cadaver discs using novel transdiscal radiofrequency electrodes. *Pain Med* 9(1):68-75, 2008.

30. Pauza K: Cadaveric intervertebral disc temperature mapping during disc biacuplasty. *Pain Physician* 11(5):669-676, 2008.

31. Petersohn JD, Conquergood LR, Leung M: Acute histologic effects and thermal distribution profile of disc biacuplasty using a novel water-cooled bipolar electrode system in an in vivo porcine model. *Pain Med* 9(1):26-32, 2008.

32. Mekhail N, Kapural L: Intradiscal thermal annuloplasty of discogenic pain: an outcome study. *Pain Practice* 4:84-90, 2004.

33. Kapural L et al: Intradiscal thermal annuloplasty for discogenic pain in patients with multilevel degenerative disc disease. *Anesth Analg* 99:472-476, 2004.

34. Cohen SP et al: Risk factors for failure and complications of intradiscal electrothermal therapy: a pilot study. *Spine* 28:1142-1147, 2003.

35. Webster BS, Verma S, Pransky GS: Outcomes of workers' compensation claimants with low back pain undergoing intradiscal electrothermal therapy. *Spine* 29:435-441, 2004.

36. Freeman BJ et al: A randomized, double-blind, controlled trial: intradiscal electrothermal therapy versus placebo for the treatment of chronic discogenic low back pain. *Spine* 30:2369-2377, 2005.

37. Pauza KJ et al: A randomized, placebo-controlled trial of intradiscal electrothermal therapy for the treatment of discogenic low back pain. *Spine J* 4:27-35, 2004.

38. Kapural L, Goyle A: Imaging for provocative discography and minimally invasive percutaneous procedures for discogenic pain. *Tech Regional Anesth Pain Med* 11(2):73-80, 2007.

39. Appleby D et al: Meta-analysis of the efficacy and safety of intradiscal electrothermal therapy (IDET). *Pain Med* 7:308-316, 2006.

40. Kapural L et al: Novel transdiscal biacuplasty for the treatment of lumbar discogenic pain: a 6-month follow-up. *Pain Med* 9(1):60-67, 2008.

41. Kapural L: Intervertebral disc cooled bipolar radiofrequency (intradiscal biacuplasty) for the treatment of lumbar discogenic pain: a 12-month follow-up of the pilot study. *Pain Med* 9(4):464, 2008.

42. Cooper AR: *Disc biacuplasty for treatment of axial discogenic low back pain—initial case series*, Glasgow, Scotland, 2007, British Pain Society Annual General Meeting.

43. Kapural L, Cata JP, Narouze S: Successful treatment of lumbar discogenic pain using intradiscal biacuplasty in previously discectomized disc. *Pain Pract* 9(2):130-134, 2009.

44. Kapural L, Sakic K, Boutwell K: Intradiscal biacuplasty (IDB) for the treatment of thoracic discogenic pain. *Clin J Pain* 26(4):354-357, 2010.

45. Komori H et al: The natural history of herniated nucleus pulposus with radiculopathy. *Spine* 21:225-229, 1996.

46. Barendse GA et al: Randomized controlled trial of percutaneous intradiscal radiofrequency thermocoagulation for chronic discogenic back pain: lack of effect from a 90-second 70 C lesion. *Spine* 26:287-292, 2001.

47. Kapural L et al: Intradiscal thermal annuloplasty versus intradiscal radiofrequency ablation for the treatment of discogenic pain: a prospective matched control trial. *Pain Med* 6:425-431, 2005.

48. Kvarstein G et al: A randomized double-blind controlled trial of intra-annular radiofrequency thermal disc therapy—a 12-month follow-up. *Pain* 145:279-286, 2009.

49. Cohen SP et al: Risk factors for failure and complications of intradiscal electrothermal therapy: a pilot study. *Spine* 28:1142-1147, 2003.

50. Freeman BJ et al: A randomized, double-blind, controlled trial: intradiscal electrothermal therapy versus placebo for the treatment of chronic discogenic low back pain. *Spine* 30:2369-2377, 2005.

51. Tehranzadeh J: Discography 2000. *Radiol Clin North Am* 36:463-495, 1998.

52. Willems PC et al: Lumbar discography: Should we use prophylactic antibiotics? A study of 435 consecutive discograms and a systematic review of the literature. *J Spinal Disord Tech* 17:243-247, 2004.

53. Guyer RD, Ohnmeiss DD: Lumbar discography; position statement from the North American Spine Society Diagnostic and Therapeutic Committee. *Spine* 20:2048-2059, 1995.

54. Fraser RD, Osti OL, Vernon-Roberts B: Discitis after discography. *J Bone Joint Surg[Br]* 69:26-35, 1987.

55. Guyer RD et al: Discitis after discography. *Spine* 13:1352-1354, 1988.

56. Thomas RW et al: A new in-vitro model to investigate antibiotic penetration of the intervertebral disc. *J Bone Joint Surg [Br]* 77:967-970, 1995.

57. Rhoten RL et al: Antibiotic penetration into cervical discs. *Spine* 37:418-421, 1995.

58. Boscardin JB et al: Human intradiscal levels with cefazolin. *Spine* 17:S145-S148, 1992.

59. Klessig HT, Showsh SA, Sekorski A: The use of intradiscal antibiotics for discography: an in vitro study of gentamicin, cefazolin, and clindamycin. *Spine* 28:1735-1738, 2003.

60. Kapural L, Cata J: Complications of minimally invasive procedures for discogenic pain. *Tech Regional Anesth Pain Med* 11(3):157-163, 2007.

61. Davis TT et al: The IDET procedure for chronic discogenic low back pain. *Spine* 29:752-756, 2004.

62. Biyani A et al: Intradiscal electrothermal therapy: a treatment option in patients with internal disc disruption. *Spine* 28:S8-14, 2003.

63. Junila J, Niinimaki T, Tervonen O: Epidural abscess after lumbar discography: a case report. *Spine* 22:2191-2193, 1997.

64. Cohen SP et al: Risk factors for failure and complications of intradiscal electrothermal therapy: a pilot study. *Spine* 28:1142-1147, 2003.

65. Djurasovic M et al: Vertebral osteonecrosis associated with the use of intradiscal electrothermal therapy: a case report. *Spine* 27:E325-328, 2002.

66. Wetzel FT: Cauda equina syndrome from intradiscal electrothermal therapy. *Neurology* 56:1607, 2001.

67. Kleinstueck FS et al: Acute biomechanical and histological effects of intradiscal electrothermal therapy on human lumbar discs. *Spine* 26:2198-2207, 2001.

68. Hsia AW, Isaac K, Katz JS: Cauda equina syndrome from intradiscal electrothermal therapy. *Neurology* 55:320, 2000.

8 Arthrodesis and Fusion for the Treatment of Discogenic Neck and Back Pain: Evidence-Based Effectiveness and Controversies

John H. Shin, Daniel J. Hoh, and Michael P. Steinmetz

CHAPTER OVERVIEW

Chapter Synopsis: Discogenic pain presents enormous challenges to both patient and pain clinician. Not only is the condition difficult to diagnose, but few of the limited treatment options provide unequivocally positive outcomes. Spinal fusion surgeries in particular have increased dramatically in recent decades, but evidence for their efficacy has been called into question. It is clear by now that discs are legitimate pain generators; but, even with evidence of a diseased or degenerated disc, other pain generators may include the surrounding muscles, tendons, and fascia. This chapter examines the literature to determine under which circumstances surgical fusion may be indicated for discogenic pain. The results are intertwined with the controversial diagnostic tool discography. In some cases, provocation discography predicts a positive outcome for fusion surgery; but in others it may produce false positives, leading to unnecessary fusion surgery with poor results. The diversity of spinal fusion techniques available further complicates the matter. As with any chronic pain condition, psychosocial factors and co-morbid conditions should be carefully considered in patient selection for any treatment.

Important Points: Discogenic pain is difficult to diagnose and treat. Current diagnostic tests, including imaging studies, do not reliably and accurately identify the source of pain in most patients. This contributes to the wealth of conflicting data in the literature. With many variables to consider, including psychosocial factors and medical co-morbidities, the identification of a pain-generating disc is often difficult. The lack of standardization of non-operative therapeutics for discogenic back pain is a major confounding variable in most prospective clinical trials.

Clinical Pearls:
- A careful and detailed patient history and physical are key to understanding the mechanism and physiology of pain.
- Fusion for discogenic pain is controversial.
- There is little evidence to suggest that fusion is associated with better clinical outcomes.

Clinical Pitfalls:
- Determining the discs responsible for pain based on imaging studies alone is inaccurate, as degeneration of multiple levels is common with age.
- Discography results should be interpreted with caution if used as a test to determine the number of symptomatic discs.

Introduction

Neck and back pain are common conditions that affect millions of people each year. Neck pain is reported to occur in as many as 66% of individuals at some point during their lifetime.[1] With the widespread use of magnetic resonance imaging (MRI), patients are increasingly being diagnosed with degenerative disc disease, prompting referrals to surgeons and pain management physicians. The clinical significance of these degenerative findings is often overstated by physicians and patients alike, leading to a cascade of interventions and treatments that may not improve their symptoms.

In the absence of radiculopathy or myelopathy, controversy exists overt the clinical significance of degenerative disc disease and its correlation with pain. Numerous diagnostic tests such as computed tomography (CT), MRI, and discography have been developed to help elucidate the etiology of nonradicular spinal pain; however, none has been shown to reliably and accurately identify the source of pain. Just as the reliability and validity of these interventions are questioned by the scientific community, so are the indications for surgery and the potential benefit of fusion for treating neck pain without any symptoms of neural compression.

Similarly, low back pain is among the leading reasons for individuals to seek medical attention. One out of 17 patients seen by general practitioners presents with low back pain, and approximately 31 million patient visits for back pain occur in the United States annually.[2] It is estimated that 70% to 85% of individuals will suffer an acute episode of low back pain in their lifetime. Although most experience near complete resolution of symptoms within several weeks, a small percentage continue to experience persistent or chronic low back pain.[3]

Persistent low back pain is a significant source of anxiety, distress, depression, and disability that affects not only the individual, but society. It is estimated that 28% of the working population in the United States will be disabled by back pain at some time during their professional life, with approximately 8% of the entire work force disabled in a given year.[3] This is a troublesome statistic since back pain is the primary cause of disability in persons less than 50 years of age, often the most productive years in a lifetime. The total socioeconomic burden of back pain, including both health care costs and lost wages, is estimated at $100 to $200 billion annually, with two thirds of this cost the result of work-related disability.[4] Of alarming concern is that, although the incidence of diagnosed chronic back pain has been stable for 30 years, the rate of disability claims has increased by 14 times that of population growth.[5]

The surgical treatment of discogenic pain is controversial, and there is no consensus from the medical literature regarding the management of these patients. In fact, there are limited data comparing nonsurgical vs. surgical treatment for discogenic neck or back pain. Because the fundamental concept of discogenic pain is debatable, the evidence comparing surgery to medical therapies for this condition is more speculative than definitive.

Spinal fusion for discogenic pain is based on the theory that pain is related to a degenerative disc causing abnormal movement across a motion segment. This has been compared to abnormal movement across other degenerative joints such as hips or knees, where degeneration causes local mechanical and chemical processes. Arthrodesis across these degenerated joints is known to successfully eliminate pain. Spine surgeons have adopted this concept and applied it toward fusing across a degenerative, abnormal motion segment to relieve pain.

Despite the lack of evidence, fusion for discogenic pain is being performed more often, and reports of successful outcomes stem mostly from small retrospective case series.[6-9] Approximately 300,000 spinal fusions are performed annually in the United States, an increase of 220% between 1990 and 2001. Of these fusion operations, approximately 75% are performed for degenerative disc disorders. National inpatient data sample identifies degenerative disc disease as the diagnosis accounting for the largest increase in lumbar fusions during this period.[5]

Critics of fusion surgery argue that current imaging and functional diagnostic modalities do not accurately identify the source of pain in most patients who lack evidence of nerve compression or neurological deficit.[10] Further, the relationship between arthrodesis and pain relief remains equivocal. Despite advancements in surgical technology, instrumentation, and osteobiologics, clinical outcomes continue to lag behind fusion rates. This lack of correlation between rates of arthrodesis and pain improvement is an argument against arthrodesis for discogenic pain.

Conversely, proponents of fusion surgery argue that patients with discogenic pain are unlike patients with radiculopathy, myelopathy, or stenosis. It is argued that patients with discogenic pain suffer from psychosocial disorders, chronic narcotic use, and prolonged disability, which negatively impact surgical outcomes. Even a modest rate of improvement in pain, narcotic use, or ability to return to work may represent a positive result for an otherwise desperate patient population that has frequently exhausted all other therapeutic resources.

This chapter reviews the current evidence for fusion and the treatment of discogenic neck and back pain. After a brief discussion regarding the pathophysiology of discogenic pain, the best available evidence on outcomes is reviewed herein.

Pathophysiology of Discogenic Pain

Discogenic pain is a controversial concept and is defined as axial spine pain without neural compression secondary to a degenerative disc. Although the exact pathophysiology is unknown, several theories have been proposed.

The two components of the intervertebral disc are the nucleus pulposus and the annulus fibrosus. The nucleus pulposus is composed of proteoglycan aggrecan molecules with 70% to 80% water content. Absorption of water into the nucleus provides disc height and resistance to compression. With loading, water diffuses out of the disc, and subsequent resorption occurs with unloading. The annulus is an interlacing collagen network that provides tensile strength in axial rotation. With bending or compression of two adjacent vertebrae, the nucleus pulposus changes volumetrically, causing bulging of the disc away from the internal axis of rotation. The annulus also functions to limit and contain expansion or herniation of the nucleus.

With aging, the disc gradually becomes less hydrated, and the concentration of proteoglycans decreases. Normal disc metabolism shifts toward catabolic processes that further deplete proteoglycans and lead to increased matrix degeneration. As a result, the disc becomes progressively dysfunctional as the nuclear material is replaced by desiccated fibrocartilaginous material. Loss of fluid results in decreased hydrostatic pressure as a mechanism for effective load transference. Thinning or microfracture of the endplates can occur, and subsequent loss of endplate vascularity reduces transport of nutrients and waste products out of the disc. With cyclical loading of the degenerated disc, radial fissures or cracks propagate through the annulus with migration of nuclear material peripherally (**Fig. 8-1, A**). With complete annular disruption, disc material can herniate into the central canal or foramen (**Fig. 8-1, B**). These degenerative processes are estimated to occur in 90% of normal individuals by 50 years of age.[10]

In 1970 Crock[11,12] first associated back pain with the pathophysiological process of disc desiccation and subsequent radial fissure formation of the annulus. He termed this entity *internal disc disruption*. It was characterized by the progressive disruption of the internal architecture of the disc while essentially maintaining the external shape such that nerve root compression did not occur. Crock hypothesized that pain was generated when degradation of the disc matrix causes release of inflammatory cytokines, which then migrate through the disrupted inner annular fibers to irritate the high concentration of sensory nerve endings in the outer annulus. His conclusion was supported radiographically by the relative absence of any nerve root compression and the high correlation of concordant pain in discs that exhibited severe radial fissures with intradiscal contrast injection.

Since then several theories regarding the relationship between degenerative disc disease and pain generation have been developed. The mechanical theory suggests that degeneration results in

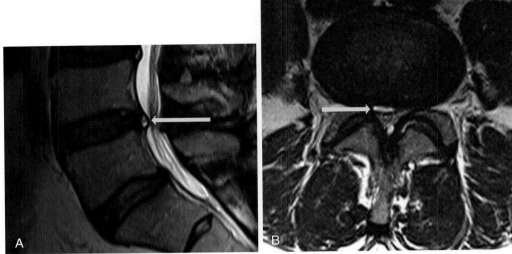

Fig. 8-1   **A,** T2 weighted sagittal magnetic resonance image (MRI) of a degenerated disc with a high intensity zone in the dorsal annulus (*arrow*) suggestive of annular disruption. **B,** T2 weighted axial MRI of a degenerated disc with a high intensity zone in the dorsal annulus (*arrow*) suggestive of annular disruption.

alteration in the biomechanical properties of the disc. As the disc degenerates and the annulus becomes disrupted, increasing instability occurs at the motion segment. Therefore with normal physiological loading the motion segment responds with excessive compression, bending, or rotation, which can trigger pain transmission in surrounding nociceptors. CT and MRI studies have quantified the response of the lumbar spine to rotatory torque and have correlated increased axial rotation in degenerated discs with pain provocation on discography.[13,14]

As the disc desiccates, it loses hydrostatic pressure, and more stress is transferred to the annulus and endplate, where pain sensitive nerve fibers are in high concentration. Increased stress to the endplate can lead to endplate fracture and disc herniation into the vertebral body, which may further propagate pain generation.

The chemical theory suggests that catabolism of the disc results in release of pro-inflammatory chemical mediators. Nitric oxide, phospholipase A₂, prostaglandin E, matrix metalloproteinases, and other cytokines have been implicated as chemical agents that infiltrate through radial fissures to irritate nociceptors present in the outer aspect of the annulus and the endplate. Proteoglycan breakdown is known to have a high concentration of the neurotransmitter glutamate, which may stimulate specific receptors in the dorsal root ganglion, resulting in pain in the absence of nerve root compression. Nociceptors are also known to be present in high concentration elsewhere within the spinal canal such as the posterior longitudinal ligament, dura, and blood vessels.

Although disc degeneration may produce pain, other structures may also produce pain, confounding the precise identification of the symptomatic pain generator. The facet joints, ligaments, fascia, nerve roots, and dura are capable of transmitting pain. Although disc degeneration may be the initial inciting pathology, one or more of these structures may in fact be the source of pain. Progressive disc disease results in increased load transference to surrounding structures such as the facet joints, ligaments, and paraspinal muscles, which may eventually exceed their capacity for resistance. Cyclical loading to these structures can lead to increased arthropathy, ligamentous hypertrophy, and muscle fatigue, which may contribute to pain. Studies performed in patients with similar presentations of low back pain have demonstrated a wide range of sources of pain, including the disc, facet joints, and sacroiliac joints.

Therefore, although the degenerated disc may be implicated in the pathophysiology of low back pain, it remains unclear whether the disc itself or other surrounding structures are the actual source of pain.

Diagnostic Controversies

Neck Pain

In patients who have discogenic neck pain refractory to conservative therapy, surgery is rarely indicated. In cases in which surgical intervention is considered, identifying a pain generator is critical yet not often possible for reasons discussed earlier.

Although imaging studies often reveal degenerative changes, including disc desiccation, loss of disc space height, and osteophyte formation, these findings usually involve multiple levels and do not localize to a single disc. Moreover, as many as 85% of asymptomatic individuals over 60 years of age exhibit degenerative changes in their cervical discs on MRI.[15,16]

Controversy regarding the validity of diagnostic testing techniques, including MRI and discography, for cervical discogenic pain continues to appear in the literature.[17,18] Cervical discography has been used by clinical practitioners in select cases as a provocative study to evaluate suspected discogenic pain.[19,20] Despite its enthusiasts, many have questioned the validity of discography for this application.[17] It has been argued that the specificity of discography is dramatically affected by the psychological profile of the patient.[17,21] Some propose that discography is not helpful in identifying the pain source or determining the predictive value of surgery.[22-25]

Conversely, there are authors who argue that discography can be used effectively in determining the source of a patient's pain.[26-28] Grubb and Kelly[28] reviewed their experience with cervical discography during a 12-year period and suggested that a reliable pattern of pain was produced by stimulation of each cervical disc. They reported a high percentage of patients who demonstrated multiple discs responsible for their axial neck pain.

Back Pain

Similar to neck pain, diagnosing the source of pain in patients with low back pain is challenging. Discogenic pain commonly occurs in patients who have a normal musculoskeletal and neurological examination. The distribution of pain is somatotopic rather than dermatomal; therefore identifying the spinal level of pathology is problematic.

Imaging findings are also generally nonspecific. Plain radiographs may show decreased disc height and sclerotic endplates (**Fig. 8-2, A**). Sclerotic endplates or bone-on-bone appearance is commonly seen with severely degenerated discs (**Fig. 8-2, B**). MRI may demonstrate dehydrated, desiccated, or collapsed discs (**Fig. 8-3, A**). However, these changes may occur in multiple discs, making it difficult to determine which level is symptomatic. Because of its sensitivity for visualizing soft tissue structures of the spine, including the discs, ligaments, joints, and neural elements, MRI is the preferred test to evaluate for nerve root compression from degenerative disc disease. The ability of MRI to detect loss of water content and disc desiccation has led to widespread use of this imaging modality. It also characterizes the effect of disc degeneration on the adjacent endplates and vertebral bodies. In the early phase the normal vertebral body bone marrow is replaced with vascularized fibrous tissue as a reparative response to injury

(**Fig. 8-3, B**). With chronic degeneration the normally red bone marrow is converted to yellow marrow as the marrow elements are replaced by fat cells, which appears to represent a chronic, stable state. Despite these findings, these changes commonly occur in asymptomatic individuals, calling into question their clinical relevance.

Despite conflicting evidence, many have adopted discography as an instrument for presurgical screening and patient selection, with the presumption that positive discography can reliably predict which patients and levels will respond favorably to fusion. Advocates of discography argue that discs demonstrating abnormal morphology and/or concordant pain provocation are likely the symptomatic levels. Therefore it is assumed that fusion across the positive discographic motion segment results in alleviation of pain. Conversely, discs with normal morphology or that do not reproduce similar pain can be reasonably excluded from surgery. As a result, many surgeons use discography not only to determine candidates for surgery but to assess how many levels to fuse.

Certain studies have demonstrated that positive discography reliably predicts positive surgical outcomes. Simmons and Segil[27]

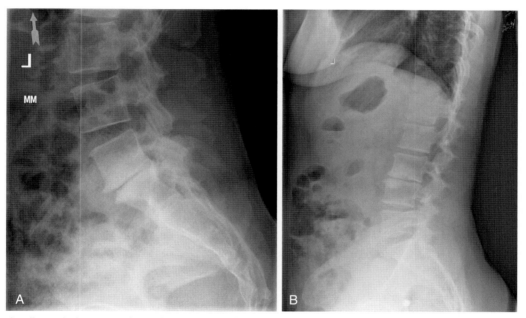

Fig. 8-2 A, Lateral radiograph demonstrating a degenerated, collapsed L5-S1 intervertebral disc space. **B,** Lateral radiograph demonstrating a degenerated L3-L4 intervertebral disc space with sclerotic endplates.

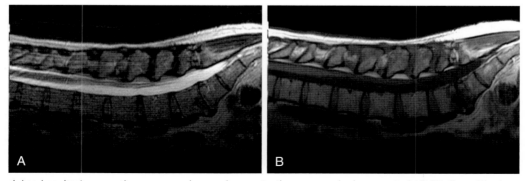

Fig. 8-3 A, T2 weighted sagittal magnetic resonance image demonstrating a severely degenerated L5-S1 disc with abnormal signal changes in the adjacent vertebral body bone marrow. **B,** T1 weighted sagittal magnetic resonance image demonstrating decreased signal in the adjacent vertebral bone marrow consistent with vascularized, fibrous tissue.

studied patients who had discography before undergoing lumbar discectomy, discectomy and fusion, or fusion alone. They found that preoperative discography demonstrated 82% diagnostic accuracy in identifying the symptomatic level. However, this study represented a heterogenous patient population, including not only patients with back pain, but those suffering from herniated discs and nerve root compression. Colhoun and associates[29] found that, among patients undergoing lumbar fusion, 89% of those with a positive preoperative discogram had significant improvement after surgery, including decreased pain, return to work, and cessation of analgesics.[29] Alternatively, patients with nondiagnostic preoperative discography had a lower rate of success after lumbar fusion, with only 52% of patients reporting a similar satisfactory postoperative outcome.

Varying degrees of success with preoperative discography have been observed. Positive clinical outcomes have been demonstrated in 64% to 86% of patients with positive discography who undergo anterior lumbar interbody fusion (ALIF).[30-32] Other studies have shown that >90% of patients with positive discography improve after posterior lumbar fusion.[33,34] Derby and colleagues[35] argue that better correlation is observed when chemically sensitive discs are identified on preoperative discography. Chemically sensitive discs provoke concordant pain under particularly low pressure injection, suggesting that pain is generated by displacing biochemical agents, which then stimulate sensory nerve endings in the outer annulus. Therefore they hypothesize that patients with chemically sensitive discs require complete discectomy with thorough removal of the offending disc for pain relief. Among patients with chemically sensitive discs, successful clinical outcome was observed in 89% of patients undergoing discectomy and interbody fusion compared to only 20% of patients undergoing dorsolateral fusion alone and 12% of patients treated without surgery. Similarly, Weatherly, Prickett, and O'Brien[36] used discography to identify painful symptomatic discs within a fused segment in patients with persistent low back pain after posterior lumbar fusion. Subsequent ventral discectomy and interbody fusion of the positive discographic levels resulted in complete resolution of pain.

However, the positive predictive value of discography for success after lumbar fusion has not borne out through multiple repeated studies. Of particular concern is that the potential for a high false-positive rate may lead to an inappropriate rise in fusion surgery and consequently an unacceptable rate of unsatisfactory outcomes. Carragee and associates[37] evaluated patients with positive single-level discography using low pressure injection, who then underwent lumbar fusion of the abnormal disc. They observed that only 27% of patients had a highly effective outcome as defined by a visual analog scale (VAS) ≤2, Oswestry Disability Index (ODI) ≤15, full return to work, and cessation of narcotics and analgesics. A minimal acceptable outcome of VAS ≤4, ODI ≤30, no narcotic use, and at least some gainful employment was reached in only 43% of patients. The authors concluded that in the "best case" calculation the adjusted positive predictive value for a minimal acceptable outcome was only 55%. Other studies have also found less promising results with successful outcomes in only 35% to 46% of patients undergoing lumbar fusion with discography as the primary diagnostic tool.[38] However, it should be noted that in one of these studies a particularly low arthrodesis rate was observed (47.9%), which may account for the unexpected poor outcomes.

Overall discography remains an imperfect instrument for diagnosing and localizing discogenic pain. Particularly discography has come into doubt as a reliable measure for predicting which patient and what levels will respond well to fusion surgery. A large degree of this lack of accuracy and consistency may be caused by discography technique and reporting of pertinent positive and negative findings.

Given the best available evidence, discography may be best indicated for correlating concordant pain in discs that are morphologically abnormal since the finding of pain provocation in otherwise normal-appearing discs appears to be clinically irrelevant. Discography may also facilitate assessing before fusion whether levels adjacent to the symptomatic level are also abnormal and may be included in the fusion construct. Last, in certain circumstances, discography may play a role in evaluating patients who have persistent back pain after posterior lumbar fusion to assess for the presence of a symptomatic disc within the fused segments.

In 2005 the Joint Section of the American Association of Neurological Surgeons/Congress of Neurological Surgeons published guidelines for the performance of fusion surgery for lumbar degenerative conditions and made recommendations regarding the diagnostic evaluation of axial low back pain.[39] In their assessment of MRI and discography, they recommended that MRI be performed initially instead of discography in evaluating chronic low back pain. They also recommended that normal-appearing discs on MRI should not undergo fusion. Conversely, surgery should not be offered based on discography alone since patients with positive discography but normal MRI had poor outcomes after fusion surgery.[40] The use of discography to determine which levels to fuse in patients with an abnormal MRI should demonstrate both concordant pain provocation and morphological abnormalities.

Psychosocial Considerations

Before considering surgery for discogenic pain, a thorough evaluation of potential psychosocial factors that may contribute to pain is imperative. Depression and anxiety are common conditions that often exacerbate the nature of these pain complaints and are easily treated. Hysteria, hypochondriasis, depression, and poor coping skills have also been shown to be predictors of suboptimal outcomes after spine surgery.[41] Physical examination may also uncover nonphysiological findings such as superficial tenderness, lumbar pain with axial loading or simulated rotation, and diminished pain when distracting patients during straight–leg raising.[42] The presence of several of these Waddell signs may suggest a pain behavior pattern that is predictive of a poor surgical outcome.

Social factors may also affect the potential for satisfactory outcome from spine surgery, including involvement in disability and workers' compensation claims, long preoperative sick leave, litigation, and reinforcement of pain behavior by family members.[43] Patients who have such negative predictors of satisfactory surgical outcome may be served best by chronic pain programs and rigorous physical and cognitive therapy. Smoking cessation is another behavioral modification strategy that should be pursued, particularly if patients are considered for fusion, since it is associated with poor fusion rates and outcomes.[44]

Discogenic Neck Pain: Surgical Outcomes Evidence

Surgery is generally not considered, except for rare cases, for patients with cervical spondylosis and isolated axial neck pain. The clinical criteria for determining surgical candidates is not clear, and several authors have proposed that surgery be recommended for one- or two-level degenerative discs associated with severe and unrelenting pain after all conservative treatment options have been exhausted. As discussed earlier, the psychological profile of the patient must be considered along with the pertinent radiographic imaging findings in these cases.

To date there are no prospective, randomized studies in the literature assessing surgical vs. nonsurgical management of discogenic neck pain. There is a paucity of clinical data referable to this topic. Much of what has been reported are retrospective case series.

Several studies have reported success with ACDF for discogenic neck pain. Whitecloud and Seago[9] reported 34 patients who underwent ACDF for discogenic neck pain confirmed with cervical discography. Follow-up was at minimum 12 months after surgery and consisted of either telephone conversation or clinical evaluation. More than 90% of the patients were in litigation secondary to either accident or workers' compensation. ACDF was performed at one level in 21 patients, two levels in nine patients, and three levels in four patients. There were eight cases of pseudarthrosis, and only two required further surgery. Of these cases, one patient improved, and the other did not despite evidence of fusion.

Outcomes were assessed using Odom's criteria, and the authors demonstrated a good or excellent result in 70%. Of the six patients who had poor results from surgery, three underwent three levels of fusion. Based on the limited data provided, the authors suggest that better outcomes may be associated with fusing fewer levels.

In a similar study Palit and associates[7] reported on 38 patients who underwent ACDF for axial neck pain with a positive discogram and mean follow-up of 53 months. All patients had failed to improve sufficiently despite aggressive conservative care that included strength training, medication, and a range of injection therapies. All patients continued to have severe pain that caused significant impairment of activities of daily living and disability. Before surgery each patient was evaluated by a psychiatrist experienced in chronic pain management. ACDF was performed at one level in 21 patients, two levels in 16 patients, and three levels in 1 patient. They reported a 79% overall satisfaction with the procedure and significant improvement in pain and function in their patients, as measured by a numerical rating scale for pain and ODI questionnaire. The mean score for neck pain before surgery was 8.3 (range, 3 to 10) and 4.1 (range, 0 to 10) after surgery. The mean score on the ODI questionnaire was 57.5 (range, 0 to 89) before surgery and 38.9 (range, 0 to 80) after surgery.

These two studies are the only studies reporting operative treatment results for patients with axial neck pain who had positive cervical discography. The quality of evidence is limited by the number of patients in each series; the nonrandomized, retrospective nature of the studies; and lack of a nonsurgical comparative group. Nonetheless these studies are often cited as evidence that surgery (i.e., anterior cervical fusion) has a role in the treatment of discogenic neck pain.

Ratliff and Voorhies[8] retrospectively reviewed their series of 20 patients with chronic axial neck pain who underwent surgery. Twelve patients underwent ACDF, and eight patients underwent a number of various posterior fusion surgeries, including foraminotomy with either spinous process wiring or lateral mass plates. Discography was not performed in each case. More than 50% of patients were involved in some form of litigation or workers' compensation case at the time of surgery. General outcomes assessment using the modified Prolo scale indicated that 85% of the patients reported satisfaction with pain relief and surgery, although only three patients returned to work.

Garvey and associates[6] retrospectively reviewed 87 patients who had undergone ACDF for neck pain with a mean follow-up of 4.4 years. Their study was an extensive outcomes analysis using the VAS, North American Spine Society Satisfaction Questionnaire, modified Roland and Morris Disability Index, and modified ODI. Discography was not performed in each case. ACDF was performed at one level in 34 patients, two levels in 32 patients, three levels in 12 patients, and four levels in 9 patients. Eighty-two percent of the patients perceived their outcome to be good, very good, or excellent. Pain improvement was reported by 93% of the patients, with a mean VAS rating 8.4 before surgery and 3.8 after surgery. Functional status improved approximately 50% on both the ODI and the modified Roland–Morris disability index.

Because of the limited data available in the literature, evidence supporting fusion for discogenic neck pain is deficient. Although these series propose that fusion may have a role in the surgical management of discogenic neck pain, the finding that fusions in each of these series were often performed at more than one disc level is disturbing. This clearly underscores the controversy surrounding identifying degenerative discs as pain generators in the cervical spine. Prospective, randomized trials comparing fusion to nonsurgical treatment are needed to provide further insight into this issue.

Discogenic Back Pain: Surgical Outcomes Evidence

The surgical treatment of low back pain caused by degenerative disc disease is controversial. This form of back pain is thought to be caused by alterations in the biomechanical and biochemical environment created by the degenerated disc. Pathological motion or stress transference to pain-generating structures under normal physiological loads can lead to pain. Disruption of the normal architecture of the disc may result in extravasation of biochemical agents that stimulate surrounding nociceptors. Lumbar fusion surgery immobilizes the motion segment and is believed to counteract these pathological processes.

The controversy with fusion surgery stems from a lack of consensus regarding the indications for surgery. Vague indications result in a heterogenous patient population undergoing fusion for back pain. In fact, many of these patients may have various causes of back pain. Therefore it is not surprising that there is wide variability with regard to the management of low back pain.

To further complicate the issue, the correlation of bony fusion, clinical outcome, and pain relief is yet to be established.[45-47] For example, studies of lumbar spondylolisthesis-related instability, which is commonly treated with arthrodesis, have failed to demonstrate a clear correlation between successful fusion and outcome. In a randomized prospective study of patients with lumbar spondylolisthesis and stenosis, dramatically increased fusion rates in patients with pedicle screw fixation did not result in a concomitant improvement in clinical outcomes.[46]

A number of clinical studies have examined outcomes after fusion surgery for low back pain attributed to degenerative disc disease. Conclusions from these studies must be drawn cautiously since the majority of studies are retrospective case series with inconsistent reporting of clinical outcomes using validated outcome measures. To date only four prospective, randomized controlled studies have compared fusion to nonsurgical treatment for back pain.

Further complicating matters, the fusion technique with best overall outcomes is unknown. Several different techniques are used and include ALIF (**Fig. 8-4, A and B**); posterior lateral interbody fusion (PLIF); transforaminal lumbar interbody fusion (TLIF) (**Fig. 8-5, A to E**); lateral interbody (**Fig. 8-6, A to C**), intertransverse posterolateral fusion (PLF), and facet fusion. The advantages and disadvantages of each of these techniques continue to be debated in the surgical literature. Adding more confusion and confounding variables to the discussion is the constantly expanding list of bone graft alternatives, including allograft and synthetic osteobiological agents. The use of segmental instrumentation and interbody

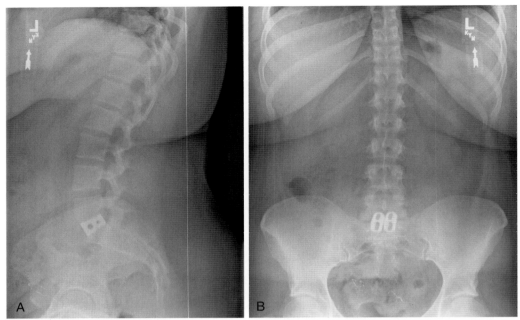

Fig. 8-4 A, Lateral radiograph demonstrating an L5-S1 ALIF with an interbody cage. **B,** Anteroposterior radiograph demonstrating an L5-S1 ALIF with two interbody cages. *ALIF,* Anterior lumbar interbody fusion.

devices also varies. With so many different surgical techniques and tools available to perform fusion surgery, it is easy to see why any consensus regarding fusion for discogenic back pain is lacking.

Anterior Lumbar Interbody Fusion, Posterior Lateral Interbody Fusion, Posterolateral, 360-Degree Fusion

Studies evaluating outcome after ALIF for discogenic back pain demonstrate high rates of clinical improvement. Newman and Grinstead[30] evaluated 36 patients who underwent ALIF with autogenous iliac crest bone graft for degenerated discs diagnosed with MRI and provocative discography. Twenty-eight patients underwent one-level fusion; eight patients had two-level fusions. Overall 86.1% of patients had a successful clinical outcome with a fusion rate of 88.9%. Failure rate observed was 13.9%. Chow and associates[48] similarly reported positive outcomes in 97 patients undergoing ALIF for degenerative disc disease. Complete relief of symptoms occurred in 60%, with an additional 29% having marked improvement in symptoms. Of note, the primary diagnosis of degenerative disc disease and which levels were symptomatic was made using only clinical history and plain radiographs in the majority of patients. Only four patients had preoperative provocation discography to facilitate assessment of the symptomatic discs. Blumenthal and associates[32] found a slightly lower rate of successful outcome after ALIF. They observed that 74% of patients with one-level discogenic disease had a positive outcome as defined by return to work and cessation of narcotic use.

Lee, Vessa, and Lee[34] studied 62 patients undergoing uninstrumented PLIF with autogenous iliac crest bone graft for chronic disabling low back pain. Symptomatic levels for fusion were determined based on provocation discography and corresponding morphological abnormalities on MRI. Overall 59.2% of patients were free of narcotic use at last follow-up. Eighty-one percent of patients had returned to work full time; over 92% of patients were used in at least some partial capacity. Seventy-two percent of patients

reported that they were completely satisfied with their surgical outcomes; 80.5% stated that they would undergo the operation again.

Parker and associates[49] assessed 23 patients who underwent instrumented PLF with iliac crest autograft for discogenic back pain. All patients underwent both MRI and discography before surgery, and the fusion levels were determined by which discs demonstrated concordant pain on provocation discography. Overall only 39% of patients had a good or excellent outcome as defined by a VAS ≤4, no analgesic use, and return to at least 75% of premorbid work status. Poor outcomes were observed in 48% of patients, who had a VAS >6, daily narcotic use, and less than 25% of previous work capacity. They noted that pseudarthrosis (22%) and unemployment for >3 months before surgery were associated with poor outcomes. Overall only 56% of patients reported that they were extremely satisfied with the surgical results.

The clinical results of combined anteroposterior or 360-degree fusion for degenerative disc disease have also been reported. Moore, Pinto, and Butler[50] studied 58 patients who underwent ALIF with instrumented posterolateral fusion for discogenic pain. With a minimum follow-up of 2 years, they observed a 95% arthrodesis rate. Eighty-six percent of patients were improved at last follow-up; 88% had returned to work. Linson and Williams[31] similarly studied patients undergoing anteroposterior fusion and reported that 80% of patients had measurable improvement in low back pain symptoms.

Leufven and Nordwell[51] studied 29 patients undergoing combined instrumented PLIF and PLF for discogenic low back pain of greater than 2 years' duration. Fusion levels were identified by positive discography. Sixty-nine percent of patients reported either no back pain or improvement of back pain symptoms; 31% described complete relief of symptoms, were off all analgesics, and had returned to full activities. Forty-eight percent of patients had a suboptimal outcome consisting of continued moderate or severe pain, some or total activity restriction, and continued daily use of analgesics. Only 62% of patients were used at follow-up, and 76% of patients stated that they would have the surgery again.

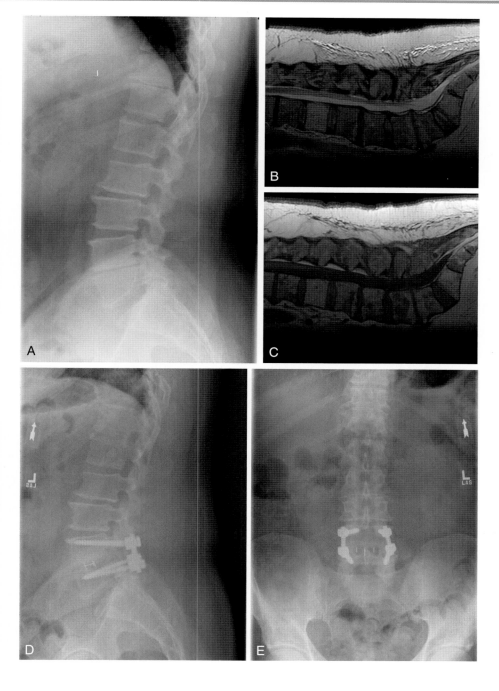

Fig. 8-5 A, Preoperative lateral radiograph demonstrating a degenerated, collapsed L4-L5 disc space. **B,** Preoperative T2 weighted magnetic resonance image of the same patient demonstrating severe L4-L5 disc desiccation with loss of T2 fluid signal within the disc. **C,** Preoperative T1 weighted magnetic resonance image of the same patient demonstrating increased signal in the adjacent L4 and L5 vertebral bone marrow consistent with chronic fat infiltration. **D,** Postoperative lateral radiograph of the same patient after L4-L5 TLIF with dorsal segmental instrumentation. **E,** Postoperative anteroposterior radiograph of the same patient after L4-L5 TLIF with dorsal segmental instrumentation. *TLIF,* Transforaminal lumbar interbody fusion.

Recently studies have also evaluated surgical outcome for the treatment of multilevel (three or more) disease, challenging the presumption that surgical fusion for degenerative disc disease is best limited to one- or two-level fusions. Suratwala and associates[52] assessed 360-degree fusion for three or more levels in patients with lumbar degenerative disc disease. Surgical procedures consisted of either ALIF or TLIF with posterior instrumentation. Diagnostic workup consisted of MRI in all patients, with 60 of 80 patients undergoing discography. Overall the authors reported a 29.5% improvement in ODI and 30.7% improvement in Roland–Morris score at a minimum of 2 years' follow-up.

Lettice and associates[53] compared patients undergoing lumbar fusion for one- or two-level discogenic disease with those with three or more affected levels.[53] Surgical procedures included PLF plus ALIF or PLIF. Symptomatic discs were identified using provocative-pressure controlled discography. They found significant improvement in SF-36 physical component scores in both groups at 1- and 2-year follow-up. The longer segment group had a higher pseudarthrosis and reoperation rate; however, the number of levels treated did not have a significant effect on overall clinical outcome as measured by SF-36.

In 2004 Geisler and colleagues[54] performed a meta-analysis of the literature to compare various fusion techniques for the treatment of discogenic low back pain.[54] They reviewed 25 papers that had a minimum of 2 years follow-up for standardized outcome measures, ODI, and VAS. They found that patients undergoing ALIF had a mean 45.5% improvement in VAS and a mean 27.9-point reduction in ODI. Similarly for 360-degree fusion (PLF plus ALIF, TLIF, or PLIF), patients demonstrated a mean 49.1% improvement in VAS and a mean 20.6 point reduction in ODI.

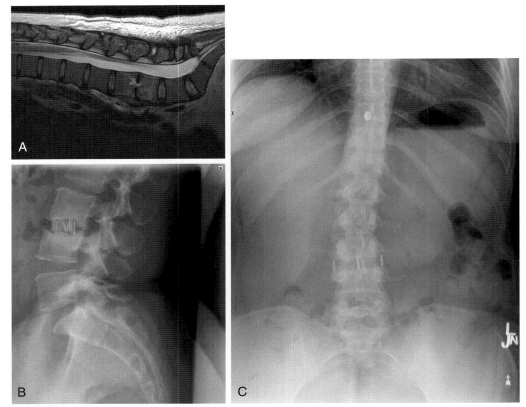

Fig. 8-6 **A,** Preoperative T2 weighted magnetic resonance image demonstrating severe disc degeneration of L3-L4 disc. **B,** Postoperative lateral radiograph of the same patient after L3-L4 lateral interbody fusion with interbody cage placement. **C,** Postoperative anteroposterior radiograph of the same patient demonstrating L3-L4 lateral interbody fusion with interbody cage placement.

In a prospective, randomized controlled trial, Fritzell and associates[55] compared patients undergoing uninstrumented PLF, instrumented PLF, and instrumented 360-degree fusion. At 2-year follow-up there was no significant difference in pain, disability, depressive symptoms, or overall rating among the three surgical groups. Although they did observe that the use of instrumentation resulted in increased fusion rates, no correlation between fusion rate and clinical outcome was demonstrated. More complications, lengthier hospitalization, increased blood loss, and new incidence of postoperative leg pain were identified in the patients undergoing pedicle screw instrumentation.

Prospective, Randomized Studies

The Oxford Center for Evidence-based Medicine classifies studies investigating medical treatment effect based on the soundness of their scientific method and the value of their clinical relevance.[56] On the basis of this classification, the majority of existing studies supporting lumbar fusion for the treatment of discogenic back pain provide only class III or IV evidence (retrospectively collected data; case-control study or case series). To date there are only four prospective, randomized controlled trials comparing lumbar fusion to nonsurgical therapy for the treatment of chronic low back pain (class I evidence).

In 2001 the Swedish Lumbar Spine Study Group published their findings comparing lumbar fusion with nonoperative treatment in patients with chronic low back pain.[57] A total of 294 patients were randomized; 222 patients underwent surgery, and 72 were treated without surgery. Inclusion criteria were patients with chronic disabling low back pain with disc degeneration. Exclusion criteria were leg pain, spondylolisthesis, spinal stenosis, fracture, infection, or tumor. Surgical patients were then randomized to uninstrumented PLF, instrumented PLF, or 360-degree instrumented fusion. Nonsurgical therapy was not standardized; the patient's treating physician decided from a range of interventions, including physical therapy, education, transcutaneous electrical nerve stimulation, epidural steroid injections, cognitive and functional training, and coping strategies.

The surgical group as a whole demonstrated a 33% reduction in back pain and 25% reduction in ODI. Sixty-three percent of surgical patients rated themselves as "much better" after surgery. Return to work was observed in 36% of surgical patients. There was also a 20% reduction in depressive symptoms in the surgical group. The nonsurgical group conversely demonstrated only a 7% reduction in back pain and 6% decrease in ODI. Only 29% of nonsurgical patients rated themselves as "much better" after treatment; only 13% returned to work. Based on these findings, the Swedish Lumbar Spine Study Group concluded that fusion surgery not only decreases chronic low back pain and disability but is superior to nonsurgical therapies.

This study received the 2001 Volvo Award for Clinical Studies, but it also sparked considerable debate. One of the main criticisms is the lack of a standardized nonsurgical treatment strategy in the nonsurgical group. Because the nonsurgical arm consisted of whichever intervention was offered by the individual treating physician, these patients were subjected to any variety of possible therapies that are not well detailed in the report. It is certainly possible that the nonsurgical group, which had already failed conservative treatment for an average duration of 8 years, were potentially randomized to a treatment arm that consisted of essentially the same continued failed therapy. As such it is not surprising that the nonsurgical group demonstrated modest (if at all) improvement in pain and disability compared to any benefit seen in the surgical group. Additional criticism arises from an unclear algorithm for diagnosing the etiology of back pain and determining the symptomatic levels.

In response to these issues, Brox and associates[58] performed a prospective, randomized controlled trial comparing instrumented lumbar fusion vs. a standardized nonsurgical treatment protocol, which had been shown to be more effective than conventional conservative care. A total of 64 patients with >1 year of low back pain and evidence of disc degeneration at L4-5 or L5-S1 were enrolled. Nonsurgical treatment consisted of an intensive 3-week program in which patients stayed at a "back hotel" and participated in physical therapy sessions three times per day, with an average total of 25 hours per week of exercises, cognitive intervention, education, and peer counseling.

Both the surgical and nonsurgical groups demonstrated significant improvements compared to baseline at 1-year follow-up in nearly all outcome measures. The surgical group had an average 15-point reduction in ODI compared to a 12-point decrease in the nonsurgical group. The surgical group had better reduction in leg pain; however, the nonsurgical group had greater improvement in finger tip–to-floor distance and fear-avoidance beliefs. No significant difference in back pain, analgesic requirements, emotional distress, life satisfaction, or return to work was observed between the surgical and nonsurgical groups. Overall both treatment strategies were considered to be effective; 70% of surgical patients and 76% of nonsurgical patients were deemed successful outcomes.

In a subsequent study the same research group performed a prospective, randomized clinical trial comparing lumbar fusion vs. the same nonsurgical treatment protocol in patients with chronic low back pain after previous disc herniation surgery.[59] A total of 60 patients were enrolled. The investigators found that the surgical group had a mean ODI reduction of 9 points compared to a 13-point decrease in the nonsurgical group. These differences were not statistically significant, and the overall success rate of the surgical group was 50% compared to 48% of the nonsurgical group. Again, the authors concluded that at 1-year follow-up lumbar fusion failed to demonstrate any significant benefit over cognitive intervention and exercise in the treatment of chronic low back pain.

The primary criticism of these two studies is that the follow-up duration was only 1 year and that both studies were significantly underpowered. Fairbank and associates[60] investigated lumbar fusion vs. an intensive rehabilitation program.[60] Three hundred forty-nine patients were randomly assigned; 176 patients underwent surgical treatment, and 173 underwent rehabilitation. The surgical procedures varied and depended on surgeon and institutional practices. The nonsurgical treatment was a standardized protocol that involved 5 days per week for 3 weeks of outpatient therapy. A total of 75 hours of intervention were performed consisting of cognitive behavioral therapy and exercises directed toward strengthening, flexibility, endurance, and aerobic conditioning. The surgical group demonstrated an average reduction in ODI of 12.5 points compared to an 8.7-point decrease in the nonsurgical group. This difference was marginal although statistically significant.

The authors concluded that the modest advantage of fusion surgery did not provide clear evidence that surgery is more

beneficial than intensive rehabilitation for the treatment of chronic low back pain. Alternatively they suggest that their study provides evidence that intensive rehabilitation with cognitive behavioral principles is a viable treatment option and alternative to fusion surgery. Critics of this study point out that 28% of nonsurgical patients crossed over to the surgical arm (i.e., patients with the worst outcomes with nonsurgical therapy ultimately had surgery). An intent-to-treat analysis was performed that was inherently biased against surgery since patients who were failing nonsurgical therapy may have gained benefit after crossing over, although this was not reflected in the final outcomes assessment.

In 2008 Mirza and Deyo[61] performed a Cochrane summary of these prospective, randomized controlled studies. They concluded that surgical treatment demonstrated improvement with an 8.9- to 15.6-point decrease in ODI, which corresponded to a 19% to 37% change from baseline. The nonsurgical group, which ranged from a nonstandardized variety of treatments to standardized protocols for intensive cognitive therapy and exercise, showed an improvement in ODI of 2.8 to 13.3 points and a 5.8 to 30.1% improvement from baseline. Their conclusion was that surgery provided a fairly modest increase in improvement compared to nonsurgical treatment for discogenic back pain. However, none of the observed differences in average back-specific disability outcome were sufficiently large enough to meet U.S. Food and Drug Administration criteria, as defined by a ≥15-point improvement in ODI, for a clinically meaningful difference between treatments.

Based on these four randomized trials, there is modest evidence that fusion for chronic discogenic back pain results in functional improvement at 1 and 2 years compared to nonsurgical treatment. Overall the data suggest that lumbar fusion surgery may be more efficacious compared to unstructured, heterogeneous nonoperative care. On the other hand, they also suggest that fusion may not be more effective than a structured rehabilitation program that includes cognitive and behavior therapy. As alluded to earlier, definitive guidelines supporting fusion over nonoperative care cannot be made because of methodological limitations of these randomized trials. Given the challenges with executing prospective, randomized surgical trials, these studies represent the best evidence currently available.

Conclusion

The surgical management of discogenic pain is challenging and controversial. The existing literature (class I, II, and III evidence) provides little support for fusion as a treatment for discogenic pain. With regard to discogenic neck pain, there are no class I data to support fusion. However, there are class I data suggesting that fusion may result in better outcomes than nonsurgical treatment for discogenic lumbar pain. Although there are better data supporting fusion for discogenic lumbar pain, the evidence is not overwhelming. Fusion may have a role in select patients; however, the limitations of the studies from which these conclusions are drawn must be considered since both surgical and nonsurgical interventions have demonstrated improvements in pain relief and back disability index measurements.

References

1. Cote P, Cassidy JD, Carroll L: The Saskatchewan Health and Back Pain Survey: the prevalence of neck pain and related disability in Saskatchewan adults. *Spine* 23:1689-1698, 1998.
2. Biyani A, Andersson GB: Low back pain: pathophysiology and management. *J Am Acad Orthop Surg* 12:106-115, 2004.

3. Manchikanti L et al: Comprehensive review of epidemiology, scope, and impact of spinal pain. *Pain Physician* 12:E35-E70, 2009.

4. Katz JN: Lumbar disc disorders and low-back pain: socioeconomic factors and consequences. *J Bone Joint Surg [Am]* 88(suppl 2):21-24, 2006.

5. Deyo RA et al: United States trends in lumbar fusion surgery for degenerative conditions. *Spine* 30:1441-1445; discussion 1446-1447, 2005.

6. Garvey TA et al: Outcome of anterior cervical discectomy and fusion as perceived by patients treated for dominant axial-mechanical cervical spine pain. *Spine* 27:1887-1895; discussion 1895, 2002.

7. Palit M et al: Anterior discectomy and fusion for the management of neck pain. *Spine* 24:2224-2228, 1999.

8. Ratliff J, Voorhies RM: Outcome study of surgical treatment for axial neck pain. *South Med J* 94:595-602, 2001.

9. Whitecloud TS, III, Seago RA: Cervical discogenic syndrome: results of operative intervention in patients with positive discography. *Spine* 12:313-316, 1987.

10. Miller JA, Schmatz C, Schultz AB: Lumbar disc degeneration: correlation with age, sex, and spine level in 600 autopsy specimens. *Spine* 13:173-178, 1988.

11. Crock HV: A reappraisal of intervertebral disc lesions. *Med J Aust* 1:983-989, 1970.

12. Crock HV: Internal disc disruption: a challenge to disc prolapse fifty years on. *Spine (Phila Pa 1976)* 11:650-653, 1986.

13. Haughton VM et al: Measuring the axial rotation of lumbar vertebrae in vivo with MR imaging. *AJNR Am J Neuroradiol* 23:1110-1116, 2002.

14. Blankenbaker DG et al: Axial rotation of the lumbar spinal motion segments correlated with concordant pain on discography: a preliminary study. *AJR Am J Roentgenol* 186:795-799, 2006.

15. Boden SD et al: Abnormal magnetic-resonance scans of the cervical spine in asymptomatic subjects: a prospective investigation. *J Bone Joint Surg Am* 72:1178-1184, 1990.

16. Matsumoto M et al: MRI of cervical intervertebral discs in asymptomatic subjects. *J Bone Joint Surg [Br]* 80:19-24, 1998.

17. Carragee EJ, Alamin TF: Discography. a review. *Spine J* 1:364-372, 2001.

18. Schellhas KP et al: Cervical discogenic pain: prospective correlation of magnetic resonance imaging and discography in asymptomatic subjects and pain sufferers. *Spine* 21:300-311; discussion 311-312, 1996.

19. Cloward RB: Cervical discography; technique, indications and use in diagnosis of ruptured cervical discs. *Am J Roentgenol Radium Ther Nucl Med* 79:563-574, 1958.

20. Shinomiya K et al: Evaluation of cervical discography in pain origin and provocation. *J Spinal Disord* 6:422-426, 1993.

21. Block AR et al: Discographic pain report: influence of psychological factors. *Spine* 21:334-338, 1996.

22. Holt EP, Jr: Fallacy of cervical discography. report of 50 cases in normal subjects. *JAMA* 188:799-801, 1964.

23. Klafta LA, Jr, Collis JS, Jr: The diagnostic inaccuracy of the pain response in cervical discography. *Cleve Clin Q* 36:35-39, 1969.

24. Klafta LA, Jr, Collis JS, Jr: An analysis of cervical discography with surgical verification. *J Neurosurg* 30:38-41, 1969.

25. Meyer RR: Cervical discography. a help or hindrance in evaluating neck, shoulder, arm pain? *Am J Roentgenol Radium Ther Nucl Med* 90:1208-1215, 1963.

26. Roth DA: Cervical analgesic discography. A new test for the definitive diagnosis of the painful-disc syndrome. *JAMA* 235:1713-1714, 1976.

27. Simmons EH, Segil CM: An evaluation of discography in the localization of symptomatic levels in discogenic disease of the spine. *Clin Orthop Relat Res* 57-69, 1975.

28. Grubb SA, Kelly CK: Cervical discography: clinical implications from 12 years of experience. *Spine* 25:1382-1389, 2000.

29. Colhoun E et al: Provocation discography as a guide to planning operations on the spine. *J Bone Joint Surg [Br]* 70:267-271, 1988.

30. Newman MH, Grinstead GL: Anterior lumbar interbody fusion for internal disc disruption. *Spine* 17:831-833, 1992.

31. Linson MA, Williams H: Anterior and combined anteroposterior fusion for lumbar disc pain: a preliminary study. *Spine* 16:143-145, 1991.

32. Blumenthal SL et al: The role of anterior lumbar fusion for internal disc disruption. *Spine* 13:566-569, 1988.

33. Schechter NA, France MP, Lee CK: Painful internal disc derangements of the lumbosacral spine: discographic diagnosis and treatment by posterior lumbar interbody fusion. *Orthopedics* 14:447-451, 1991.

34. Lee CK, Vessa P, Lee JK: Chronic disabling low back pain syndrome caused by internal disc derangements. The results of disc excision and posterior lumbar interbody fusion. *Spine* 20:356-361, 1995.

35. Derby R et al: The ability of pressure-controlled discography to predict surgical and nonsurgical outcomes. *Spine* 24:364-371; discussion 371-372, 1999.

36. Weatherley CR, Prickett CF, O'Brien JP: Discogenic pain persisting despite solid posterior fusion. *J Bone Joint Surg [Br]* 68:142-143, 1986.

37. Carragee EJ, Lincoln T, Parmar VS, Alamin T: A gold standard evaluation of the "discogenic pain" diagnosis as determined by provocative discography. *Spine* 31:2115-2123, 2006.

38. Wetzel FT et al: The treatment of lumbar spinal pain syndromes diagnosed by discography: lumbar arthrodesis. *Spine* 19:792-800, 1994.

39. Resnick DK et al: Guidelines for the performance of fusion procedures for degenerative disease of the lumbar spine. Part 6. Magnetic resonance imaging and discography for patient selection for lumbar fusion. *J Neurosurg Spine* 2:662-669, 2005.

40. Gill K, Blumenthal SL: Functional results after anterior lumbar fusion at L5-S1 in patients with normal and abnormal MRI scans. *Spine* 17:940-942, 1992.

41. Epker J, Block AR: Presurgical psychological screening in back pain patients: a review. *Clin J Pain* 17:200-205, 2001.

42. Waddell G et al: Nonorganic physical signs in low-back pain. *Spine* 5:117-125, 1980.

43. Mannion AF, Elfering A: Predictors of surgical outcome and their assessment. *Eur Spine J* 15(suppl 1):S93-S108, 2006.

44. Andersen T et al: Smoking as a predictor of negative outcome in lumbar spinal fusion. *Spine* 26:2623-2628, 2001.

45. Resnick DK et al: Guidelines for the performance of fusion procedures for degenerative disease of the lumbar spine. Part 12. Pedicle screw fixation as an adjunct to posterolateral fusion for low-back pain. *J Neurosurg Spine* 2:700-706, 2005.

46. Fischgrund JS et al: Volvo Award winner in clinical studies: degenerative lumbar spondylolisthesis with spinal stenosis: a prospective, randomized study comparing decompressive laminectomy and arthrodesis with and without spinal instrumentation. *Spine* 22:2807-2812, 1997.

47. Bjarke Christensen F et al: Long-term functional outcome of pedicle screw instrumentation as a support for posterolateral spinal fusion: randomized clinical study with a 5-year follow-up. *Spine* 27:1269-1277, 2002.

48. Chow S et al: Anterior spinal fusion or deranged lumbar intervertebral disc. *Spine* 5:452-458, 1980.

49. Parker LM et al: The outcome of posterolateral fusion in highly selected patients with discogenic low back pain. *Spine* 21:1909-1916; discussion 1916-1917, 1996.

50. Moore KR, Pinto MR, Butler LM: Degenerative disc disease treated with combined anterior and posterior arthrodesis and posterior instrumentation. *Spine* 27:1680-1686, 2002.

51. Leufven C, Nordwall A: Management of chronic disabling low back pain with 360 degrees fusion: results from pain provocation test and concurrent posterior lumbar interbody fusion, posterolateral fusion, and pedicle screw instrumentation in patients with chronic disabling low back pain. *Spine* 24:2042-2045, 1999.

52. Suratwala SJ et al: Functional and radiological outcomes of 360 degrees fusion of three or more motion levels in the lumbar spine for degenerative disc disease. *Spine* 34:E351-E358, 2009.

53. Lettice JJ et al: Does the number of levels affect lumbar fusion outcome? *Spine* 30:675-681, 2005.

54. Geisler FH et al: Neurological complications of lumbar artificial disc replacement and comparison of clinical results with those related to

lumbar arthrodesis in the literature: results of a multicenter, prospective, randomized investigational device exemption study of Charite intervertebral disc. Invited submission from the Joint Section Meeting on Disorders of the Spine and Peripheral Nerves, March 2004. *J Neurosurg Spine* 1:143-154, 2004.

55. Fritzell P et al: Chronic low back pain and fusion: a comparison of three surgical techniques: a prospective multicenter randomized study from the Swedish lumbar spine study group. *Spine* 27:1131-1141, 2002.

56. Oxford Centre for Evidence-based Medicine Levels of Evidence and Grades of Recommendation, 2009.

57. Fritzell P et al: 2001 Volvo Award Winner in Clinical Studies: Lumbar fusion vs. nonsurgical treatment for chronic low back pain: a multicenter randomized controlled trial from the Swedish Lumbar Spine Study Group. *Spine* 26:2521-2532; discussion 2532-2534, 2001.

58. Brox JI et al: Randomized clinical trial of lumbar instrumented fusion and cognitive intervention and exercises in patients with chronic low back pain and disc degeneration. *Spine* 28:1913-1921, 2003.

59. Brox JI et al: Lumbar instrumented fusion compared with cognitive intervention and exercises in patients with chronic back pain after previous surgery for disc herniation: a prospective randomized controlled study. *Pain* 122:145-155, 2006.

60. Fairbank J et al: Randomised controlled trial to compare surgical stabilisation of the lumbar spine with an intensive rehabilitation programme for patients with chronic low back pain: the MRC spine stabilisation trial. *Br Med J* 330:1233, 2005.

61. Mirza SK, Deyo RA: Systematic review of randomized trials comparing lumbar fusion surgery to nonoperative care for treatment of chronic back pain. *Spine* 32:816-882, 2007.

9 Nucleus Pulposus Replacement and Motion-Sparing Technologies

Alberto Di Martino, Andrea Luca, Angela Lanotte, and Vincenzo Denaro

CHAPTER OVERVIEW

Chapter Synopsis: Because discogenic pain can arise or worsen with movement of diseased or degenerated disc segments, it makes sense that minimizing movement might alleviate pain. This chapter examines several "motion-sparing" techniques that may relieve discogenic pain and prevent degeneration from affecting neighboring segments. Spine arthroplasty—in which the joint is rebuilt—and nucleus pulposus replacement are two such techniques. Although minimally invasive, the prosthesis implanted for pulposus replacement still requires rigorous attention to issues that may arise with long-term use. The aim of the prosthesis is to mimic the intervertebral disc as closely as possible—biomechanically and biochemically—to support proper spacing of the spine and thereby retain motion. Both nucleus pulposus replacement and arthroplasty are indicated for specific types of discogenic pain, which are outlined here. The chapter also provides details about the various total disc and nucleus pulposus replacement devices currently available. Implants are specialized for lumbar or cervical replacement. As with any surgical treatment, each procedure comes with its own risks and possible complications.

Important Points:
- Nucleus pulposus and disc replacement implants are currently used in clinical practice to address the issue of discogenic pain.
- The goals of these new technologies are to slow progression or prevent adjacent disc level degeneration, restore normal pressure loads at the diseased level, and improve overall spinal biomechanics.
- Nucleus pulposus replacement is minimally invasive; the aim of this approach is to avoid intervertebral motion.
- Rigorous evaluation of the new devices still needs to be completed, and the issues of long-term implant and procedure-related complications must still be addressed.
- Strict adherence to appropriate patient selection criteria and knowledge of contraindications and limitations of these procedures are ideal to improve clinical results and meet patients' expectations.

Clinical Pearls:
- Long-term stability, endurance, and strength of the prostheses are unknown for the majority of implants.
- Proper selection of the patients remains the mainstay for this kind of surgery in order to achieve good clinical results.
- When performing cervical arthroplasty surgery, patients with cervical disc herniations and radiculopathy seem to have better clinical outcomes compared to those with myelopathy.
- The protective role of disc implants on adjacent segment disc degeneration still remains to be proved.

Clinical Pitfalls:
- A wide spectrum of complications related to the use of nucleus pulposus replacement and cervical spine arthroplasty devices have been described in the literature.
- Patients with preoperative kyphotic sagittal alignment tend to worsen their symptoms with motion-sparing implants, and may benefit from fusion surgery instead.
- Since this technology is becoming easier to use and more appealing, frequency of the complications related to implants performed by less experienced surgeons may increase.
- The role of facet joints in determining the stability of the spinal segment and potential stability of disc implants cannot be overemphasized.

Introduction

In recent years there has been a big push toward improving and using motion-sparing technologies that aim to minimize soft tissue dissection and preserve the spinal segment motion. Cervical and lumbar spine arthroplasty and nucleus pulposus (NP) replacement currently represent valid alternatives to standard surgical procedures for the treatment of discogenic pain.

Motion preservation technologies have gained attention as an alternative to spinal fusion primarily for two reasons: possible prevention of adjacent level disc degeneration and preservation of segmental motion at the affected level.

However, the long-term stability, endurance, and strength of the prostheses are unknown for the majority of implants. Researchers currently are trying to understand at what point in the life span of the spinal arthroplasty implant problems will develop. When these problems occur it is not certain what strategies for revision are most likely to resolve the problems for non-fusion technologies.

In this chapter we focus on the current clinical evidence for NP replacement devices and cervical and lumbar arthroplasty implants and provide an analysis of current indications and complications.

Anatomy

The intervertebral disc consists of three components: an inner gelatinous NP, an outer annulus fibrosus (AF), and vertebral endplates (EPs) located superiorly and inferiorly. The AF is a circular layer consisting of concentric lamellae that are resistant to tensile strength; its tensile strength resistance is caused by an abundance of type I collagen. In these lamellae, collagen fibers run obliquely between the lamellae of the annulus in alternating directions. The NP consists of proteoglycan and water gel held together loosely by an irregular network of fine type II collagen and elastin fibers. The major proteoglycan of the NP is aggrecan,[1] which provides the osmotic properties needed to resist compression. The intervertebral disc is avascular, and consequently it is nourished through the vessels in the subchondral bone adjacent to the hyaline cartilage of the EP by passive diffusion.[2] Cells of the nucleus and inner annulus are supplied by the blood vessels of the vertebral body and the distinct capillary network that penetrates the subchondral plate. The nutrients then diffuse from these capillaries across the cartilaginous EPs and through the dense NP to the target cells.[3]

NP and AF cells maintain the normal metabolism of the discs by controlling production of cytokines, enzymes, and growth factors. NP cells produce proteoglycan and collagen. A monomer of proteoglycan consists of a protein core linked to extended polysaccharide chains such as keratan sulphate and chondroitin sulphate. Each monomer is bound to hyaluronic acid by a link protein. Aggrecan represents about 70% of the NP and 25% of the AF. It has high osmotic pressure arising from the water retained within the NP and tends to inflate the collagen framework.[4] This balance is responsible for the ability of the disc to retain fluid within the matrix, resulting in high viscoelasticity. The high concentration of aggrecan and its associated fluid enable the tissue to support compressive loads without collapsing; through this mechanism, loads are transferred equally to the AF and vertebral body during the flexion and extension of the spine.[5]

The equilibrium of water content also depends on the loads applied to the intervertebral disc; when loads are applied to the disc, the water of the NP is directed to the adjacent EPs; the converse occurs after unloading. This pumping mechanism enhances delivery of the nutrients to the nucleus.[6]

Disc degeneration in humans can occur as early as the third decade of life.[7] However, disc degeneration does not always cause pain. In one study, degeneration appeared in at least one intervertebral disc in 35% of subjects between 20 and 39 years of age, and in all of the study subjects 60 to 80 years of age.[8] Aging, obesity, smoking, vibration from transportation, excessive axial loads, and other factors may accelerate degeneration of intervertebral discs.[9,10] The degree of disc degeneration appears to be correlated with the patient's age. Although many studies have been carried out to show such a relationship, no distinct cause has been established.[11,12] Although all of a person's discs are the same age, discs in the lower lumbar segments are more vulnerable to degenerative changes than those in upper lumbar segments, suggesting a prevalent role of mechanical loading over aging.[13]

Cervical disc degeneration, typically associated with the development of calcified disc herniation, is a slower process than that which occurs in the lumbar spine, where frank disc herniation or disc degeneration occurs. Damage to the AF that occurs in progressive disc degeneration or after surgical discectomy causes a gradual loss in disc height, leading to changes in the biomechanical characteristics of the remaining disc.[14] Such mechanical changes may ultimately place additional stress on the facet joints and lead to circumferential spinal segment degenerative changes.[15-17]

Several other factors have been reported to cause disc degeneration. Growth factors such as transforming growth factor, insulin-like growth factor, and basic fibroblast growth factor stimulate the NP or AF cells to produce more extracellular matrix and inhibit the production of matrix metalloproteinases.[18] Since an increase in the level of the basic fibroblast growth factor and transforming growth factor promotes the repair of the degraded matrix,[19-21] it is likely that a decrease in the concentration of these growth factors is associated with degeneration of the intervertebral disc. Decreased anabolism or increased catabolism of senescent cells also may promote degeneration.[22]

Basic Science

Artificial intervertebral disc characteristics should resemble those of native discs biomechanically to preserve both segmental motion and global stability. The vertebral column consists of 24 separate vertebrae and the sacrum, connected by a complex system of facet joints, intervertebral discs, ligaments, and muscles. Simple replacement of one section of the vertebral column may adversely affect the entire system. It is estimated that the spine undergoes approximately 100 million flexion cycles in a lifetime,[23] not taking into account the slight motions that occur with breathing, estimated to be about 6 million a year.[24] Thirty million cycles appear to be the optimal life span of an implant, and 10 million cycles are considered the minimum.[25]

As opposed to peripheral joints, the stability of which is essentially achieved by ligamentous structures, the disc provides a major part of its own stability. For instance, the alternating collagen fibers in the annulus create a very efficient system for controlling and restricting rotation.

Design goals for successful disc replacement prostheses include approximation of size and motion of a physiological disc to avoid distraction or overloading of the facet joints. Physiological motion is complex and unlikely to be replicated by a simple hinge joint with a fixed center of rotation. The intervertebral disc joint controls the majority of range of motion (ROM) in compression, flexion, and lateral bending; whereas the facet joints dictate axial rotation and extension. During spinal flexion almost all of the resistance comes from the anterior column. In the lumbar spine, normal discs allow 8 to 13 degrees of ROM at each level.[26] The total ROM for lateral bending (right to left) at each level is also significant; approximately 10 degrees for upper lumbar discs and approximately half of that for lower lumbar discs. This lateral bending is resisted primarily by the disc. Because of the resistance from the facet joints, the ROM for extension and axial rotation are comparatively less than the ROM for other movements.

Because of the requirement for stability and mobility, lumbar spinal movement is complex. Translation and rotation are possible in three orthogonal planes.[27] The disc is the main constraint to motion, but it also allows a certain amount of movement.[28] In upper lumbar motion segments, lateral bending is the predominant motion. In the lower lumbar spine and lumbosacral motion segment, flexion and extension are the prevalent motions.[29] In addition, 2 to 4 mm of anterior translation in the sagittal plane is normal for the lumbar spine vertebrae.[27] Finally, the center of rotation for each lumbar motion segment changes with flexion, lateral bending, and rotation.[30] In addition, the movements of axial rotation and lateral bending are coupled in the lumbar spine.[31] Physiological lordosis allows the facet joints in the lumbar spine to bear axial loads (up to 16% in some studies).[32]

The cervical spine is the most mobile segment of the spine. Total cervical spinal movement ranges between 130 and 145 degrees of flexion and extension, 90 degrees of lateral flexion, and 160 to 180 degrees of axial rotation bilaterally. Sagittal flexion-extension motion is mainly sustained by the C0-C2 segment, whereas the other cervical spinal segments are only responsible for a few degrees of segmental ROM (around 10 to 20 degrees per level).[33,34] In addition, the segmental and global cervical spinal ROM decreases with increasing age; in fact, significant loss of movement in all planes is found in healthy asymptomatic individuals between 50 and 54 years of age compared with those between 35 and 39 years of age.[35] ROM is also inversely affected by increase in body weight and decrease in the level of physical activity.[36] Moreover, a healthy cervical spine moves more than one afflicted with degenerative disc disease or radicular compression.[37,38] Consequently, immobilization of a single spinal segment seems to have little effect on the global ROM of the cervical spine, especially in patients in whom the spine was stiff before surgery. Further studies are required to better understand cervical spine kinetics and to attempt to reproduce physiological ROM with cervical spine arthroplasty (CSA).[39,40]

When considering replacement of the NP, implants are intended to replace the extruded or surgically removed intervertebral disc or the degenerated disc before definitive collapse. The principal biomechanical function of the NP prosthesis is to maintain or restore the physiological height of the intervertebral disc space, the mobility and load-bearing function of the spine, and the normal mechanical behavior of the AF. It has been demonstrated that removal of the NP is associated with an increase in spinal mobility ranging between 38% and 100%.[41] Moreover, removal of the nucleus leads to outward bulging of the outer region of the annulus and bulging of its inner region toward the center of the disc with axial loading.[42] These factors cause circumferential tears in the AF and may further decrease annular ability to resist shearing forces. Nuclear replacement procedures are intended to restore the biomechanical function of the annulus by placing annular fibers under tension. To achieve this result, the nucleus replacement device must maintain and recreate the functional characteristics of the NP. Furthermore, the same device should be able to bear a considerable load before it fails; implant components should have a stiffness similar to that of a native disc to avoid stress shielding, atrophy, and bone resorption that may lead to subsidence and extrusion of an implant.[43] It is of utmost importance that the modulus of the

component material is comparable to the vertebral EPs because modular mismatches can lead to EP subsidence, especially if the stresses applied to the implant are greater than the strength of the bone. Conversely, if the stresses are lower, the changes in stress distribution may result in the remodeling of the vertebral body.[44]

Indications/Contraindications

The indication for NP replacement is lumbar discogenic back pain unresponsive to active conservative treatment for a minimum of 6 months.[43] Klara and Ray[45] described the indications for the prosthetic disc nucleus (PDN) device as back pain, with or without leg pain, related to degenerative disc disease that is refractory to nonoperative treatment. Patients with a disc space height of less than 5 mm were excluded because of the difficulty of implanting the device in such a narrowed disc space. It appears that such implants could be helpful in managing the pain from very early stages of symptomatic disc disruption or as an adjunct to discectomy to maintain disc space height and motion at the surgical level. Additional selection criteria include: posterior disc height of more than 5 mm (because of the implantation device height currently available); a symptomatic pathology restricted to one level between L2 and S1; an age range between 18 and 65 years; and, finally, the absence of any associated severe vertebral pathology. Some exclusion criteria are: previous spinal surgery; spinal problems at more than one level; globular disc; central disc herniation; pronounced Schmorl's nodules at the involved level; EP lesions; significant spinal, foraminal, or lateral recess stenosis; symptomatic degenerated facet joints; degenerative spondylolisthesis greater than grade I; lytic spondylolisthesis; severe osteoporosis; bone tumors or congenital bony abnormalities; active infection; and the presence of malignant tumors.[46]

CSA is currently indicated in the treatment of radiculopathy and myelopathy at one or two levels and, although unproven, is used by some of the authors in the treatment of three or more symptomatic disc levels or levels adjacent to an arthrodesis. Arthroplasty use in the management of axial pain presumed secondary to disc degeneration is unknown but would not be expected to be better than fusion. More data are required to specifically expand the clinical indications. Contraindications are instability, significant facet arthrosis, osteomyelitis, and infections. Patients with spondylosis and preexisting ankylosis may not retain motion and may benefit significantly from joint arthroplasty. In the current prospective studies, lumbar arthroplasty is performed to manage chronic severe disabling discogenic low back pain isolated to one or two levels that has been unsuccessfully treated without surgery for a minimum of 6 months. In addition, the spine should be stable and free from significant facet arthrosis. Patients should be able to tolerate an anterior approach. Contraindications include significant psychosocial symptoms, obesity greater than two standard deviations above the bodies mass index, osteoporosis, and infection. Nuclear replacement has a more limited role. It is thought to be indicated early in the degenerative cascade before significant loss of height and EP changes.[47]

Current contraindications that can be considered common to both the cervical or lumbar spine surgeries include: arthritis of facet joints, preoperative instability, systemic diseases (osteoporosis and inflammatory diseases), previous posterior surgery, advanced age, and ossification of the posterior longitudinal ligament. Currently there is a debate regarding the role of CSA in the presence of myelopathy. Many of the authors still use these devices in patients with either myelopathy or radiculopathy, but in some cases clinical outcomes in patients with myelopathy are not as good as in radiculopathy patients. Nonetheless, randomized clinical studies are required to address this issue.[33]

Patients who are good candidates for lumbar arthroplasty are young, active patients with chronic lower back pain and discogenic pain reproduced by provocative discography. Definitely, before considering disc replacement the patient should have failed to improve after an appropriate course of nonoperative care, including active rehabilitation, activity modification, medication, and spinal injections. The patient should have pain related to disc disruption or degeneration. Mainly at the lumbar spine, computed tomography (CT) and provocative or analgesic discography are helpful in determining if the disc is the pain generator and which level(s) should be replaced. There are several possible uses for artificial discs that are still under investigation such as treatment of a disc level adjacent to a previously fused segment or painful disc levels in patients with scoliosis. Facet joint abnormality is considered a contraindication to disc replacement; and, since the pain originating from the facets is not treated, there may be increased risk for the development of joint hypertrophy, resulting in painful facet disease.

Bertagnoli and Kumar[48] defined criteria based on disc height, condition of the facet joints, the number of levels treated surgically, degeneration of other spinal segments, and the condition of the posterior elements. They defined a prime candidate for the procedure to be a patient with a disc height of more than 4 mm, no facet joint changes, single-level disc problem, no adjacent segment degeneration, and intact posterior elements; as many as 98% of these patients reported a certain degree of satisfaction after surgery.

Historical Review and Equipment

The aim of disc replacement is to implant a device that is safe and durable and that functions similarly to a normal disc (i.e., maintains a proper intervertebral spacing, allows for motion, and provides stability). In addition, the prosthesis must be designed so it can be implanted safely and removed if necessary in case of revision surgery.

As suggested by Cummings, Robertson, and Gill,[49] the stability and success of a prosthesis depends on its design, the technique used by the surgeon, immediate postoperative stable interface, and, ideally, subsequent biological end growth of bone to ensure long-term stability. The device should have significant strength and durability, be biomechanically and biochemically compatible, and not be associated with subsidence or migration into adjacent bone.

Therefore biomechanical and tribological characteristics of the implants play a leading role in the success of the procedure and should be well known and carefully selected.

According to Szpalski and associates,[50] two fundamental principles can be differentiated in the success of a discal replacement device: the reproduction of the viscoelastic properties of the disc and the imitation of its motion characteristics. The devices targeting the first principle are usually made from various silicones or polymers (injected as polymers or in monomer form and polymerized in situ) coupled with a mechanical system (springs or piston).

The implants built to mimic the motion characteristics of the discs are usually mechanical devices (metal and sometimes polyethylene couples) based on the basic principles of peripheral joint prostheses. In between are some other devices that combine both principles.

Because of the plethora of disc replacement designs available, several nomenclature systems have been proposed over time based on the materials, design, type of fixation, and kinematics. Currently, there are two basic types of disc designs: *NP replacements* and *total disc replacements*.

Lumbar Implants

Nucleus Pulposus Replacement The first preliminary experiences with partial lumbar disc replacement consisted of the injection of polymethyl methacrylate (PMMA) or silicone into the NP space.[51,52] In 1966 Fernstrom[53] reported his experience with a stainless steel spherical endoprosthesis. These pioneering procedures did not achieve acceptable clinical results; in particular, in most of the cases, the device developed by Fernstrom showed evident radiological subsidence, which was probably related to the poor clinical outcome. Although the results of these early experiences were poor, they provided a solid basis for further improvement of a nuclear replacement.

The development of new technologies and materials with a better understanding of the biomechanical properties of the disc brought a significant push in this field. Pursuing an "ideal" device capable of reproducing the biological properties of the disc, the use of synthetic viscous materials called *hydrogels* was extensively studied. One of the most important characteristics of these materials is the ability to absorb and release water, depending on the applied load, mimicking the hydrophilic properties of the native NP tissue.[54,55] Many hydrogel-based nucleus replacement devices have been developed; they can be classified into two main groups. The first includes so-called *contained devices* and devices with predefined geometry; the second are uncontained or injectable devices.

One of the most extensively studied nucleus replacement devices is the PDN (Raymedica, Inc., Bloomington, Minn).[56] It is a hydrogel pellet contained in a polyethylene jacket. The hydrogel component can absorb as much as 80% of its weight in water because of the hydroactive action of its main constituents (polyacrylamide and polyacrylonitrile). Water absorption allows for restoration and maintenance of the original disc height. The outer polyethylene jacket prevents unlimited swelling, minimizes the horizontal spreading, and reduces the risk of consequent fractures of the contiguous vertebral EPs.[57]

The NeuDisc (Replication Medical, Inc., New Brunswick, NJ) is a hydrogel device similar to the PDN device; it expands preferentially in the axial direction using the same mechanism. In contrast to the PDN, the NeuDisc is not surrounded by an outer polyethylene jacket but by structured layers located inside the device.[58] The NeuDisc can be placed in situ using minimally invasive techniques.

The DASCOR (Disc Dynamics Inc., Eden Prairie, Minn) is another contained device filled with an injectable cool polyurethane polymer; in this case a balloon avoids unlimited spreading of the polymer.[58]

The Newcleus (Zimmer Spine, Warsaw, Ind), previously used in other fields (cardiovascular surgery), is an unconstrained elastic memory-coiling spiral made of polycarbonate urethane that functions mainly as a spacer. The Newcleus can be placed in situ using minimally invasive techniques.

The Aquarelle (Stryker Corp., Kalamazoo, Mich), a polyvinyl alcohol hydrogel nucleus replacement, has also been tested extensively. The device is implanted in a hydrated state and provides uniform pressure across the EP. In contrast to the PDN device, the lifting force is much less, reducing the risk of EP fracture.

An alternative to the aforementioned devices are other substances injected as void fillers. The SINUX ANR (J&J DePuy, Raynham, Mass) is a liquid polymethylsiloxane polymer that completely cures into a viscoelastic mass within a few minutes after injection.[58] The BioDisc (Cryolife, Inc., Kennesaw, Ga) is an injectable device consisting of a mixture of serum albumin and glutaraldehyde. The NuCore IDN (Spine Wave Inc., Shelton, Conn) is a tissue-engineered device; it avoids the risk of transmitting or causing diseases. The Gelifex (Gelifex, Inc., Philadelphia, Pa) is a polymer that is liquid at room temperature and hardens once implanted.

Lumbar Disc Replacement   The Link SB Charité III, now in its third generation, has emerged as the most commonly implanted lumbar total disc replacement. It was designed in former East Germany in the early 1980s by Schellnac and Büttner-Jans and was first implanted by Zippel in 1984.[59] Because the first generation had an unacceptably high rate of implant migration and metal fatigue fractures, it was improved over time. The Link SB Charité III (Waldermar Link, Hamburg, Germany), the third generation design, has been used since 1987, with more than 5000 implanted worldwide to date. It consists of two metal (cobalt-chrome) EPs with a sliding polyethylene core between them. There is a metal wire around the circumference of the core to aid in imaging. The device is anchored to the adjacent vertebral bodies by ventral and dorsal teeth on the surfaces of the EPs.

It is a nonconstrained device that attempts to mimic normal disc biomechanics by permitting translation and rotation.

In the same time frame Steffee developed a lumbar one-piece implant, the Acroflex, consisting of two titanium plates with a rubber core attached between them. This device, implanted in only six patients, is no longer used because of concerns about a possible carcinogenic agent in the rubber.

Another disc device used in Europe since 1990 is the ProDisc (Spine Solutions, New York, NY). It is a semi-constrained device and consists of three pieces: two metal EPs and a polyethylene core that is fixed to the inferior EP once the device is implanted.

Other implants have been designed and are in various stages of testing. The Maverick disc (Medtronic Sofamor Danek, Minneapolis, Minn) is a metal-on-metal design with anchoring keels similar to the ProDisc (**Fig. 9-1**). The Flexcore is another disc that uses a unique biomechanical design involving seven preassembled pieces that include a conical internal specialized spring.

Cervical Implants

Although still in the early stages of development, cervical disc replacement seems to have a more promising future in the treatment of cervical disc disease than current fusion techniques.

According to the artificial cervical disc nomenclature of the Cervical Spine Study Group, the implants currently are classified into three types: nonarticular, uniarticular, or biarticular. With reference to the material, the implants may be classified as metal-on-metal, metal-on-polymer (ultrahigh molecular-weight polyethylene), ceramic-on-polymer, and ceramic-on-ceramic. They may also be classified according to whether they are modular (having replaceable components) or not. In some cases a supplemental vertebral body screw fixation is required, whereas other devices are press fitted. The implants may be further classified into the following categories: constrained, semi-constrained, or unconstrained.[60]

In spite of the number of different disc replacement designs, only a few have reached the level of clinical implantation. In 1964 Reitz and Joubert[61] reported the placement of spherical endoprostheses (Fernstrom type) in the cervical spines of patients with intractable headaches and cervicobrachialgia. In 1985 Alemo-Hammad[62] described the insertion of methyl methacrylate after anterior cervical discectomy in five patients. During the 1990s other studies investigated the use of PMMA in cervical disc replacement. In a small 1998 study with good clinical results Cummings, Robertson, and Gill[49] reported on the use of the Bristol cervical disc, a two-piece stainless steel disc device that is screwed to the anterior portion of the adjacent vertebral bodies.

Although several other devices have been implanted, clinical results in large numbers of patients with long-term follow-up have been reported for only three implants: the Bryan Cervical Disc (Medtronic Sofamor Danek, Memphis, Tenn), the Prestige (Medtronic Sofamor Danek), and the Prodisc-C (Synthes-Spine, Paoli, Pa). The Bryan Cervical Disc consists of two titanium alloy shells that contain a polyurethane nucleus; the shells are fixed to the bone by a porous titanium layer, and the device is enclosed by a flexible polyurethane membrane forming a closed articular space. It allows for ROM in all planes. The Prestige cervical disc (Medtronic Sofamor Danek) is a stainless steel, metal-on-metal semiconstrained–bearing surface. The EPs are grit blasted to promote osteointegration. The Prodisc-C prosthesis (Synthes-Spine, Paoli, Pa) is a metal polyethylene ball-in-socket design with two metal fins; the material used is an interface ultrahigh–molecular weight polyethylene inlay; the superior and inferior plates are made of cobalt-chrome alloy, with the titanium surface facing the bony side. Another

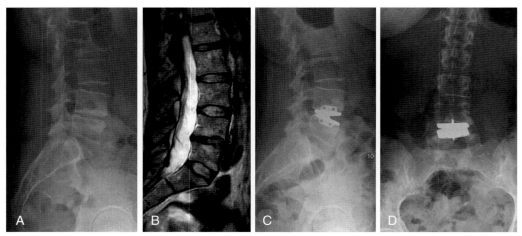

Fig. 9-1   T.G., age 53 years, before surgery complaining of lumbar discogenic pain at L4-L5, as shown by radiographs **(A)** and MRI **(B)**. **(C, D)** Six-week postoperative radiographs showing implant of Maverick lumbar disc replacement device (Medtronic Sofamor Danek, Minneapolis, Minn). *MRI*, Magnetic resonance imaging.

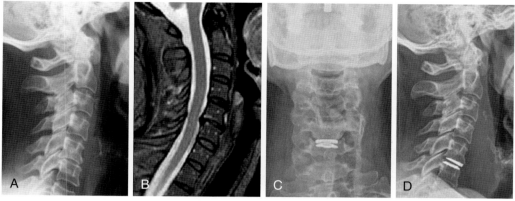

Fig. 9-2 W.S., age 52 years, before surgery complaining of neck axial pain without radiculopathy at C5-C6 level. Symptoms were confirmed by preoperative radiographs **(A)** and MRI **(B)**. **(C,D)** Six-week postoperative radiographs showing implant of Discover cervical disc replacement device (DePuy Spine, Raynham, Mass). *MRI*, Magnetic resonance imaging.

similar implant, the Discover artificial cervical disc (DePuy Spine, Raynham, Mass), has been available in the European Union since 2007. It consists of a ball-and-socket design constructed from titanium and polyethylene (**Fig. 9-2**). Preliminary data show its safety and its ability to positively impact pain, ROM, disc height, and adjacent level disease.

Surgical Technique

The surgical approach for cervical disc replacement is not particularly difficult. The patient is placed in a supine position with the head slightly extended. A mild reverse Trendelenburg position allows for better drainage. Fluoroscopic guidance is recommended to confirm the targeted disc level. Usually a transverse incision provides good exposure to the surgical field.

A standard Smith-Robinson approach via fascial dissection exposes the appropriate surgical area. Once it has been identified and confirmed, the disc is removed, and all osteophytes resected. The decompression itself has to be meticulous and should include all of the osteophytes arising from the uncinate processes and posterior longitudinal ligament, particularly in the case of a symptomatic neurological compression. Care must also be taken to maintain the midline orientation that is essential for correct positioning of the device.

The vertebral EPs are prepared by removing the cartilage until the surface of subchondral bone is exposed. This may be performed using a high-speed bur or curette. Once the targeted interspace preparation is complete and all of the bony irregularities have been filed, the appropriate size of prosthesis should be defined by the trial device. Positioning of the prosthesis should be monitored constantly with fluoroscopy to ensure that the device is implanted properly. Abnormal positioning of the device could severely compromise its functionality.

Most of the currently available lumbar disc prostheses are placed by an anterior approach, the same one generally used for anterior lumbar interbody fusion. Surgical details may vary from implant to implant and are frequently based on surgeon's preferences. Frequently a small midline laparotomy allows for adequate exposure of the lumbar spine by an anterior retroperitoneal approach. The transperitoneal approach may be considered for obese patients or in revision cases. The L5-S1 level is the easiest segment to approach. Fluoroscopic guidance helps to confirm the appropriate surgical level. Once it has been identified and

confirmed, a standard anterior discectomy is carefully performed. Care should be taken to preserve the integrity of the EPs. PLL needs to be preserved, if possible.

A slight distraction of the disc space is required. Sizing the implant is usually performed before placing the definitive prosthesis. Fluoroscopy is strongly suggested to evaluate the central position of the implant. Gradual release of the distraction and new radiographs complete the procedure.

Minimally invasive approaches to lumbar disc arthroplasty have also been developed. Disc nucleus replacement is usually performed through a minimally invasive approach; a small incision is generally required (4 to 5 mm).

In situ curing polymers are introduced into the nucleotomized cavity in a liquid state and harden after their implantation. The polymers should have a fast polymerization time to avoid leakage and because most monomers are toxic if absorbed in high doses.

Risks and Avoidance of Complications

Some of the complications reported for cervical disc replacement are related to the surgical approach.[63] They include prevertebral hematoma, dural tear during decompression, epidural hematoma, neurological deficit, and deterioration secondary to disc arthroplasty as result of inadequate root decompression at the neural foramen. Neurological symptoms after cervical disc replacement may include radicular pain, limb weakness, and reduction in sensation.[64] Esophageal injury, usually caused by improper placement of self-retainer retractor blades, is quite uncommon but may result in retropharyngeal abscess or mediastinitis. Some authors recommend a left-sided approach to the cervical spine to reduce the risk of recurrent laryngeal nerve injury. After surgery, Horner's syndrome has been described as a potential complication of the anterior approach as a result of iatrogenic injury of the sympathetic nerve and stellate ganglion.

Other complications can be caused by the implant itself; prevertebral ossification with ankylosis has been widely reported in the literature.[65] Age, sex (male more commonly than female), preoperative spondylosis and segmental ankylosis, and incorrect implantation technique have been described as risk factors. Experience with hip arthroplasty suggests a decrease in this risk with the administration of nonsteroidal antiinflammatory drugs for 2 to 3 weeks after surgery.[66]

Postoperative kyphosis has been reported as a complication after cervical disc replacement. Reduction in physiological lordosis, cervical kyphosis (segmental or total), and inadequate preparation of the EPs have also been suggested as risk factors.[64,67,68]

Adjacent vertebral fracture and subsidence can also occur, especially in osteoporotic patients. To minimize this risk, careful attention to EP preparation and design of the prostheses is required. In fact, this complication is invariably related to the footprint of the device, which should be as large as possible to better share the axial load, and the integrity of the EPs.[63,64,69] In addition, failure of the device has been reported as a possible complication of cervical disc replacement. It includes loss of segmental mobility and loosening or migration of the implant.[63,70]

In the lumbar spine, complications resulting from the surgical approach may be challenging to treat. Care should be taken to avoid violation of the peritoneum, bowel (quite rare), and urethral injuries (usually caused by inappropriate exposure). Major blood vessel injuries are rare during the procedure (2% to 4%) but potentially catastrophic; self-retaining retractors should constantly be under direct control. In addition, before mobilizing the iliac vessels or the aorta, proximal and distal control should be obtained. The left iliolumbar vein can be avulsed if not ligated before mobilizing the left common iliac vein.

Another potential risk of this procedure is the retrograde ejaculation that occurs for iatrogenic injuries of the hypogastric plexus. The use of monopolar electrocautery overlying the L5-S1 interspace has been associated with an increased incidence of retrograde ejaculation and should be avoided.

Neurological complications are quite rare. Epidural hematoma, nerve root syndromes with radiculopathies, and dural tears or compression of the thecal sac represent possible postoperative conditions requiring revision surgery.

Patients who have had previous posterior surgery should be apprised of the risk of postoperative radicular pain. Nerve root traction by postoperative fibrosis may limit the surgeon's ability to restore disc height and may require posterior surgery for root decompression if the pain is persistent.

In lumbar disc replacement surgery the incidence of spontaneous ankylosis after total disc replacement can be as high as 60% at 17 years.[71] Postoperative bracing or inactivity have been suggested as risk factors. Lemaire and associates[72] reported a rate of 2% of adjacent-level disease requiring surgical treatment.

Implant failure and subsequent migration, poor osteointegration, subsidence, and debris formation are all potential complications that may occur.

Extrusion of the injected material represents one of the most common complications of NP replacement.[43] Several different device shapes, materials, and scaffolds have been developed over time to minimize these complications. Patient weight, disc size, and postoperative rehabilitation protocol are important parameters for evaluation in the perioperative setting to reduce the risk of extrusion.[45,73]

Despite the strenuous research aimed at developing new materials capable of perfectly mimicking the biomechanical properties of the annulus, all of these devices pose a risk of intravertebral migration.

Clinical Outcomes
Nucleus Pulposus Replacement   NP replacement devices have been widely used in clinical practice; the first clinical studies in the 1990s reported encouraging clinical results. Since these reports, many further changes have been adopted to improve these results (i.e., the device has been modified in its shape, dimension,

and biomechanical properties to achieve an "ideal" device that imitates the normal disc). Surprisingly an increase in device migration was reported with the use of the new implants. To overcome the migration problem, the shape of the device was changed to a trapezoid with anterior and posterior wedges. These secondary modifications somewhat improved the clinical success rate. Several authors[45,74,75] reported a significant reduction in the rate of complications. In 2003 Ray and Schonmayr[74] presented their results with NP replacement devices in 300 patients showing impressive improvements after surgery, with a dramatic drop in the Oswestry Disability Index score from 50 to less than 10. Despite the positive clinical results, a high rate of displacement still represents the biggest limitation of this procedure.

Total Disc Replacement   The first prospective, multicenter clinical trial of the Bryan Cervical Disc replacement for single-level degenerative disease was published in 2002[76]; it showed significant movement preservation 1 year after surgery in 21 patients (87.5%). The complications reported were related to the surgical technique and migration of the device. Similar results have been published in subsequent studies with a longer follow-up and using bilevel implants; the movement was preserved in 79 of the 90 patients with a single-level implant and in 42 of the 49 with bilevel implants, providing good clinical results.[63] In another study on 14 subjects, the Bryan Cervical Disc preserved the ROM at the replaced levels 2 years after implantation.[77]

Recently the Bryan Cervical Disc has been implanted in patients with myelopathy, despite reports[78] suggesting better clinical results in patients with radiculopathy. Patients with myelopathy are less likely to regain normal function than those with radiculopathy.

Several other studies compared clinical outcomes of anterior cervical discectomy with fusion to outcomes of total cervical disc replacement. In a study of 115 patients with single-level cervical disc disease randomized to Bryan Cervical Disc implantation or anterior cervical discectomy and fusion with allograft and plate, it was found that the cervical disc replacement group compared favorably to discectomy with fusion during long-term follow-up.[79]

A multicenter study reported clinical results in 463 patients randomized to receive Bryan Cervical Disc replacement (242 patients) or anterior discectomy and fusion with allograft and plating (221 patients),[80] 424 of whom were available at a 2-year follow-up. Overall success, defined as a 5-point improvement in Neck Disability Index score and absence of serious adverse reaction related to the implant or surgical procedure, was achieved in 200 patients who received disc replacement and 161 of those who underwent fusion. Complications occurred in 75 patients in the disc replacement group and 61 in the discectomy and fusion study group. In most cases complications resulted from the general medical condition of the patient. The frequency of secondary procedures at the surgical level was not different between the groups.

Multi-center comparison studies are also available for other devices. One, involving 541 patients with single-level degenerative disc disease, compared the use of the Prestige ST cervical disc replacement (276 patients) to anterior discectomy and fusion (265 patients).[81] After 2 years the arthroplasty group showed better clinical and neurological outcomes, a lower rate of revisions, and lower frequency of adjacent disc degenerative disease. A recent study comparing the results of the Prodisc-C with those of anterior discectomy and fusion showed no complications related to the use of the implant, no adjacent disc degeneration, and positive clinical results at 3 years follow-up in both study groups.[82] No significant differences in the clinical outcomes were detected when the device was used at one or more levels.[83]

In 2003 de Kleuver, Oner, and Jacobs[84] conducted a systematic review of the literature on total disc replacement in the lumbar spine. They found that in short-term follow-up, clinical outcomes of disc replacement appeared to be comparable to those of arthrodesis. However, considering the lack of persuasive studies, they concluded that, despite the long-term clinical use, there were insufficient data to adequately evaluate functional performance of total disc replacement.

In 2006 another systematic review was published. According to Freeman and Davenport,[85] the Charité lumbar disc replacement system proved its effectiveness in treatment of mechanical lower back pain associated with single-level degenerative disc disease. The same device maintained optimal flexion and extension ROM at least 24 months after surgery. It seems that both pain control and ROM depend on correct placement of the device.

Studies analyzed could prove neither the effectiveness of total disc replacement in preventing adjacent level disc degeneration nor its role when used at the adjacent disc level with previous arthrodesis. Moreover, those studies do not clearly define the role of therapeutic multilevel disc replacement.

Conclusions

In conclusion, several NP and disc replacement systems are currently used in clinical practice for the treatment of discogenic pain. NP replacement procedures have gained wide interest because of their minimally invasive nature and their promise to minimize and control intervertebral motion. Cervical and lumbar disc arthroplasties are currently studied prospectively. Careful long-term trials are needed to fully define the role of these technologies in the management of lumbar degenerative disc disease.

The goals of these new technologies are to slow adjacent disc degeneration, restore normal loads to the diseased area, and improve global spinal biomechanics. Rigorous clinical evaluations of these new devices must still be completed. Knowledge of contraindications and limitations and strict adherence to indications for these procedures are essential to improve clinical results and meet patients' expectations.

References

1. Borgesen SE, Vang PS: Herniation of the lumbar intervertebral disk in children and adolescents. *Acta Orthop Scand* 45:540-549, 1974.
2. Key JA: Intervertebral-disc lesions in children and adolescents. *J Bone Joint Surg [Am]* 32:97-102, 1950.
3. Roberts S et al: Transport properties of the human cartilage endplate in relation to its composition and calcification. *Spine* 21:415-420, 1996.
4. Lowrey JJ: Dislocated lumbar vertebral epiphysis in adolescent children: report of three cases. *J Neurosurg* 38:232-234, 1973.
5. Parisini P et al: Lumbar disc excision in children and adolescents. *Spine* 26:1997-2000, 2001.
6. Bao QB et al: The artificial disc: theory, design and materials. *Biomaterials* 17:1157-1167, 1996.
7. Denaro V editor: *Stenosis of the cervical spine*, Berlin, 1982, Springer Verlag.
8. Boden SD et al: Abnormal magnetic-resonance scans of the lumbar spine in asymptomatic subjects: a prospective investigation. *J Bone Joint Surg [Am]* 72:403-408, 1990.
9. Zhang YG et al: Features of intervertebral disc degeneration in rat's aging process. *J Zhejiang Univ Sci B* 10:522-527, 2009.
10. Zhang Y et al: Advances in susceptibility genetics of intervertebral degenerative disc disease. *Int J Biol Sci* 4:283-290, 2008.
11. Buckwalter JA: Aging and degeneration of the human intervertebral disc. *Spine* 20:1307-1314, 1995.
12. Nachemson A et al: In vitro diffusion of dye through the end-plates and the annulus fibrosus of human lumbar intervertebral discs. *Acta Orthop Scand* 41:589-607, 1970.
13. Miller JA, Schmatz C, Schultz AB: Lumbar disc degeneration: correlation with age, sex, and spine level in 600 autopsy specimen. *Spine* 13:173-178, 1988.
14. Fornasier VL et al: Intervertebral disc degeneration—an autopsy study. *Eur J Orthop Surg Traumatol* 10:159-165, 2000.
15. Brinckmann P, Grootenboer H: Change of disc height, radial disc bulge, and intradiscal pressure from discectomy: an in vitro investigation on human lumbar discs. *Spine* 16:641-646, 1991.
16. Frei H et al: The effect of nucleotomy on lumbar spine mechanics in compression and shear loading. *Spine* 26:2080-2089, 2001.
17. Natarajan RN et al: Effect of annular incision type on the change in biomechanical properties in a herniated lumbar intervertebral disc. *J Biomech Eng* 124:229-236, 2002.
18. Seki S et al: A functional SNP in CILP, encoding cartilage intermediate layer protein, is associated with susceptibility to lumbar disc disease. *Nat Genet* 37:607-612, 2005.
19. Risbud MV et al: Towards an optimum system for intervertebral disc organ culture: TGF-b3 enhances nucleus pulposus and annulus fibrosus survival and function through modulation of TGFb-R expression and ERK signaling. *Spine* 31(8):884-890, 2006.
20. Peng B et al: Possible pathogenesis of painful intervertebral disc degeneration. *Spine* 31:560-566, 2006.
21. Doita M et al: Immunohistologic study of the ruptured intervertebral disc of the lumbar spine. *Spine* 21:235-241, 1996.
22. Roberts S et al: Senescence in human intervertebral discs. *Eur Spine J* 15(suppl 3):S312-316, 2006.
23. White AA, Panjabi MM: The basic kinematics of the human spine. *Spine* 3:12-20, 1978.
24. Kostuik JP: Intervertebral disc replacement. In Bridgwell KH, De Wald RL, editors: *The textbook of spinal surgery*, Philadelphia, 1997, Lippincott-Raven, pp 2257-2266.
25. Kostuik JP et al: Design of an intervertebral disc prosthesis. *Spine* 16:S256-S260, 1991.
26. Adams MA, Hutton WC: Mechanics of the intervertebral disc. In Golsh P, editor: The biology of the intervertebral disc, vol 2, Boca Raton, Fla, 1988, CRC Press, pp 39-72.
27. Simon SR: Kinesiology. In Simon SR, editor: *Orthopaedic basic science*, Rosemont, Ill, 1994, American Academy of Orthopaedic Surgeons, pp 519-622.
28. Benzel E, editor: *Biomechanics of spine stabilization*, Rolling Meadows, Ill, 2001, American Association of Neurological Surgeons.
29. Pope MH, Frymoyer JW, Lehmann TR: Structure and function of the lumbar spine. In Pope MH et al, editors: *Occupational low back pain: assessment, treatment, and prevention*, St Louis, 1991, Mosby, pp 95-113.
30. Rolander SD: Motion of the lumbar spine with special reference to the stabilizing effect of posterior fusion: an experimental study on autopsy specimens. *Acta Orthop Scand* (suppl 90):1-144, 1966.
31. Pope MH et al: Experimental measurements of vertebral motion under load. *Orthop Clin North Am* 8:155-167, 1977.
32. Adams MA, Hutton WC: The mechanical function of the lumbar apophyseal joints. *Spine* 8:327-330, 1983.
33. Denaro V: Cervical spinal disc replacement. *J Bone Joint Surg [Br]* 91-B(6):713-719, 2009.
34. Panjabi MM et al: Mechanical properties of the human cervical spine as shown by three-dimensional load–displacement curves. *Spine* 26:2692-2700, 2001.
35. Alaranta H et al: Flexibility of the spine: normative values of goniometric and tape measurements. *Scand J Rehabil Med* 26:147-154, 1994.
36. Castro WH et al: Noninvasive three-dimensional analysis of cervical spine motion in normal subjects in relation to age and sex: an experimental examination. *Spine* 25:443-449, 2000.
37. Dvorak J et al: In vivo flexion/extension of the normal cervical spine. *J Orthop Res* 9:828-834, 1991.
38. Dvorak J et al: Clinical validation of functional flexion/extension radiographs of the cervical spine. *Spine* 18:120-127, 1993.

39. Chang UK et al: Changes in adjacent level disc pressure and facet joint force after cervical arthroplasty compared with cervical discectomy and fusion. *J Neurosurg Spine* 7:33-39, 2007.

40. Liu F, Stinton S, Komistek RD: Mathematical model of detrimental effects of cervical spine fusion. *J Bone Joint Surg [Br]* 90-B(suppl 1):185, 2008.

41. Eysel P et al: Biomechanical behaviour of a prosthetic lumbar nucleus. *Acta Neurochir (Wien)* 141:1083-1087, 1999.

42. Meakin JR, Hukins DW: Effect of removing the nucleus pulposus on the deformation of the annulus fibrosus during compression of the intervertebral disc. *J Biomech* 33:575-580, 2000.

43. Di Martino A et al: Nucleus pulposus replacement: basic science and indications for clinical use. *Spine* 30:16(suppl):S16-S22, 2005.

44. Meakin JR: Replacing the nucleus pulposus of the intervertebral disk: prediction of suitable properties of a replacement material using finite element analysis. *J Mater Sci Mater Med* 12:207-213, 2001.

45. Klara PM, Ray CD: Artificial nucleus replacement: clinical experience. *Spine* 27:1374-1377, 2002.

46. Korge A, et al: A spiral implant as nucleus prosthesis in the lumbar spine. *Eur Spine J* 11(suppl 2):S149-S153, 2002.

47. Anderson PA, Rouleau JP: Intervertebral disc arthroplasty. *Spine* 2779-2786, 2004.

48. Bertagnoli R, Kumar S: Indications for full prosthetic disc arthroplasty: a correlation of clinical outcome against a variety of indications. *Eur Spine J* 11(suppl 2):S131-S136, 2002.

49. Cummings BH, Robertson JT, Gill SS: Surgical experience with an implanted artificial cervical joint. *J Neurosurg* 88:943-948, 1998.

50. Szpalski M et al: Spine arthroplasty: a historical review. *Eur Spine J* 11(suppl. 2):S65-S84, 2002.

51. Hamby WB, Glaser HT: Replacement of spinal intervertebral discs with locally polymenting methyl methacrylate. *J Neurosurg* 16:311-313, 1959.

52. Nachemson AL: Some mechanical properties of the lumbar intervertebral disc. *Bull Hosp Joint Dis* 23:130-132, 1962.

53. Fernstrom U: Arthroplasty with intercorporal endoprosthesis in herniated disc and in painful disc. *Acta Chir Scand* 357(suppl):154-159, 1966.

54. Ambrosio L, DeSantis R, Nicolais L: Composite hydrogels for implants. *Proc Inst Mech Engl* 212(2):93-99, 1998.

55. Iatridis JC et al: Is the nucleus pulposus a solid or a fluid? Mechanical behaviours of the nucleus pulposus of the human intervertebral disc. *Spine* 21(10):1174-1184, 1996.

56. Ray CD: Lumbar interbody threaded prostheses: flexible, for an artificial disc and rigid, for a fusion. In: Brock M, Mayer HM, Weigel K, editors: *The artificial disc*, Berlin, 1991, Springer-Verlag, pp 53-67.

57. Ray CD: The PDN prosthetic disc-nucleus device. *Eur Spine J* 11(suppl 2):137-142, 2002. Epub 2002.

58. Viscogliosi AG, Viscogliosi JJ, Viscogliosi MR: *Beyond total disc: the future of spine surgery, Spine Industry Analysis Series*, New York, 2004, Viscogliosi Bros, LLC, pp 131-198.

59. Buttner-Janz K: *The development of the artificial disc: SB Charité.* Dallas, 1992, Hundley & Associates.

60. Mummaneni PV, Haid RW: The future in the care of the cervical spine: interbody fusion and arthroplasty. *J Neurosurg Spine* 2:155-159, 2004.

61. Reitz H, Joubert MJ: Intractable headache and cervico-brachialgia treated by complete replacement of cervical intervertebral discs with a metal prosthesis. *S Afr Med J* 38:881-884, 1964.

62. Alemo-Hammad S: Use of acrylic in anterior cervical discectomy: technical note. *Neurosurgery* 17:94-96, 1985.

63. Goffin J et al: Intermediate follow-up after treatment of degenerative disc disease with the Bryan cervical disc prosthesis: single level and bi-level. *Spine* 28:2673-2678, 2003.

64. Denaro V et al: Degenerative disk disease. In Denaro L, D'Avella D, Denaro V, editors: *Pitfalls in cervical spine surgery (avoidance and management of complications)*, Berlin Heidelberg, 2010, Springer-Verlag, pp 121-163.

65. Leung C et al: Clinical significance of heterotopic ossification in cervical disc replacement: a prospective multicenter clinical trial. *Neurosurgery* 57:759-763, 2005.

66. Tortolani PJ et al: Computed tomography (CT) scan assessment of paravertebral bone after total disc replacement: temporal relationships and the effect of NSAID, 2003 (abstract), Cervical Spine Research Society Congress, Scottsdale, AZ.

67. Sekhon LH: Cervical arthroplasty in the management of spondylotic myelopathy: 18-month results. *Neurosurg Focus* 17:8, 2004.

68. Kim SW et al: Effects of a cervical disc prosthesis on maintaining sagittal alignment of the functional spinal unit and overall sagittal balance of the cervical spine. *Eur Spine J* 17:20-29, 2008.

69. Fong SY et al: Design limitations of Bryan disc arthroplasty. *Spine J* 6:233-241, 2006.

70. Sasso RC et al: Motion analysis of Bryan cervical disc arthroplasty versus anterior discectomy and fusion: results from a prospective, randomized, multicenter, clinical trial. *J Spinal Disord Tech* 21:393-399, 2008.

71. Putzier M et al: Charité total disc replacement: clinical and radiographical results after an average follow-up of 17 years. *Eur Spine J* 15:183-195, 2006.

72. Lemaire JP et al: Clinical and radiological outcomes with the Charité artificial disc: a 10-year minimum follow-up. *J Spinal Disord* 18:353-359, 2005.

73. Carl A, Ledet E, Yuan H, et al: New developments in nucleus pulposus replacement technology. *Spine J* 4(suppl 6):325-329, 2004,

74. Ray CD, Schonmayr R: *Two-year follow-up on PDN device disc replacements patients*, 1998 (abstract), North American Society Spine Society. San Francisco, California.

75. Schönmayr R et al: Prosthetic disc nucleus implants: the Wiesbaden feasibility study: 2-year follow-up in ten patients. *Riv Neuroradiol* 12(suppl 1):163-170, 1999.

76. Goffin J et al: Preliminary clinical experience with the Bryan cervical disc prosthesis. *Neurosurgery* 51:840-845, 2002.

77. Pickett GE et al: Effects of a cervical disc prosthesis on segmental and cervical spine alignment. *Neurosurg Focus* 17:E5, 2004.

78. Lafuente J et al: The Bryan cervical disc prosthesis as an alternative to arthrodesis in the treatment of cervical spondylosis: 46 consecutive cases. *J Bone Joint Surg [Br]* 87-B:508-512, 2005.

79. Sasso RC et al: Artificial disc versus fusion: a prospective, randomized study with 2-year follow-up on 99 patients. *Spine* 32:2933-2940, 2007.

80. Heller JG et al: Comparison of Bryan cervical disc arthroplasty with anterior cervical decompression and fusion. *Spine* 34:101-107, 2009.

81. Mummaneni PV et al: Clinical and radiographic analysis of cervical disc arthroplasty compared with allograft fusion: a randomized controlled clinical trial. *J Neurosurg Spine* 6:198-209, 2007.

82. Delamarter RB et al: Cervical disc replacement: over 3-year prospective randomized clinical outcomes and range of motion follow-up with the Prodisc-C prosthesis, Cervical Spine Research Society, 2006 (abstract), Palm Beach, FL.

83. Bae HW et al: 1 versus 2 versus 3-level cervical artificial disc replacements: a prospective report of clinical outcomes with the Prodisc-C device, Proceedings of the Cervical Spine Research Society, 2006 (abstract), Palm Beach, FL.

84. de Kleuver M, Oner FC, Jacobs WCH: Total disc replacement for chronic low back pain: background and a systematic review of the literature. *Eur Spine J* 12:108-116, 2003.

85. Freeman BJ, Davenport J. Total disc replacement in the lumbar spine: a systematic review of the literature. *Eur Spine J* Aug;15(suppl 3):S439-S447, 2006.

10 Cervical and Thoracic Discogenic Pain: Therapeutic Nonsurgical Options

James L. North

CHAPTER OVERVIEW

Chapter Synopsis: Although the predominant therapies for discogenic pain involve surgery, nonsurgical alternatives are increasingly becoming available. This chapter surveys these techniques with a focus on cervical and thoracic discogenic pain. The most conventional of these options is injection of steroids into the disc; outcomes evidence is mixed. Annuloplasty and nucleoplasty use radiofrequency technique to modify disc tissue. Some other less conventional techniques have been used only in lumbar spine. For example, biochemical ablation can be achieved by injecting the enzyme papain, which digests the proteoglycan molecule. Ozone injection is thought to relieve inflammation by improving microcirculation in the disc, and injection of methylene blue has been shown to relieve lumbar discogenic pain by destroying sensory nerve endings. Development and improvement of nonsurgical interventions for discogenic pain is likely to continue in the coming years.

Important Points:
- Cervical and thoracic discogenic pain is far less studied than lumbar disease.
- Interventional treatment for cervical and thoracic disc disease is largely anecdotal.

Clinical Pearls:
- Cervical discography is approached from the anterior right side.
- Thoracic discography involves advancing the needle into the center of the disc on a course that bisects the two articulations of the head of the rib.

Clinical Pitfall:
- Myelopathic symptoms such as bowel and bladder changes, lower extremity weakness, altered balance, and hyperreflexia point toward significant central disc herniation.

Cervical and Thoracic Discogenic Pain

Neck pain is a near ubiquitous complaint. Fortunately most neck pain is self-limited. Neck pain that limits activities is not uncommon, with 12-month prevalence estimates ranging from 2% to 11%.[1] However, when neck pain becomes chronic, diagnosis of the pain generator may prove difficult. The source is more obvious when accompanied by radicular symptoms. The source of axial neck pain is often limited to myofascial, facetogenic, discogenic, and often a combination of all three.[2] Posterior thorax pain is a much rarer entity than cervical and lumbar pain. A common cause of thoracic back pain is reflex muscle spasm radiating from an original lumbar pain source. Thoracic discs, facets, and myofascia are all possible sources of upper to midback pain. Of discogenic pain complaints 36% are of cervical origin, compared to only 4% in the thoracic regional. Obviously the remaining 62% involve the lumbar region.[3,4]

Clinical Presentation

Discogenic neck and upper back pain usually manifests in axial pain that may progress to involve radiculopathy. The disc may herniate, resulting in compression of the adjacent nerve root or cord segment. It may manifest an annular fissure (**Fig. 10-1**), resulting in chemical irritation of the adjacent nerve root or cord segment. The disc itself may prove painful, with neoinnervation of the annulus. History elements that suggest discogenic pain in the neck include pain with flexion, prolonged sitting, and protruded head positions. Physical examination findings that suggest cervical discogenic pain include decreased range of motion (ROM) and referred pain patterns (**Fig. 10-2**).[5] If radiculopathy is present, compression tests such as the Spurling and shoulder abduction tests have a high specificity but low sensitivity.[6] Sensory, motor, and reflex tests are helpful in cervical radiculopathy diagnosis. Myelopathic symptoms such as bowel/bladder changes, lower-extremity weakness, altered balance, and hyperreflexia point toward significant central disc herniation.

History elements that suggest thoracic discogenic pain are similar: flexion, prolonged sitting/standing, and Valsalva maneuvers. Physical examination findings that suggest thoracic discogenic pain manifestation include decreased ROM and referred pain patterns. Thoracic radiculopathy may manifest in altered sensory

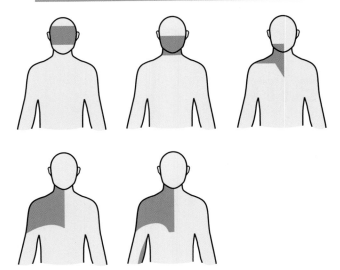

Fig. 10-1 Posterior view. Pain caused in varying distributions secondary to provocative cervical discography. Adapted from Grubb SA et al: Cervical discography: clinical implications from 12 years of experience, *Spine* 25:1382-1389, 2000.

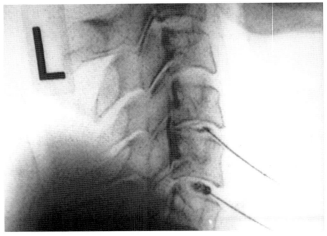

Fig. 10-2 Cervical discography. Lateral fluoroscopic view demonstrating a posterior annular tear at C4-C5 with epidural leak of the contract and a normal nucleogram at C5-C6.

testing; however, motor and reflex testing is not readily interpreted. Visceral complaints have been manifestations of thoracic disc herniations often diagnosed only after an extensive cardiac, pulmonary, and gastrointestinal workup.

Establishing Diagnosis

Cervical Discogenic Pain

The primary role of plain radiographs in the evaluation of cervical pain is to evaluate for fracture, tumors, or infection.[7] Magnetic resonance imaging (MRI) has become the gold standard in imaging the disc, but there is a high incidence of degenerative findings in otherwise pain-free subjects. Careful comparison with physical examination and MRI findings is a must. Electromyography (EMG)/nerve conduction study (NCS) can be helpful in isolating difficult or complex clinical scenarios. EMG/NCS may not confirm painful compression of a nerve if motor nerves are not yet involved.

Selective nerve root blocks (SNRBs) are helpful in this situation. I prefer local anesthetic–only blocks since there have been numerous cases of cerebellar infarcts when steroids have been injected close to the cervical nerve roots.

Cervical Discography

A thorough chapter devoted to discography is included in this reference. Cervical discography requires adaptations of standard lumbar discography techniques. First, the patient is supine rather than prone. An anterolateral angle is used with a right-sided approach favored, since the esophagus typically has a more left-sided deviation in the cervical spine. Care must be taken to ensure not damaging important vascular and nervous structures. Retraction of the carotid/jugular/vagus complex is done with the nondominant hand. Manipulation of this complex may result in an intense vagal response. Smaller volumes, 0.25 to 0.5 mL, are injected since the cervical nucleus pulposus contains little volume.[8]

Cervical-specific complications from discography include myelopathic precipitations if a central disc herniation is augmented and infectious events from improper needle placement. Although discitis is a feared complication, it is extremely rare. Recent systematic review demonstrated an incidence of discitis of 22 out of 14133 cervical disc injections.[9]

Thoracic Discogenic Pain

Plain radiography is the next step beyond a history and physical examination. Radiographic evidence of disc space narrowing, osteophyte formation, and abnormally impressive kyphosis are signs of disc degeneration. Disc calcification is most commonly seen with degenerative disc disease of the thoracic region. MRI is invaluable for ascertaining thoracic disc anatomy and potential disease; however, it is not a functional test, with a known high rate of false positives.

Thoracic Discography

A thorough chapter devoted to discography is included in this text. Thoracic discography is very similar to lumbar discography from technique standpoint, with a few notable exceptions.

Thoracic intervertebral discs have a small yet well-defined nucleus pulposus. It is more centrally located and surrounded by a denser annulus than the lumbar discs. This stresses the need for central needle placement in all planes. The needle is advanced into the center of the disc on a course that bisects the two articulations of the head of the rib. The nerve root is typically superior to the needle trajectory. The normal thoracic discs may be injected with a volume of 0.5 mL to 0.6 mL without causing pain.[10] Normal discogram volumes are in the 0.5- to 1-mL range.

Thoracic specific complications from discography include myelopathy precipitations if a central disc herniation is augmented and infectious events from improper needle placement and pneumothorax.

Interventional Treatment of Cervical and Thoracic Discogenic Pain

Nonsurgical interventional treatments for cervical and thoracic discogenic pain for the most part have been limited to radicular focus. Epidural steroid injections in both the thoracic and cervical regions are frequently used to treat radicular pain. The studies are mixed on their effectiveness; and prospective, randomized studies are needed to solve this debate.[11] A recent study demonstrated no significant difference in outcome if steroids were used in an interlaminar cervical epidural injection intended to treat radiculitis; the group that received steroids and the group that did not both gained significant improvement.[12] There are no studies in the literature on the usefulness of thoracic epidural injections.

Decompression of Cervical and Thoracic Disc Herniation

Percutaneous discectomy is accomplished by the physical removal of disc material rather than ablation. Automated devices have been developed to remove disc material from the center of the disc, in theory providing room for a herniated disc to resorb to its original, unherniated position. Stryker, Laurimed, Richard Wolf, and Clarus Medical all have some derivative of a percutaneous disc removal system. Each has clearance from the U.S. Food and Drug Administration through the 510(k) process for the labeled intended use "for percutaneous discectomies in the lumbar, thoracic, and cervical region of the spine."

The Stryker system Dekompressor involves placing a cannula percutaneously into the center of the disc. The nucleus is removed using an Archimedes principle; essentially a probe with a rotating screw is placed into the cannula, allowing for nucleus material to be "pumped" out of the disc. Variable amounts of disc material can be removed by making several passes in different planes within the disc.

Unfortunately studies have been equivocal on the use and success of the Stryker system when compared to the more accepted microdiscectomy. There are very little data beyond case series in the cervical and thoracic region.

Annuloplasty and Nucleoplasty

Annuloplasty and nucleoplasty are techniques that use energy—from lasers, radio waves, or plasma fields—to vaporize disc tissue. Although approved for contained cervical and thoracic disc herniations, most of the literature and experience is in the lumbar spine. "Controlled ablation," or coblation, is a technique in which a strong electrical field is generated between electrodes; the resulting plasma field disrupts soft tissue molecular bonds (**Fig. 10-3**). This reduces

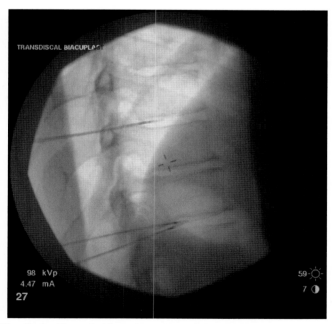

Fig. 10-3 Thoracic biacuplasty. Lateral view demonstrating needle placement in the posterior annulus at T7-T8 and T10-T11. Radiofrequency ablation of the posterior annulus is accomplished with a bipolar technique.

the nucleus material to a mixture of gases that exit the disc via the introducer.

Birnbaum[13] demonstrated a randomized study of cervical disc nucleoplasty using the coblation technique. A total of 26 patients were treated with coblation and followed for 2 years. This group was compared to a randomized 30-patient control group that was treated with only conservative medical and physical therapy. The two-year average visual analog scale (VAS) was 2.3 in the coblation group vs. 8.4 in the control group.

Li and associates[14] reported a prospective study of 126 consecutive patients with 126 contained cervical disc herniations treated with percutaneous cervical decompression using the SpineWand nucleoplasty technique.[14]

Intradiscal Injection Therapy

Chymopapain has a colorful history as an intradiscal injectate. An enzyme derived from the papaya fruit, chymopapain catalyzes the hydrolytic cleavage of glycosaminoglycans from proteoglycan aggregates in the disc. This results in nucleus pulposus contraction secondary to decreased hydration. Although evidence is strong in the lumbar spine, no thoracic or cervical experience with chymopapain injection exists in the literature at this time.

Ozone

Intradiscal ozone therapy is postulated to reduce inflammation, affect mucopolysaccharides-water interaction, and/or improve microcirculation. Several European centers provided most of the data on intradiscal ozone injection as a treatment for lumbar discogenic/radicular pain.[15] No thoracic or cervical experience with ozone injection exists in the literature at this time.

Methylene Blue

Much recent attention has been focused on a single-site success in treating lumbar discogenic pain with intradiscal methylene blue injection. Intradiscal methylene blue is postulated to destroy the sensory nerve ending within a degenerated and painful disc.

Peng[16] reported a randomized placebo-controlled trial of methylene blue in chronic lumbar discogenic pain, with largely positive results. Peng's technique was described as a typical double-needle discogram; however, after placing the contrast, 1 mL of 1% methylene blue was injected, followed by 1 mL of 1% lidocaine. No thoracic or cervical experience with methylene blue injection exists in the literature at this time.

Summary

In summary, cervical and thoracic disc disease is a less common complaint than lumbar disease. The nonsurgical interventional treatments for cervical and thoracic disc disease have been poorly studied, but recent advances in lumbar disc disease treatment hopefully will be applied to these regions as well.

References

1. Hogg-Johnson S et al: The burden and determinants of neck pain in the general population: results of the Bone and Joint 2000-2010 Task Force in Neck Pain and its associated disorders, *Spine* 33(suppl 4):S39–S51, 2009.
2. Rao R: Neck pain, cervical radiculopathy, and cervical myelopathy: pathophysiology, natural history, and clinical evaluation, *J Bone Joint Surg [Am]* 84:1872-1881, 2002.
3. Hult L: Cervical, dorsal and lumbar spinal syndromes: a field investigation of a nonselected material of 1200 workers in different

occupations with special reference to disc degeneration and so-called muscular rheumatism, *Acta Orthop Scand* 7(suppl):1-102, 1954.

4. McKenzie RA: *The cervical and thoracic spine: mechanical diagnosis and therapy*, Wakainae, New Zealand, 1990, Spinal Publications.

5. Grubb SA, Kelly CK: Cervical discography: clinical implications from 12 years of experience, *Spine* 25:1382-1389, 2000.

6. Viikari-Juntura E, Porras M, Laasonen EM: Validity of clinical tests in the diagnosis of root compression in cervical disc disease, *Spine* 14(3):253-257, 1989.

7. White AA, Panjabi MM: *Clinical biomechanics of the spine*, ed 2, Philadelphia, 1991, Lippincott; pp 85-125.

8. Singh V: The role of cervical discography in interventional pain management, *Pain Physician* 7:249-255, 2004.

9. Kapoor SG et al: Systematic review of the incidence of discitis after cervical discography, *Spine J* 10(issue 8):739-745, 2010.

10. Wood KB et al: Thoracic discography in healthy individuals: a controlled prospective study of magnetic resonance imaging and discography in asymptomatic and symptomatic individuals, *Spine* 24:1548-1555, 1999.

11. Huston CW: Cervical epidural steroid injections in the management of cervical radiculitis: interlaminar versus transforaminal: a review, *Rev Musculoskelet Med* 2(1):30-42, 2009.

12. Manchikant IL et al: The effectiveness of fluoroscopic cervical interlaminar epidural injections in managing chronic cervical disc herniation and radiculitis: preliminary results of a randomized, double-blind, controlled trial, *Pain Physician* 13:223-236, 2010.

13. Birnbaum K: Percutaneous cervical disc decompression, *Surg Radiol Anat* 31:379-387, 2009.

14. Li J et al: Percutaneous cervical nucleoplasty in the treatment of cervical disc herniation, *Eur Spine J* 17:1664-1669, 2008.

15. Muto M: Treatment of herniated lumbar disc by intradiscal and intraforaminal oxygen-ozone (O_2-O_3) injection, *J Neuroradiol* 31:183-189, 2004.

16. Peng B et al. A randomized placebo-controlled trial of intradiscal methylene blue injection for the treatment of chronic discogenic low back pain, *Pain* 149:124-129, 2010.

11 Disc Herniations: Injections and Minimally Invasive Techniques

Thomas M. Larkin, Michael DeMarco, José Suros, and Steven P. Cohen

CHAPTER OVERVIEW

Chapter Synopsis: Discogenic pain can result from various perturbations of the disc itself, ranging from simple dehydration to herniation outside the vertebral column. Exposure of the central nucleus pulposus of the disc can trigger an inflammatory immune response and provoke painful mechanical sensitization. Mechanical damage can also cause sensory nerve apoptosis, leading to chemically mediated hyperalgesia in neurons of the dorsal root ganglia. The minimally invasive therapies discussed in this chapter are aimed at both of these pain-generating conditions. With a bulging or contained herniated disc, the nucleus pulposus material does not escape the spinal column. Sequestrated or uncontained herniations with pulposus tissue escape must be considered differently in choosing a course of treatment. According to studies of outcomes, epidural injection of steroids into the disc can alleviate discogenic pain, but only for certain types and cases. Cytokine inhibitors target tumor necrosis factor-alpha (TNF-α) and other inflammatory mediators. Although associated with some serious risks, preemptive treatment with a TNF-α inhibitor in an animal model prevented pain behaviors and neurodegeneration. Therapies such as ozone injection also appear to target these chemical pain generators. Percutaneous decompression of disc material provides another therapeutic avenue, with many different techniques now available. Chemonucleolysis uses the enzyme papain to decrease the volume of the disc and has shown positive outcomes in terms of pain relief. This chapter surveys the risks and complications associated with each procedure.

Important Points:
- The diagnosis of a herniated disc starts with a complete history and physical examination. The addition of radiological studies should serve to confirm the diagnosis.
- Pain and neurological symptoms from a disc herniation are the end result of a combination of both chemical and mechanical factors.
- A disc herniation is one of the end results of a more chronic degenerative cascade that occurs with disc aging.

Clinical Pearls:
- It is important to understand the different types of disc herniations that exist—contained vs. extruded—and how they affect the response to interventions.
- Success with percutaneous disc techniques depends on proper patient selection. Familiarity with MRI imaging and discography help in making the diagnosis of a contained disc herniation with an intact outer annulus fibrosis.
- An extruded disc herniation creates pain via both chemical and mechanical factors while a contained disc tends to create radicular pain via mechanical influences alone.
- Epidural injections of steroids, TNF-α, and in rare cases use of oxygen-ozone therapy are the preferred modes of treatment of the chemical changes associated with extruded disc herniations.
- The use of TNF-α inhibitors has shown promise for treating disc herniations but the more recent blinded clinical studies have been less favorable than the initial studies.
- Percutaneous disc decompression techniques are viable treatment options for treating radicular pain secondary to the compressive mechanical forces that are exerted on nerve roots by contained bulging disc herniations.
- All percutaneous lumbar disc decompression techniques are based on the same theory. The technical aspects of disc coblation, the lumbar decompressor, LASE, and PLDD all are similar in nature and require the same skill sets.
- Chymopapain is the only decompressive disc treatment that can be used for contained and non-contained disc herniations so long as they are not extruded or sequestered.

Clinical Pitfalls:
- All lumbar disc interventions have risk. Most notably they are associated with infections, bleeding, direct nerve trauma, and neurovascular injury. They should not be attempted for weak indications.
- The performance of percutaneous disc decompression techniques requires at least a moderate degree of familiarity with intradiscal procedures, notably discography. This should be mastered by the provider before he/she attempts the more invasive intradiscal therapies.
- Lumbar epidural steroid injections are the most commonly performed lumbar injections for disc herniations, but the efficacy of this procedure remains a point of controversy.

Establishing the Diagnosis

In 1934 the syndrome of "disc herniation" was born when Mixter and Barr[1] first proclaimed that a posterior rupture of the intervertebral disc that allowed nuclear material to escape and compress the adjacent spinal nerve root(s) was a common cause of back and leg pain, a condition commonly known as *sciatica*.

Determining the presence of a disc herniation starts with a careful history. A herniated disc can lead to radiculopathy, radicular pain, or referred pain. Radiculopathy describes neurological changes such as numbness, weakness, and diminished reflexes with or without the presence of pain. Radicular pain is pain that typically follows a dermatomal pattern with or without the presence of sensory or motor deficits. Referred pain is pain that spreads into the lower limbs and is perceived in regions innervated by nerves other than those that innervate the site of noxious stimulation.[2]

The patient may describe an acute onset of this pain or a period of heavy activity that preceded the development of symptoms, but radiculopathy in the elderly often occurs without a specific inciting event. Sneezing, coughing, or bending usually intensifies the pain. However, in a clinical setting the classic findings of radiculopathy are not always present. Often what emerges is an incomplete pattern of spread or spread that overlaps various dermatomes. Signs and symptoms that could indicate cauda equina syndrome include progressive weakness of the extremity, erectile dysfunction, or bowel or bladder dysfunction.

Anatomy

The lumbar spine serves two basic and vital functions. The first is that it provides the structural framework that houses the spinal cord and spinal nerves. The second is that it provides a mechanical support for the entire axial skeleton. The lumbar spine is composed of five motion segments. Each motion segment consists of the vertebral body, intervertebral disc, pedicles, zygapophyseal joints, posterior lamina, and spinous process. These structural elements are supported by a vast array of ligaments that help maintain the stability of the spine (**Fig. 11-1**).

The intervertebral disc has three basic structural components: the nucleus pulposus (NP), annulus fibrosus (AF), and vertebral endplate (VE). The AF and NP are the major structural components of the disc; the VE is responsible for metabolic functions. The NP comprises the gelatinous center of the disc. Under normal conditions the NP equally shares load bearing with the AF. The NP has a high water content, secondary proteoglycans, and aggregate molecules that trap and hold water. Surrounding the NP is the AF, which is fibrous in nature. The annulus is made up of 15 to 25 concentric sheets of collagen known as lamellae. In the normal disc it is the interplay between the nucleus and annulus that allows the disc to distribute very high axial loads equitably.

Nutritional support of the intervertebral disc comes via diffusion of nutrients across the VE. The healthy disc is the largest avascular structure in the body. As a result, it is prone to ischemia in the event of injury to the endplate.

The normal disc is innervated in the outer one third of the annulus by fibers from the sinuvertebral nerve, which also supplies nociceptive input from the dural sac and nerve root sleeve. Branches of the gray rami communicantes have also been identified in the anterolateral annulus.[3,4]

As the disc degenerates and internal fissures develop, nociceptive fibers may invade into deeper layers of the AF, sometimes reaching the NP itself. These fibers travel along with vascular structures toward the center of the disc.[5] Once the fissure has penetrated to the nucleus, inflammatory mediators contained within the NP now are exposed to nervous elements. This process, known as *internal disc disruption*, has been theorized as a major component of chronic low back pain.[6]

A gradual weakening of the outer annulus occurs with aging and endplate disruption. In the normal disc axial loads are distributed evenly across the AF and NP. However, in the case of internal disc disruption, the nucleus no longer evenly shares weight-bearing loads with the annulus. This may cause a generalized disc bulging that is evenly distributed across the annular fibers, or a unilateral bulging. Alone or in combination with other age-related changes (facet arthropathy, ligamentum flavum hypertrophy), this can lead to nerve root compression. Under high mechanical stress the outer annular fibers may disrupt entirely, allowing nuclear material to be displaced outside of the disc itself, resulting in an extruded or sequestered disc herniation (**Fig. 11-2**).[7]

Basic Science

The intervertebral disc is immunogenic. This is because, after embryonic development is complete, the avascular NP no longer has exposure to the immune system. Thus, when NP is introduced outside of the confines of the annulus, it is capable of inducing an autoimmune, inflammatory response.[8]

Several inflammatory mediators have been identified in the intervertebral disc in laboratory models designed to duplicate the chemical effects of disc herniation. These inflammatory mediators include phospholipase A_2, prostaglandin E_2, interleukin 1-α, interleukin 1-β, interleukin-6, tumor necrosis factor-α, and nitrous oxide (NO).[9,10]

Animal studies in which autologous NP and AF were placed on or even adjacent to nerve roots demonstrate that it is the nuclear material that induces the chemical radiculitis. The application of NP to nerve roots has been shown to induce axonal and myelin sheets alterations, increased vascular permeability, and decrease intraneural blood flow. Not surprisingly, studies evaluating antagonists to various inflammatory mediators have shown them to abate or prevent hyperalgesic responses in animal models.[11,12]

There are equally compelling studies involving the effects of mechanical compression. Direct compression of the nerve root

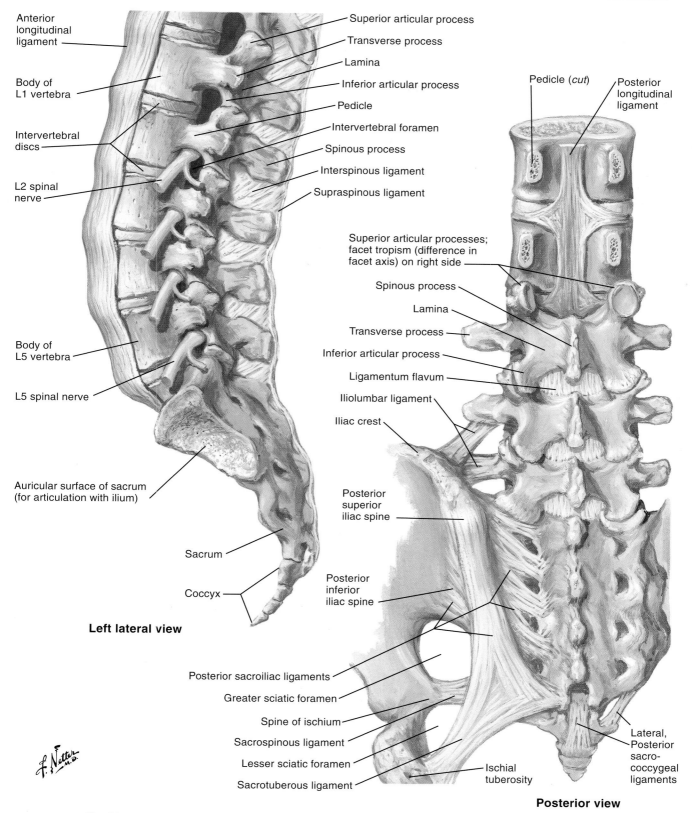

Anterior longitudinal ligament

Body of L1 vertebra

Intervertebral discs

L2 spinal nerve

Body of L5 vertebra

L5 spinal nerve

Auricular surface of sacrum (for articulation with ilium)

Sacrum

Coccyx

Left lateral view

Superior articular process

Transverse process

Lamina

Inferior articular process

Pedicle

Intervertebral foramen

Spinous process

Interspinous ligament

Supraspinous ligament

Pedicle (*cut*)

Posterior longitudinal ligament

Superior articular processes; facet tropism (difference in facet axis) on right side

Spinous process

Lamina

Transverse process

Inferior articular process

Ligamentum flavum

Iliolumbar ligament

Iliac crest

Posterior superior iliac spine

Posterior inferior iliac spine

Posterior sacroiliac ligaments

Greater sciatic foramen

Spine of ischium

Sacrospinous ligament

Lesser sciatic foramen

Sacrotuberous ligament

Ischial tuberosity

Lateral, Posterior sacro-coccygeal ligaments

Posterior view

Fig. 11-1 Spinal anatomy. Netter illustration from www.netterimages.com. ©Elsevier Inc. All rights reserved.

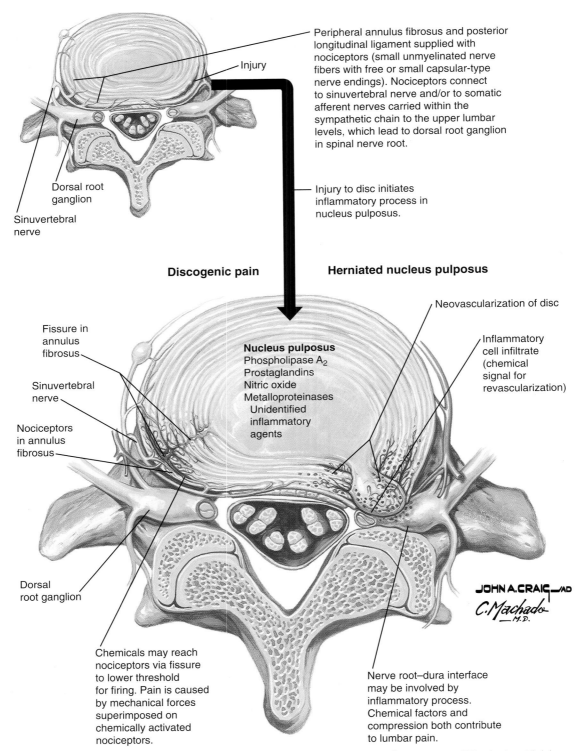

Injury

Peripheral annulus fibrosus and posterior longitudinal ligament supplied with nociceptors (small unmyelinated nerve fibers with free or small capsular-type nerve endings). Nociceptors connect to sinuvertebral nerve and/or to somatic afferent nerves carried within the sympathetic chain to the upper lumbar levels, which lead to dorsal root ganglion in spinal nerve root.

Dorsal root ganglion

Sinuvertebral nerve

Injury to disc initiates inflammatory process in nucleus pulposus.

Discogenic pain

Herniated nucleus pulposus

Neovascularization of disc

Fissure in annulus fibrosus

Nucleus pulposus
Phospholipase A_2
Prostaglandins
Nitric oxide
Metalloproteinases
Unidentified inflammatory agents

Inflammatory cell infiltrate (chemical signal for revascularization)

Sinuvertebral nerve

Nociceptors in annulus fibrosus

Dorsal root ganglion

Chemicals may reach nociceptors via fissure to lower threshold for firing. Pain is caused by mechanical forces superimposed on chemically activated nociceptors.

Nerve root–dura interface may be involved by inflammatory process. Chemical factors and compression both contribute to lumbar pain.

JOHN A. CRAIG—MD
C. Machado—M.D.

Fig. 11-2 Pathophysiology of disc-related pain. Netter illustration from www.netterimages.com. ©Elsevier Inc. All rights reserved.

both proximal and distal to the dorsal root ganglion (DRG), with or without extruded NP, results in pain-related behaviors in animal models. These pain-related behaviors are affected by a variety of factors, most notably apoptosis.[13,14] Mechanical compression can produce apoptosis of the more severely injured neurons, which leads to retrograde transport of inflammatory mediators to the DRG, thereby inducing mechanical allodynia. This may be further exacerbated by diminished blood flow caused by edema and direct compression of the neuronal microvasculature. This explains why a disc bulge without extrusion can still produce neuropathic pain.

Imaging

Plain films as a stand-alone tool have a limited role in the diagnosis and management of lumbar radiculopathy, having been supplanted by more advanced imaging. However, in some instances a plain

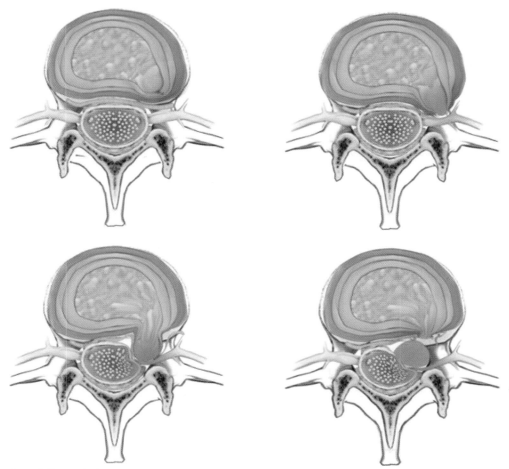

Fig. 11-3 Classification of disc pathology. From Weiner BK, Patel R: The accuracy of MRI in the detection of lumbar disc containment, *J Orthop Surg Res* 3:46, 2008.

radiograph can help identify bony abnormalities that can lead to radicular pain such as facet arthropathy, spondylolisthesis, and reduced disc height. On a similar note, the role of myelography has changed over the past few decades from the principal means of diagnosing a herniated disc(s) to a secondary role, usually in combination with computed tomography (CT) in patients who cannot undergo magnetic resonance imaging (MRI).

As noted previously, CT is still used today for diagnosing disc herniations, primarily in patients with prior instrumented surgery and those who cannot have MRI (e.g., patients with spinal cord stimulators or pacemakers). In contrast to plain radiographs, CT does allow for imaging of soft tissues and disc contours. The limitations of CT imaging include high radiation exposure and inferior image quality compared to MRI.

MRI remains the modality of choice in diagnosing lumbar disc herniations. Its benefits include excellent resolution of the disc itself and the surrounding nerves, ligaments, and bony structures. The downside is that MRI is relatively sensitive in demonstrating degenerative changes, which can result in the detection of pathology in segments that are not pain generators.[15]

The nomenclature for describing disc abnormalities on MRI can be ambiguous. For example, there is no defined set of descriptors for grading or defining lumbar disc herniations. Perhaps more important, when considering whether percutaneous therapies are indicated, there is a need to establish whether or not a disc herniation is contained. MRI evaluations have been shown to be only 70% accurate in making an accurate diagnosis of a contained

vs. noncontained disc herniation.[16] Frequently discography can provide valuable information regarding whether or not a disc herniation is contained with the outer fibers of the annulus intact and pathology that is amenable to percutaneous interventions.[17]

For the purposes of this chapter, disc herniations are classified as contained and noncontained disc herniations and then divided into the following four categories (**Fig. 11-3**)[7]:

1. Disc protrusion: The disc protrusion has intact annular fibers and posterior longitudinal ligament (PLL). It is a contained disc herniation.
2. Subannular extrusion: The disc bulge has disrupted the inner annular fibers but has not ruptured the outermost portion of the annulus or the PLL. It is considered a contained disc herniation.
3. Transannular extrusion: The disc material has now extruded past the outer annular fibers and PLL. It is a noncontained disc herniation.
4. Sequestrated disc: This is a free fragment of disc material without a tail into the remainder of the disc. It is a noncontained disc herniation.

Epidural Steroid Injections (Interlaminar, Transforaminal, and Caudal)

The rationale behind epidural steroid injection (ESI) is that higher concentrations of corticosteroid are delivered to the inflamed nerve

Table 11-1: Selecting Candidates for Epidural Steroid Injections

Favorable Prognosis	Unfavorable Prognosis
Radiculopathy caused by herniated nucleus pulposus	Degenerative disc disease or spinal stenosis (short duration of benefit)
Short duration of symptoms	Pain >6 months in duration
Leg pain > back pain	Back pain > leg pain
Intermittent pain	Constant pain
Neuropathic descriptors (e.g., shooting, burning, electrical-like)	Nociceptive descriptors (e.g., aching, throbbing, dull)
Absence of psychopathology	Psychological overlay (e.g., somatization disorder, depression, poor coping skills, catastrophization)
Active lifestyle, good physical shape	Sedentary lifestyle, obesity, or deconditioning
Self-employed	On disability or with secondary gain issues
Young age	Older age, concomitant spinal pain generators
Isolated, single-level pathology	Multilevel pathology
No previous or previously successful interventions	Previous spine surgery or multiple failed interventions

root(s) than with oral or parenteral routes, resulting in enhanced pain relief and reduced side effects. ESIs have been studied predominantly in patients with radicular pain (**Table 11-1**), which is most commonly caused by a disc herniation. There are three ways to access the epidural space: the caudal, interlaminar, and transforaminal approaches. The interlaminar and transforaminal techniques can be used in the cervical, thoracic, and lumbar spine. The caudal epidural space is accessed via the sacral hiatus and thus is reserved for lumbosacral symptomatology.

Indications/Contraindications

The indications for ESI are the source of ongoing controversy. Historically they have been used to treat conditions as diverse as phantom pain, peripheral neuropathy, complex regional pain syndrome, and pelvic pain. However, their principal use is for the treatment of radiculopathy.

How many ESIs should be performed is also subject to debate. The practice of limiting injections to 3 in 6 months is not based on sound evidence in the form of prospective studies.[18] Rather, the law of diminishing returns and the cumulative risk of steroid-related side effects and complications dictates an inverse relationship between the number of injections and the added benefit for each successive injection. Thus, although limiting the number of injections would appear to be prudent, the exact number and timing of injections need to be determined from clinical trials.

The need for repeat injections should be dictated by the patient's response to the initial injection. If a patient obtains complete relief with one injection, a second injection can be done on an as-needed basis. If he or she has incomplete relief with the initial injection, a second injection at the same or different site can be repeated in as early as 1 week, although most people wait at least 2 weeks before repeating the procedure. No relief from the first injection warrants reevaluation; if a decision is made to repeat the ESI, either switching the route (i.e., transforaminal instead of interlaminar or intervertebral level) may be beneficial. There are no data to justify an automatic series of ESIs. Most interventionalists limit the use of ESIs to three or four in a 6-month period. The literature suggests that patients who respond to ESI usually require between one and three injections.[18,19]

Risk and Complication Avoidance

The recovery period immediately following ESIs is generally less than 10 minutes. Immediate adverse effects include increased pain from the pressure exerted on the nerves during injection, which typically resolves within hours. Other minor complications include vasovagal reactions, which are more common in females and during cervical spine procedures, weakness or numbness, and transient low back pain. Adverse effects associated with corticosteroids include weight gain, water retention, flushing (hot flashes), mood swings, insomnia, elevated blood sugar levels in patients with diabetes, and suppression of the hypothalamic-pituitary-adrenal axis.

Epidural injections are subject to the same generic complications associated with any procedure such as bleeding, infection, and inadvertent puncture of the adjacent structures (e.g., the dura, kidneys, and blood vessels). Nevertheless, the rare complications that do occur can produce devastating complications such as meningitis, epidural abscess, and epidural hematomas.[20]

The complication that has received most interest of late is inadvertent spinal cord infarction after transforaminal ESI. There have also been at least 10 cases of this occurring after lumbar transforaminal ESI. Some cases have occurred at levels as low as S1. The most prominent theory as to the etiology of this complication is that there is inadvertent puncture of a spinal radiculomedullary artery. The largest of these vessels, the artery of Adamkiewicz, frequently projects into the lumbar spine as low as the L3 level. Unrecognized injection of particulate steroids into one of these arteries can cause occlusion of blood flow to the spinal cord, leading to infarction. Methods to reduce the risk of this complication include using continuous fluoroscopy or subtraction angiography during injection, minimizing manipulation of the needle, administering a nonparticulate steroid such as dexamethasone, injecting through a catheter inserted through the needle, and using a test dose of local anesthetic before injection.[21]

Epidural hematomas typically develop over a period of hours. The risk of epidural hematoma is less than 2 in 10,000 but increases in the presence of active anticoagulation, bleeding diathesis, and traumatic injection. Epidural hematomas classically present with severe low back pain and spasm along with progressive neurological deterioration. It is critical to recognize this complication within 8 hours because delayed intervention exponentially worsens prognosis.[22]

Although rare, there is a small risk of either bacterial meningitis or epidural abscess associated with ESI. The actual infectious risk from ESI is not well known since most literature is in the form of retrospective studies evaluating spinal anesthetics or continuous epidural catheters. The risk of meningitis secondary to intrathecal injection is estimated to be around 1 in 50,000.[22]

Anticoagulant Therapy

Regarding anticoagulant therapy, Raj and associates[23] provided an exhaustive review for the American Society of Interventional Pain Physicians (ASIPP) of not just medication but patient and procedurally-related factors involved in assessing and minimizing the risk of bleeding complications.[23] Horlocker and associates[24] were more liberal in arriving at guidelines for the American Society of Regional Anesthesia and Pain Medicine (ASRA). **Table 11-2** contains a simplified list of recommendations regarding anticoagulants. These do not address specific patient factors associated with bleeding.

Outcomes Evidence

A key shortcoming in evaluating the evidence for ESI is that many studies evaluating the efficacy of interlaminar injections were done without fluoroscopic guidance. Previous studies have demonstrated high rates (8.8% to 70%) of false loss of resistance for blind (without fluoroscopic guidance) ESIs, which may be higher in the cervical region.[25,26] Even when the epidural space is successfully accessed, blinded injections may not deliver the medication to the area of pathology. In a study conducted in 50 patients with failed back surgery syndrome, Fredman and colleagues[26] found that 5 mL of blindly administered injectate reached the targeted area only 26% of the time.

Multiple reviews have been written about the efficacy of ESIs.[27-30] These reviews are limited by reviewer bias (reviews conducted by people who perform epidural injections tend to be more favorable than those done by people who do not), the inclusion of studies with small sample sizes, serious methodological flaws, inadequate outcome measures, and heterogeneity with respect to route of injection and use of fluoroscopy. In one of the earliest reviews, Koes and associates[27] illustrated the difficulty of properly evaluating the literature in a systematic review of 12 randomized clinical trials with disparate methodological qualities, half of which were deemed positive. The primary care physicians who conducted this review concluded that the benefits of epidural steroids, if any, seem to be of short duration. A similar review conducted 4 years later by a French task force of rheumatologists determined that 8 of 13 randomized studies demonstrated no measurable benefit.[31] The authors of this analysis concluded that no determination could be made regarding the efficacy of epidural steroids for sciatica. The main weaknesses in the studies analyzed in these reviews were that none used fluoroscopic guidance and all used an interlaminar approach, which is probably clinically inferior to transforaminal ESIs.

In recent European guidelines for the management of low back pain, Airaksinen and colleagues[32] concluded that epidural corticosteroid injections should be considered only for radicular pain, if a contained disc prolapse is the cause of the pain, and if the corticosteroid is injected close to the site of pathology. They further noted that injections should be fluoroscopically guided toward the ventral epidural space. These recommendations are in direct contrast with those outlined in a recent report by a subcommittee of the American Academy of Neurology that concluded that lumbosacral ESIs for radicular pain do not improve function, provide long-term pain relief (>3 months), or obviate the need for surgery.[33] The authors found insufficient data to draw a conclusion for cervical ESI.

Table 11-2: Anticoagulant Therapy and Neuraxial Procedures			
	Duration of Effects	**Recommended Hold Time**	**Special Factors**
Aspirin	7-10 days	7-10 days	ASRA not contraindicated; ASIPP says to hold
Nonsteroidal antiinflammatory drugs	3-5 days	3-5 days	ASRA not contraindicated; ASIPP says to hold
COX-2 inhibitors	None	None	
Nonaspirin antiplatelet medications (ticlopidine [Ticlid], clopidogrel [Plavix])	Ticlopidine 14-21 days Clopidogrel 7-10 days	Ticlopidine 14 days Clopidogrel 7 days	Required with platelet receptor antagonists such as abciximab (ReoPro), eptifibatide (Integrilin)
Warfarin	At therapeutic levels: 3-5 days	5 days	Check INR before proceeding; INR <1.4
Heparin intravenous	Variable and dose dependent	4 hours after last heparin dose	
Heparin subcutaneous	Variable and dose dependent	No contraindication with twice daily dosing under 10,000 units	Can hold needle placement until 4 hours after last dose; effects of doses more than 10,000 units unknown
Low–molecular-weight heparin	Variable and dose dependent	Hold for 12 hours with standard dosing, 24 hours with higher dosing	Increased risk of bleeding with concomitant use of antiplatelet medications
Herbal medications	Garlic 7 days Ginkgo 36 hours Ginseng 24 hours	Not available	Recommendations not available; potential side effects

ASIPP, American Society of Interventional Pain Physicians; *ASRA*, American Society of Regional Anesthesia and Pain Medicine; *INR*, international normalized ratio.

Recent systematic reviews by Abdi and associates[28] and Boswell and associates[34] reached different conclusions. The authors found strong evidence for short-term pain relief and functional improvement for lumbar transforaminal, cervical interlaminar, and caudal ESI and moderate evidence for long-term relief. The evidence supporting lumbar interlaminar injections was strong for short-term improvement but limited for long-term benefit.

The randomized controlled trials that have evaluated caudal, interlaminar, and transforaminal ESIs (TFESIs) to date carry major flaws in that fluoroscopic guidance was not used in most of the early studies and most were conducted in patients hospitalized for their pain.

One small randomized controlled study conducted by an orthopedic group found that lumbar TFESIs decreased the need for decompression surgery for up to 5 years since most of the patients who underwent lumbar TFESI elected not to undergo decompression surgery.[35]

Fluoroscopic guidance and method of injection (interlaminar vs. transforaminal) appear to account for most of the heterogeneity among the systematic reviews. The reviews with heterogeneity among methods of injection did not find a clinical benefit for the procedure,[26,33] whereas those with stratified trials based on the method of injection found evidence to support transforaminal and caudal ESIs performed with fluoroscopic guidance.[28,34] Considering that transforaminal and caudal ESI more reliably deliver medication to the ventral epidural space, this finding is not surprising.[25] Transforaminal injections have also been found to be clinically superior to interlaminar ESI in two head-to-head comparisons.[36,37] Transforaminal ESIs appear to afford better and longer-lasting relief than interlaminar and caudal ESI; however, the added benefit must be balanced against the higher risk.

TNF-α Inhibitors

Cytokines play a prominent role in the development of radiculopathy. Consequently there has been growing interest in using cytokine inducers and inhibitors for the treatment of the pain from herniated discs. Cytokines known to be involved in the pathological changes associated with herniated discs include tumor necrosis factor–alpha (TNF-α), interleukin (IL)-1, IL-6, and IL-8. After disc injury, IL1-β promotes matrix degeneration, and the administration of an IL-1 antagonist has been shown to prevent subsequent disc degeneration.[38] TNF-α inhibitors appear to be involved in promoting thrombus formation, intraneural edema, and reduced nerve conduction velocity.[39] However, the preemptive administration of TNF-α inhibitors in experimental models of herniated discs have been shown to prevent pain behaviors and reduce neurodegeneration.[40]

Outcomes Evidence

The first studies treating sciatica used either subcutaneous or intravenous infusions; and, although the earlier pilot studies showed favorable results, more recent blinded studies failed to demonstrate success.[41-43]

This has led to the promotion of targeted injections with TNF-α inhibitors as treatment for sciatica. There have been three studies evaluating local administration of etanercept (Enbrel) for discogenic pain. In the first randomized, double-blind, placebo-controlled study by Cohen and associates,[44] the intradiscal administration of etanercept was not found to be more effective than placebo. In a later double-blind, placebo-controlled pilot study conducted in patients with acute radiculopathy, a strong trend toward improvement in leg and back pain was found in the transforaminal etanercept treatment groups compared to groups

given placebo. Unlike epidural steroids, the dosages of etanercept used in these studies were significantly lower than those used for parenteral administration.[44] Etanercept was superior to placebo when used for treatment of sciatica.[45] In a randomized controlled study by Kume and associates,[46] evaluating the caudal administration of 25 mg etanercept, the treatment group had significantly lower pain scores than the placebo group 1 day after the injection. One month after treatment both groups demonstrated significant improvement, with no between-group differences noted.

Risk and Complication Avoidance

The risks associated with injection of TNF-α inhibitors are similar to those risks associated with standard epidural steroid injections. Although the cumulative dosage of local etanercept is significantly less than for parenteral administration, the immunosuppressive effects at these dosages have not been established. Larger and more stringent efficacy and safety studies should be conducted before routine use in humans can be advocated.

Percutaneous Disc Decompression Techniques

Treating radicular pain secondary to contained disc herniations with standard surgical techniques results in poorer outcomes than surgery for extruded or sequestered discs.[47] Alternative techniques have been developed to address this problem. The first of these was chymopapain (Chymodiactin) chemonucleolysis, introduced in 1964. In 1975 a paper on percutaneous lumber discectomy was presented, launching the development of a succession of devices designed to mechanically extract disc material.[48]

The theoretical basis for percutaneous disc decompression (PDD) relies on two basic assumptions: that a bulging disc exerts pressure on a nerve root or DRG; and that removal of contained nuclear material will result in a precipitous drop in intradiscal pressure, leading to the retraction of annular fibers away from the nerve. Therefore, for PDD techniques to work, the following criteria must be met: the presence of a bulge in a disc with intact outer annular fibers and enough volume to produce this continuing outward pressure on the annulus (**Table 11-3**).

Case, Choy, and Altman[49] showed that a large rise in pressure regularly results from a small increase in volume, confirming the biomechanical basis for the benefits of disc decompression. However, the effects of PDD may not be caused solely by biomechanical changes. There is mounting evidence that these procedures may alter cytokine release. Increased production of IL-8 and decreased release of IL-1 have been demonstrated with nucleoplasty, and oxygen-ozone therapy has been shown to decrease production of TNF-α, IL-1β, and IL-6.[50,51]

Automated Percutaneous Lumbar Discectomy (Nucleotome)

The Nucleotome (Clarus Medical, Minneapolis, MN) was the first PDD device, released in 1985.[52] The Nucleotome uses an automated reciprocating shaver and continuous irrigation to remove disc nucleus. The benefit of this device is that generally it can remove a larger amount of disc material than similar products (e.g., Stryker Dekompressor, Allendale, NJ) and it requires a less elaborate and expensive setup than techniques requiring lasers (**Figs. 11-4 and 11-5**).

Technique

The Nucleotome procedure is performed on a fluoroscopy table with the patient positioned in either the prone or lateral decubitus

Table 11-3: Indications and Contraindications for Percutaneous Disc Decompression

Indications	Contraindications
Back and/or leg pain for 3 months in a patient with a contained disc herniation	Extruded (with the exception of chymopapain) or sequestered disc herniation
Well-maintained disc height of greater than 60%	Progressive neurological deficits or cauda equina syndrome
Radicular pain in a specific dermatomal distribution that correlates with MRI or CT findings	Disc height less than 50%
Unilateral leg pain greater than low back pain	Calcified disc herniations
Imaging studies that show a subligamentous contained disc herniation	Severe lateral recess or central spinal stenosis
The radicular pain or paresthesias should correlate with the nerve root being compromised on imaging.	A disc herniation; takes up more than 50% of the spinal canal
Mild weakness, hypoesthesia, and hyporeflexia may or may not be present but should follow the nerve root distribution.	Patient is unwilling to agree to the procedure; should be performed under local anesthesia or conscious sedation to allow patient monitoring for signs of segmental spinal nerve irritation; general anesthesia contraindicated
The patient should have had an adequate trial of conservative treatments, including relative rest, physical therapy, oral medications, and epidural steroid injections.	Conditions that would put patient at risk such as pregnancy, malignancy, or ongoing infection

CT, Computed tomography; *MRI*, magnetic resonance imaging.

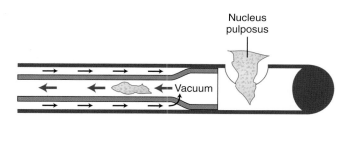

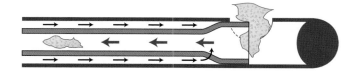

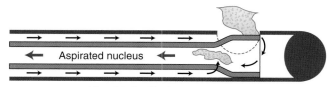

Fig. 11-4 Nucleotome action.

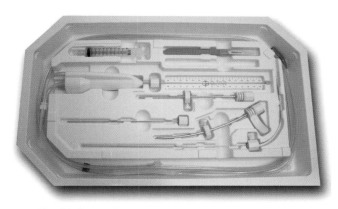

Fig. 11-5 Nucleotome tray. ©2010 Clarus Medical LLC.

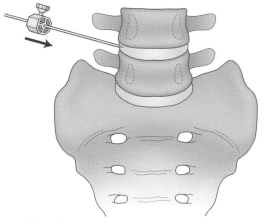

Fig. 11-6 Insertion of the guide needle.

position. A 3-mm skin incision is made at the entry point, and the guide needle is inserted on the side of the herniation into the center of the disc (**Figs. 11-6** and **11-7**). Once the correct position is confirmed, the knob attached to the guide needle is removed.

With careful attention not to further advance the guide needle, the straight cannula and tapered dilator are advanced over the guide needle until the dilator (2 mm longer than the cannula) makes contact with the outer wall of the annulus. The dilator is then removed, and the cannula is advanced 2 mm to make contact with the annulus. Once the cannula position is confirmed fluoroscopically, the stop can be lowered to the skin level and secured in

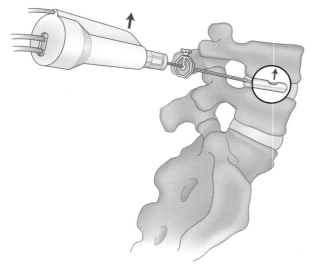

Fig. 11-7 Insertion of the Nucleotome into the disc.

place. A curved cannula/dilator can be used in place of the straight cannula/dilator at the L1-L5 disc levels.

A trephine is placed over the guide needle and through the cannula until it makes contact with the annulus. The trephine is rotated in a clockwise motion to make a shallow circular incision or crater on the wall of the annulus into which the cannula nestles. After the annulus is incised, the cannula stop is loosened, and the combined cannula and trephine are advanced until the distal end of the cannula is about 5 mm inside the disc annulus. The cannula stop is secured against the skin, and the trephine removed from the operating channel of the cannula. After the Nucleotome probe is inserted into the cannula and the seal nut is locked into place, proper probe placement is confirmed using anteroposterior (AP) and lateral views.

The manufacturer recommends initiating treatment at the maximum cutting rate to prevent clogging. Later the rate can be decreased to facilitate greater removal of disc material. Removed nuclear material can be visualized via the aspiration line. Since the NP is avascular, the aspirate should be bloodless. If blood is observed, the cannula may be against the annulus.

Slight changes in angulation of the cannula in the plane of the disc can be made to reach the different parts of the disc. The probe is worked within the disc space until no further material can be obtained. The manufacturer's surgical technique guide reports that this process is normally completed in 20 to 30 minutes.

Outcomes

There have been over 80 published studies to date on automated percutaneous lumbar discectomy (APLD), but most have been disregarded in systematic reviews because of flawed methodology. The results of these reviews have been mixed. In a review of interventional techniques, Boswell and colleagues[53] concluded that there was moderate evidence for short-term and limited evidence for long-term relief following APLD. In a more recent review using strict inclusion criteria by Hirsch and associates evaluating 11 studies,[54] APLD was given a "strong positive" recommendation.

However, two older reviews were not as positive in their conclusions. Gibson and Wadell[55] found that three clinical trials evaluating APLD provided moderate evidence that it is less effective than standard discectomy or chymopapain. In an earlier technology assessment a panel included four randomized studies that all showed negative results.[56]

Complications

Teng and associates[57] reported a complication rate of 0.06% (nine cases of discitis) in 1582 procedures. In another study evaluating over 1000 patients, Maroon and Allen[58] reported on only one muscular hematoma and two cases of discitis, for a complication rate of 0.002%. To minimize complications, aseptic technique should be adhered to, frequent fluoroscopy used, and deep sedation avoided.

A recent study by Carragee and colleagues[59] noted that percutaneous discography is linked to an increased rate of disc herniations and disc degeneration in both symptomatic and asymptomatic discs. This effect was primarily attributed to the mechanical damage that occurs with the disc puncture itself; there was a nonsignificant increase in the overall effect when larger-bore cannulae were used. Therefore the possibility remains that any of the percutaneous disc treatments described in this chapter have the potential to increase the overall rate of disc degeneration of the treated disc.

Percutaneous Lumbar Laser Discectomy

In mid-February 1986 Peter Ascher and Daniel Choy performed the first percutaneous laser disc decompression (PLDD) procedure in Graz, Austria. Thus PLDD technology has been available for the past 25 years. Despite its long history, it has failed to gain widespread popularity at least in part because of several factors:

1. Insurance companies still consider this an experimental technique.
2. The learning curve is relatively steep to become adept at the procedure.
3. There is fierce competition with other percutaneous treatments.
4. It is less effective than open surgical microdiscectomy.

The purported benefits of percutaneous lumbar laser discectomy (PLLD) compared to other forms of PDD are that it can be used with (or without) endoscopic guidance and can easily remove larger volumes of disc material than some of the other techniques described. PLLD involves targeted decompression of the annulus while preserving the healthy nucleus and anterior annulus as much as possible.[60] The mechanism of action is through the use of laser energy to vaporize NP.

Equipment

Multiple systems are available for laser discectomy. These include Nd:YAG, Ho:YAG, and KTP/532 lasers. There have been no direct comparisons between the different types of systems, which makes it difficult to determine superiority.[61]

One system known as LASE (Clarus Medical, Minneapolis, MN) incorporates endoscopy, continuous irrigation, a steerable catheter, and a working channel that allows for the use of surgical forceps and direct laser ablation of the NP. The system uses a Ho:YAG laser that provides an added safety feature because of the shallower depth of penetration (**Figs. 11-8 to 11-10**).

Technique

The initial preparatory steps for disc access have been described previously in the chapter.

The flexible guiding needle is advanced into the center of the disc. After correct position is confirmed using AP and lateral fluoroscopy, the dilator is locked onto the working channel by twisting the hub of the dilator clockwise. The working channel and dilator are then passed over the flexible guiding needle and advanced to

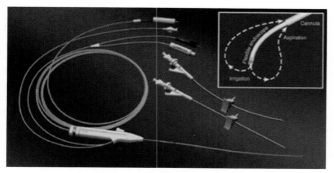

Fig. 11-8 LASE. ©2010 Clarus Medical LLC.

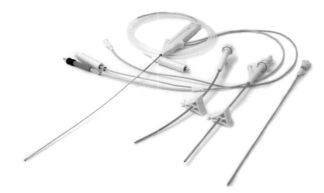

Fig. 11-9 LASE set. ©2010 Clarus Medical LLC.

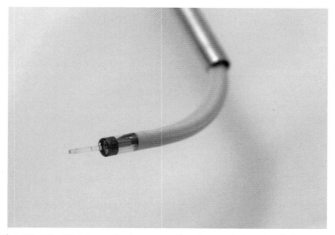

Fig. 11-10 The laser device extending beyond the tip of the introducer. ©2010 Clarus Medical LLC.

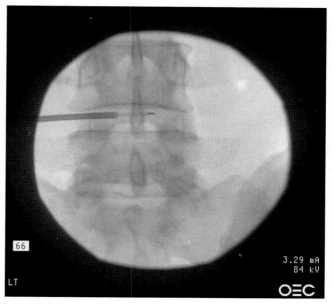

Fig. 11-11 Posterior-anterior view of the LASE device within the disc. ©2010 Clarus Medical LLC.

contact the outer edge of the annulus, taking care not to advance the guide needle.

The dilator is removed, and the trephine is placed over the guide needle and through the working channel until it contacts the AF. The trephine is rotated in a clockwise motion to make a circular incision on the wall of the annulus to provide an entry point to the nucleus by the LASE device. The trephine is removed, and the dilator is reattached to the working channel.

The working channel/dilator pair should be advanced gently so the distal tip lies inside the outer edge of the annulus. After the skin stopper is lowered and secured and the dilator and guide needle removed, the LASE endoscope is inserted down to the nucleus (**Fig. 11-11**).

The laser settings can be adjusted to desired levels. The training manual notes that the maximum recommended "average power setting" is 30 watts. This may best be achieved with an energy setting of 2.0 joules/pulse at a rate of 15 pulses/second. However, it may be more comfortable to begin the procedure at a lower power setting. Constant irrigation and aspiration must be maintained throughout the procedure to avoid clogging and thermo-coagulation and to promote safety and patient comfort.

Outcomes

Although there are no randomized controlled studies examining PLDD, there are over 30 observational and retrospective studies. All of these studies were positive, with overall success rates ranging from 56% to 87%. The criticisms related to PLDD have been mainly directed at the dearth of better quality studies.

The results of evidence-based reviews on PLDD have been mixed. Gibson and Wadell[55] concluded that the results of the extant literature were fair but that PLDD was not superior to open surgical techniques. Schenk and associates[62] noted that, despite its long history, scientific proof of efficacy remained relatively poor, although the potential medical and economic benefits of PLDD were too high to justify discarding on the sole basis of insufficient scientific proof. Other reviews have been more positive. Boswell and colleagues[63] determined that the evidence was moderate for short-term and limited for long-term relief for PLDD. In a more recent analysis focusing solely on laser disc decompression, Singh and associates[64] gave a favorable recommendation to the technique in carefully selected patients.

Complications

The most common complication related to PLDD is the same as for other percutaneous disc interventions—spondylodiscitis, which can be further classified into aseptic and septic. Aseptic discitis is believed to be the result of heat damage, occurring in between 0.3% and 1.2% of subjects.[65] In a retrospective analysis involving 658 cases, Mayer, Brock, and Stern[66] reported intraoperative and postoperative complication rates of 1.1% and 1.5%, respectively. These included discitis and injuries to nerve root, vascular structures, and transverse processes.

Stryker Dekompressor System

The Stryker Dekompressor (Allendale, NJ) is a self-contained single-use probe intended for percutaneous discectomies in the lumbar, thoracic, and cervical spine. The device contains a drill with a spiral-tipped probe (**Fig. 11-12**) that acts via Archimedes' principle to remove nuclear material from the center of protruding discs that are focally contained. Differences between this device and other percutaneous technologies include a smaller gauge and simplicity of use. The main drawback is that it removes less disc material than the other previously described procedures. Unlike the LASE system, it also contains a fixed probe that is more difficult to redirect within the nucleus (**Fig. 11-13**).

Technique

Using standard discographic procedures, the introducer and stylet are inserted into the disc. The stylet is removed, and the probe tip is advanced into the introducer until it extends one full turn beyond the cannula. The collection chamber is attached to the cannula.

The Dekompressor is then turned on, and the probe is slowly advanced under live fluoroscopy at a rate of approximately 1 cm/10 sec. A green depth marker secured at the skin marks the depth of the anterior annulus nucleus boundary. After 3 minutes the probe may be removed and inspected for NP tissue. The procedure can be repeated after cleaning the probe, depending on the volume of tissue needed and observed. The manufacturer recommends discontinuing the procedure when:

- The physician believes that sufficient material has been removed.
- The collection chamber is full.
- No material is present on the probe following 3 minutes of activation.
- A maximum of 10 minutes of operation has expired.

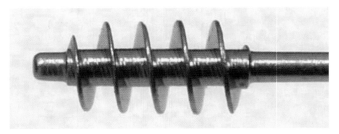

Fig. 11-12   The spiral-tipped probe. ©2010 Stryker Corporation.

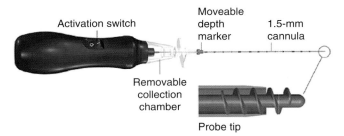

Fig. 11-13   The Stryker Dekompressor. ©2010 Stryker Corporation.

Outcomes

There is a paucity of literature regarding the Dekompressor device. A recent review identified only four studies, with two from the same cohort of patients. Only half of the studies met the minimal criteria for quality. As a result, the recommendation for use was favorable but weak.

In an observational study involving 64 patients, Lierz, Alò, and Felleiter[67] reported an average decrease in pain scores from 7.3 to 2.1 after 12 months, with 80% of the study patients able to reduce their pain medications. In an earlier observational study performed in 50 patients, Amoretti and associates[68] reported a >70% decrease in pain in 72% of cases. Of note, better outcomes were obtained in more lateral disc herniations.

Risk and Complication Avoidance

Although none of the published studies dealt specifically with complications, the same risks exist as for other percutaneous procedures. There is also one report of a probe disconnecting from the parent unit, requiring surgical removal.[69]

Radiofrequency Coblation (Plasma Discectomy)

"Coblation" is short for "controlled ablation" and is composed of two processes: ablation of tissues followed by coagulation. When first introduced, coblation technology was used for arthroscopic surgery, but a plethora of other indications (e.g., tonsillectomies, facial resurfacing) soon followed. These indications were further expanded to the treatment of spinal pain in 1999 when ArthroCare Spine (Austin, Tex) received U.S. Food and Drug Administration (FDA) clearance for its first spine system, a procedure using the Perc-D catheter.

The mechanical basis for the use of coblation technology is the same as for other PDD devices (i.e., a small decrease in intradiscal volume substantially reduces pressure within the disc and surrounding tissues). The temperatures attained during the procedure are relatively low, between 40° and 70°C, thereby reducing the risk of heat-related damage. During the ablation phase an electric field is generated between electrodes. With current flowing through an electrically conductive solution (i.e., saline), a voltage is introduced across the electrodes, exciting electrolytes in the solution and creating a plasma field. This plasma field contains charged particles with sufficient energy to break soft tissue molecular bonds, creating elemental molecules and low-molecular-weight gases as by-products. These by-product gases (e.g., oxygen, nitrogen, hydrogen, carbon dioxide) exit the disc through the introducer needle.[70]

Indications/Contraindications

The indications for radiofrequency (RF) coblation discectomy are essentially the same as noted for other PDD. More recently this technique has also been used to treat discogenic low back pain, albeit with a lesser degree of effectiveness.

Technique

Using standard discographic procedures, the supplied 17-gauge Crawford introducer needle is placed into the disc space. The spine wand is then inserted inside the cannula until the tip is at the end. At this point a circumferential marker is used to determine the proximal limit of the wand. The wand is subsequently advanced until it contacts the anterior annular border, after which the adjustable depth-stop is secured to make sure that the wand does not penetrate the annular fibers. Decompression can now begin. There are two modes on the machine: ablation and coagulation. Ablation is applied while the wand is advanced forward at a rate of 0.5 mL/

sec. As the needle is withdrawn at the same rate, the coagulation mode is used. A total of six channels is usually created at the two, four, six, eight, ten, and twelve o'clock positions, although some people elect to generate more.

Outcomes Evidence

Several reviews have been published on RF coblation. A systematic review by Manchikanti and associates[71] evaluating five studies containing a total of 332 patients with at least 1-year follow-up reported an average of 71% pain relief (range 56% to 80%). The authors concluded that there was weak evidence supporting nucleoplasty for radicular low back pain secondary to a disc herniation.

A more recent systematic review published in the same journal was even more favorable. Gerges, Lipsitz, and Nedeljkovic[72] evaluated 14 trials in which nucleoplasty was performed to treat discogenic pain. In contrast to the review by Manchikanti and colleagues, this article included studies with as little as 2-week follow-up and patients who were experiencing only axial pain. They concluded that there was strong evidence to support nucleoplasty for pain secondary to a contained disc herniation.

In contrast to these two reviews written by interventionalists, a review by the American Pain Society (noninterventionalists) was less auspicious. They concluded that there was "good or fair evidence" that percutaneous intradiscal RF thermocoagulation was not effective.[73]

Risk and Complication Avoidance

In an observational study involving 49 patients, Bhagia and associates[74] found the only complications to be procedure-related pain, increased low back pain, and paresthesias. Smuck and colleagues[75] reported a single case of epidural fibrosis after nucleoplasty. In addition to the aforementioned complications, the same risks exist for nucleoplasty as for other procedures.

Chymopapain

History

Chemonucleolysis using chymopapain was the first percutaneous intradiscal therapy for herniated NP. First isolated in 1941, chymopapain is a proteolytic enzyme derived from the crude latex of *Carica papaya*. In 1963 Lynan Smith[76] demonstrated dissolution of the NP while leaving the annulus intact and the following year reported positive results in human trials. Long accepted as a viable alternative to surgery, its use became controversial because of cases of fatal anaphylaxis and permanent neurological deficits. In 2003 it was placed on the FDA's "discontinued drug product list," which states that it was "not removed for reasons of safety or effectiveness."[77]

Indications

Chemonucleolysis is somewhat different from other PDD techniques in that the disc herniation can be contained or noncontained, as long as it is neither sequestered nor fragmented. Outcomes are improved if nerve root tension signs are present.[78,79] Additional levels can be injected if the same criteria apply. It has been shown to be safe and effective in patients ages 60 to 80, provided there is adequate hydration of the disc.[80]

Contraindications

Aside from the contraindications previously mentioned, prior treatment with chymopapain is thought to sensitize the patient and increase the likelihood of an allergic reaction; however, repeat treatments have been shown to be safe and effective.[81,82]

Equipment/Technique

Patients are screened for chymopapain allergy using the Chymo-FAST test before the procedure. It is a test for the chymopapain-specific immunoglobulin (Ig)E antibodies thought to mediate anaphylaxis. Positive tests were found in 0.94% of 11,658 patients.[83] Patients also receive pretreatment with H_1 and H_2 blockers for 24 hours. Prophylactic steroids have also been advocated but are of questionable benefit.[84] Large-bore intravenous access, 100% oxygen, and adequate hydration can help mitigate an anaphylactic reaction.

Chymopapain is available in 4000- and 10000-unit vials. A 4000-unit amount is reconstituted with 2 mL of sterile water. Bacteriostatic water may inactivate the enzyme. Alcohol used to cleanse the vial stopper must be allowed to air dry before proceeding with reconstitution because residual alcohol may also inactivate the enzyme. After chymopapain is reconstituted, the solution should be used within 2 hours. Unused portions of the solution must be discarded.[85] A study comparing 2000 to 4000 units found no difference in outcomes at 12 months compared to 4000 units. But there was no decrease in side effects, including back pain.[80] Although the maximum dosage is 10,000 units, doses as low as 500 units per disc have been advocated.[86]

Chymopapain is potentially toxic in the subarachnoid space, especially when mixed with iodinated contrast. It disrupts small blood vessels, causing subarachnoid hemorrhage. The use of discography during chymopapain administration is controversial; some recommend it to reduce the chance of diffuse epidural extravasation, whereas others believe that it increases risk. A saline acceptance test is an alternative to confirm an intact annulus, but epidural leakage is not a contraindication to chemonucleolysis.[87] If epidural leakage is present, the medication should be injected very slowly over a 5- to 10-minute period to allow for adequate binding of the enzyme to the proteins. Intradiscal antibiotics are not injected because they might inactivate the enzyme, and needles should be restyletted before removal.

Patient Management/Evaluation

Physical therapy can begin as soon as tolerated. Modalities such as hot packs, cold packs and electrical stimulation may help with postprocedure muscle spasms. Oral analgesics, nonsteroidal anti-inflammatory drugs, and muscle relaxants are all appropriate after the procedure. Walking and sidestroke swimming have been advocated by some.[82] Patients can return to light activity by 2 weeks and full activity as early as 6 weeks.

Outcomes

Chemonucleolysis is well acknowledged to be an effective treatment for sciatica caused by herniated discs. A meta-analysis by Couto, Castilho, and Menezes[88] identified five placebo-controlled studies, four of which were positive. In the lone negative study, a nonsignificant trend for superior pain relief was noted in the treatment group, which persisted for longer than one year.[89] In comparative-effectiveness studies comparing chemonucleolysis with chymopapain or collagenase, three of four trials found significant benefit for both treatments with no difference between the two treatments, whereas one favored chymopapain. In studies comparing chymopapain to surgery, seven studies favored surgery, three showed no difference between groups, and one reported chymopapain to be superior. A larger review evaluating 28 retrospective trials found a positive response rate of 75%.[90]

In a study comparing long-term follow-up of patients who have undergone postchymopapain laminectomy vs. patients who have undergone repeat laminectomy, better results were obtained in patients who received chemonucleolysis.[91] A cost-effectiveness study by Ramirez and Javid[92] found chymopapain treatment to be significantly less expensive, with reoperation rates comparable between groups. Another study conducted in 104 patients suggested that intraoperative chymopapain during lumbar microdiscectomy reduced the rate of recurrent disc herniation.[93] Ideal candidates for chymopapain chemonucleolysis are leg pain worse than back pain, focal protrusion (rather than diffuse bulge), young age, and shorter duration of symptoms.

Risks/Complications

Nordby, Fraser, and Javid[82] reviewed the records of 135,000 patients treated with chymopapain chemonucleolysis over a 9-year period. One hundred twenty-one adverse events were reported to the FDA. There were seven cases of fatal anaphylaxis, and an all-cause mortality rate of 0.019%. Other serious adverse events included acute transverse myelitis, multiple sclerosis, recurrent disc herniations, Guillain-Barré syndrome, and meningitis. In the 31 neurological events (0.024%), complete or partial recovery occurred in 19 patients.

In 1990 Bouillet[87] reviewed 43,662 cases from 316 departments in Europe and the United States. The overall complication rate was 3.7%. Of these cases 1% resolved without treatment, including allergic reactions, voiding difficulties, and temporary neurological deficits; 0.14% resolved with treatment, including deep venous thrombosis, pulmonary embolus, and ileus. There were 0.44% "severe" complications. These included discitis, anaphylaxis, meningitis, pancreatitis, and cauda equina syndrome. No deaths were reported.

Life-threatening anaphylaxis is a known side effect of chymopapain with an incidence rate of <1%. Since 1982 there has been a reduction in the incidence of anaphylaxis as a result of avoiding chemonucleolysis in patients with IgE antibodies to chymopapain, prophylactic use of H_1 and H_2 blockers, preoperative fluids, and physician education.[94]

Oxygen-Ozone Therapy

Although not yet FDA-approved in the United States, oxygen-ozone therapy has been widely used in Europe since the mid-1990s. Oxygen-ozone therapy exploits the chemical properties of ozone. Among the many biological properties attributed to ozone are bactericidal effects, immunomodulation, direct analgesia, and antiinflammatory effects.[95]

Ozone is a known toxic compound. In addition to being well documented as an atmospheric pollutant, it has also has been shown to cause damage to the lungs with prolonged exposure. This is because, when surface tissue molecules are exposed to ozone, a chemical reaction occurs that results in the formation of reactive oxygen-containing compounds such as hydrogen peroxide, hydroperoxides, and other free radicals. In high concentrations these can overwhelm the natural antioxidant defense system of the body, leading to tissue damage. The principle behind medical ozone uses is that lesser amounts of oxidative stress exert positive effects on exposed tissues such as improved O_2 delivery, immune activation, release of autacoids, NO and growth factors, and up-regulation of antioxidant enzymes.[96]

The histological effects of ozone are based on interactions with proteoglycans. When ozone contacts disc tissue, a cascade occurs, resulting in the release of free radicals and subsequent tissue damage. The immediate result of this process is the contraction of nuclear material and activation of fibroblasts, which in turn leads to further scarring and reduction in volume. Histologically, the NP

after ozonolysis shows scarring and desiccation. This suggests that the oxidative stress within the confines of the anaerobic disc is far greater than that which normally occurs within blood. The analgesic and antiinflammatory effects that occur after ozone exposure may be partially caused by decreased release and activation of cytokines, bradykinins, prostaglandins, and other pain-inducing substances.[97]

Indications/Contraindications

Indications for oxygen-ozone therapy are similar to those for other PDD techniques. However, because ozone therapy does not rely exclusively on reduction in intradiscal volumes, it has also been advocated as a treatment for extruded discs and degenerative spondylosis.[98] The ideal candidates for this procedure are patients with a disc herniation and annular tear, in which case the gas migrates out through the rupture, exposing the herniated NP and inflamed nerve root to the oxygen-ozone mixture. The contraindications to ozone-oxygen therapy are the same as for other PDD procedures.

Technique

The initial preparatory steps for disc access have been described previously in the chapter.

Using standard discographic technique, a 22-gauge spinal needle is inserted into the center of the disc. Unlike discography, it is not recommended that contrast be injected because the limited disc volume may make it difficult or impossible to inject the ozone-oxygen solution.

At this point the ozone gas is prepared. The machine is connected to an oxygen source, and ozone is created through ionization of oxygen. Most machines are set up to administer preset medical doses, typically 25 to 40 mcg/mL of ozone in oxygen. The optimal volume depends on the condition and capacity of the disc itself. If there is a lumbar annular tear, approximately 4 mL of gas is released into the disc, and another 8 mL outside the disc in the area of the herniation. In the absence of an annular tear, only a limited amount of gas can be injected into the disc. Smaller volumes are used for cervical disc herniations.

Once the solution is prepared, it must be injected quickly because the ozone within the mixture rapidly degrades back to oxygen (typically at a rate of 2 mcg/mL every 20 seconds). The gas is injected at a steady rate until resistance is felt, after which it may be "pumped in" gently for a few more seconds. The usual time it takes to complete the injection is approximately 15 seconds. Once the disc itself has been filled with the gaseous ozone solution, the needle can be withdrawn into the epidural space, and an additional 8 mL of solution injected.

Ozone usually takes about 2 weeks for a clinical benefit to be realized. If the patient is in severe, acute pain, some practitioners elect to administer concomitant ESIs (**Figs. 11-14** and **11-15**).

Patient Management/Evaluation

After treatment it is recommended that the patient rest in a recumbent position for the next 2 hours to allow the gas to diffuse throughout the disc and dissolve into the interstitial fluid. At discharge patients are instructed to resume normal activity gradually.

Outcomes Evidence

Most clinical studies relating to the use of ozone-oxygen therapy have come out of Europe, in particular Italy, where both intradiscal and intramuscular injections of ozone-oxygen are relatively commonplace.

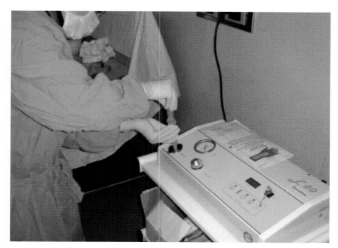

Fig. 11-14 Withdrawing the ozone from the generator. Courtesy Minimus spine.

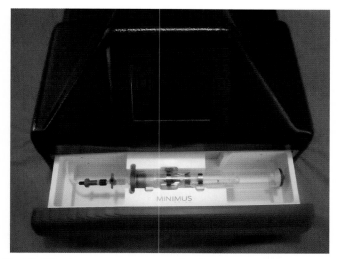

Fig. 11-15 An ozone generator and syringe. Courtesy Minimus spine.

Andreula and associates[95] prospectively studied 600 patients with lumbar disc herniations to receive either intradiscal ozone alone or intradiscal ozone and periganglionic steroids. In both groups the treatment was considered a success (good or excellent outcomes), but higher rates of success were reported in the steroid group (70.3% vs. 78. 3% at 6 months).[95] In a later study by Galluci and associates[99] (n = 159), the authors found that the combination of ozone treatment with intradiscal and transforaminal steroids was superior to steroids alone (74% vs. 47% success rate at 6 months).

A retrospective study by Muto and colleagues[100] in 2900 patients with lumbar disc herniations showed success rates of 75% to 80% for soft disc herniation, 70% for multiple-disc herniations, and 55% for failed back surgery syndrome.[100]

Wu and associates[101] showed comparable effects for ozone combined with collagenase and open surgery for noncontained lumbar herniated discs. In the ozone group success rates at 3 and 12 months were 86% and 89%, respectively, vs. 93% and 95% in the surgical group.

Interestingly, similar results have been obtained with intramuscular injections of ozone. In a placebo-controlled study by Paoloni and associates,[102] 60 patients with axial low back pain with or without lower extremity radiation secondary to a herniated disc received either triweekly injections of 20 mL ozone into the paraspinal muscles or sham injections for 5 weeks. The treatment arm showed a "pain-free" success rate of 61% at 6 months vs. 33% for the sham treatment. The authors concluded that the beneficial effect was achieved through the inhibition of proinflammatory cytokines.

Risk and Complication Avoidance

Ozone is a toxic compound if given in high enough doses. If toxic doses are given, the normal antioxidant capacity of the body becomes overwhelmed, and cell damage and death can ensue. The dosages prescribed for ozone therapy have been defined experimentally and are well within our antioxidative capacity. To date no complication has been attributed to ozone toxicity.

The complications that have occurred were attributable to disc access and misplaced injectate. These include two cases of infection, with one resulting in septicemia and death.[103,104] In addition there was one reported case of pneumocephalus secondary to intrathecal spread of ozone, resulting in a thunderclap headache that resolved over several days.[105]

Conclusions

It is estimated that between one third and one half of all cases of spinal pain are neuropathic in nature. Among the various etiologies of radiculopathy, herniated discs account for a majority in the nonelderly population. There is currently no safe and reliable treatment for neuropathic spinal pain. Medications, both complementary and alternative, tend to have small effect sizes, and surgery is a major endeavor that may not significantly alter the long-term course of the condition. Outcomes for standard decompression surgery are also poorer for small, contained disc herniations than for larger extrusions or sequestrations, which forms the rationale for PDD techniques. The strongest evidence for nonsurgical interventions is for ESIs, which in carefully selected patients may reduce the need for surgery. The epidural administration of TNF inhibitors is a promising field, but more research must be done before it can be recommended for widespread human use. There is compelling evidence to support chemonucleolysis for disc herniations, but its use must be weighed against the low risk of catastrophic complications, which can be minimized with proper screening, preventive measures, and physician education. More research is needed to identify the ideal candidates for the other PDD techniques and to better determine effectiveness.

References

1. Mixter W, Barr J: Rupture of the intervertebral disc with involvement of the spinal canal. *N Engl J Med* 211:210-215, 1934.
2. Bogduk N: On the definitions and physiology of back pain, referred pain, and radicular pain. *Pain* 147(1-3):17-19, 2009. Epub Sept 16, 2009. Review.
3. Bogduk N: The lumbar disc and low back pain. *Neurosurg Clin North Am* 2:791-806, 1991.
4. Ohtori S et al: Sensory innervation of the dorsal portion of the lumbar intervertebral disc in rats. *Spine* 24:2295-2299, 1999.
5. Inoue G et al: Exposure of the nucleus pulposus to the outside of the annulus fibrosus induces nerve injury and regeneration of the afferent fibers innervating the lumbar intervertebral discs in rats. *Spine* 31:1433-1438, 2006.
6. Coppes MH et al: Innervation of "painful" lumbar discs. *Spine* 15:22(202):2342-2349, 1997.
7. Weiner BK, Patel R: Licensee BioMed Central Ltd. *J Orthop Surg* 3:46, 2008. Epub *J Orthop Surg* Oct 2, 2008.

8. Elves MW, Bucknill T, Sullivan MF: In vitro inhibition of leucocyte migration in patients with intervertebral disc lesions. *Orthop Clin North Am* 6(1):59-65, 1975.

9. Takahashi H et al: Inflammatory cytokines in the herniated disc of the lumbar spine. *Spine* 21(2):218-224, 1996.

10. Kang JD et al: Toward a biochemical understanding of human intervertebral disc degeneration and herniation: contributions of nitric oxide, interleukins, prostaglandin E2, and matrix metalloproteinases. *Spine* 22(10):1065-1073, 1997.

11. Freemont AJ: The cellular pathobiology of the degenerate intervertebral disc and discogenic back pain. *Rheumatology (Oxford)* 48(1):5-10, 2009. Epub 2008.

12. Olmarker K, Rydevik B: Selective inhibition of tumor necrosis factor-alpha prevents nucleus pulposus-induced thrombus formation, intraneural edema, and reduction of nerve conduction velocity: possible implications for future pharmacologic treatment strategies of sciatica. *Spine* 26:863-869, 2001.

13. Sekiguchi M et al: Comparison of neuropathic pain and neuronal apoptosis following nerve root or spinal nerve compression. *Eur Spine J* 18(12):1978-1985, 2009. Epub June 19, 2009.

14. Shubayev V, Myers RR: Axonal transport of TNF-alpha in painful neuropathy: distribution of ligand tracer and TNF receptors. *J Neuroimmunol* 114:48-56, 2001.

15. Jensen MC et al: Magnetic resonance imaging of the lumbar spine in people without back pain. *N Engl J Med* 331(2):69-73, 1994.

16. Mirzai H et al: The results of nucleoplasty in patients with herniated disc: a prospective study of 52 consecutive patients. *Spine J* 7(1):88-92, 2007.

17. Weiner BK, Patel R: The accuracy of MRI in the detection of lumbar disc containment. *J Orthop Surg Res* 3:46, 2008.

18. Cluff R et al: The technical aspects of epidural steroid injections: a national survey. *Anesth Analg* 95:403-408, 2002.

19. Riew KD et al: The effect of nerve-root injections on the need for operative treatment of lumbar radicular pain: a prospective, randomized, controlled, double-blind study. *J Bone Joint Surg (Am)* 82-A(11):1589-1593, 2000.

20. Bogduk N et al: Complications of spinal diagnostic and treatment procedures. *Pain Med* 6:S11-S34, 2008.

21. Kennedy DJ et al: Paraplegia following image-guided transforaminal lumbar spine epidural steroid injection: two case reports. *Pain Med* 10(8):1389-1394, 2009. Epub Oct 26, 2009.

22. Kane RE: Neurologic deficits following epidural or spinal anesthesia. *Anesth Analg* 60:150-161, 1981.

23. Raj PP et al: Bleeding risk in interventional pain practice: assessment, management, and review of the literature. *Pain Physician* 6:3-52, 2004.

24. Horlocker TT et al: Regional anesthesia in the patient receiving antithrombotic or thrombolytic therapy: American Society of Regional Anesthesia and Pain Medicine Evidence-Based Guidelines. ed 3. *Reg Anesth Pain Med* 35(1):64-101, 2010.

25. Stojanovic MP et al: The role of fluoroscopy in cervical epidural steroid injections. *Spine* 27(5):509-514, 2002.

26. Fredman B et al: Epidural steroid for treating "Failed back surgery syndrome": is fluoroscopy really necessary? *Reg Anesth Pain Med* 88:367-372, 1999.

27. Koes B et al: Efficacy of epidural steroid injections for low back pain and sciatica: a systematic review of randomized clinical trials. *Pain* 63:279-288, 1995.

28. Abdi S et al: Epidural steroids in the management of chronic spinal pain: a systematic review. *Pain Physician* 10:185-212, 2007.

29. Peloso PM et al: Medicinal and injection therapies for mechanical neck disorders: a Cochrane systematic review. *J Rheumatol* 33(5):957-967, 2006.

30. Nelemans P et al: Injection therapy for subacute and chronic benign low back pain. *Spine* 26:501-515, 2001.

31. Rozenberg S et al: Efficacy of epidural steroids in low back pain and sciatica. *Revue du Rhumatisme* 66:79-85, 1999.

32. Airaksinen O et al: Chapter 4: European guidelines for the management of chronic nonspecific low back pain. *Eur Spine J* 15:S192-S300, 2006.

33. Armon C et al: Assessment: use of epidural steroid injections to treat radicular lumbosacral pain. *Neurology* 2007;68:723-729, 2007.

34. Boswell MV et al A systematic review of therapeutic facet joint interventions in chronic spinal pain. *Pain Physician* 10:229-253, 2007.

35. Riew KD, Park JB, Cho YS et al. Nerve root blocks in the treatment of lumbar radicular pain. *J Bone Joint Surg [Am]* 88-A(8):1722-1725, 2006.

36. Thomas E et al: Efficacy of transforaminal versus interspinous corticosteroid injection in discal radiculargia—a prospective, randomised, double-blind study. *Clin Rheumatol* 22:299-304, 2003.

37. Schaufele MK, Hatch L, Jones W: Interlaminar versus transforaminal epidural injections for the treatment of symptomatic lumbar intervertebral disc herniations. *Pain Physician* 9(4):361-366, 2006.

38. Hoyland JA, Le Maitre C, Freemont AJ: Investigation of the role of IL-1 and TNF in matrix degradation in the intervertebral disc. *Rheumatology (Oxford)* 47(6):809-814, 2008.

39. Olmarker K, Rydevik B: Selective inhibition of tumor necrosis factor-alpha prevents nucleus pulposus–induced thrombus formation, intraneural edema, and reduction of nerve conduction velocity: possible implications for future pharmacologic treatment strategies of sciatica. *Spine* 26(8):863-869, 2001.

40. Olmarker K, Nutu M, Størkson R: Changes in spontaneous behavior in rats exposed to experimental disc herniation are blocked by selective TNF-alpha inhibition. *Spine* 28(15):1635-1641, 2003.

41. Genevay S, Stingelin S, Gabay C: Efficacy of etanercept in the treatment of acute, severe sciatica: a pilot study. *Ann Rheum Dis* 63(9):1120-1123, 2004. Epub Apr 28, 2004.

42. Tobinick E, Davoodifar S: Efficacy of etanercept delivered by perispinal administration for chronic back and/or neck disc-related pain: a study of clinical observations in 143 patients. *Curr Med Res Opin* 20(7):1075-1085, 2004.

43. Korhonen T et al: The treatment of disc-herniation-induced sciatica with infliximab: one-year follow-up results of FIRST II, a randomized controlled trial. *Spine* 31(24):2759-2766, 2006.

44. Cohen SP et al: A double-blind, placebo-controlled, dose-response pilot study evaluating intradiscal etanercept in patients with chronic discogenic low back pain or lumbosacral radiculopathy. *Anesthesiology* 07(1):99-105, 2007.

45. Cohen SP et al: Randomized, double-blind, placebo-controlled, dose-response, and preclinical safety study of transforaminal epidural etanercept for the treatment of sciatica. *Anesthesiology* 110(5):1116-1126, 2009.

46. Kume et al: Presented at the 9th Annual European Congress of Rheumatology, Paris, France, June 2008.

47. Carragee EJ et al: Clinical outcomes after lumbar discectomy for sciatica: the effects of fragment type and annular competence. *J Bone Joint Surg [Am]* 85-A:102-108, 2003.

48. Hijikata S: Percutaneous nucleotomy: a new concept technique and 12 years' experience. *Clin Orthop Relat Res* 238:9-23, 1989.

49. Case RB, Choy DS, Altman P: Intervertebral disc pressure as a function of fluid volume infused. *J Clin Laser Med Surg* 13:143-147, 1985.

50. O'Neill CW et al: Percutaneous plasma decompression alters cytokine expression in injured porcine intervertebral discs. *Spine J* 4(1):88-98, 2004.

51. Chang JD et al: Ameliorative effect of ozone on cytokine production in mice injected with human rheumatoid arthritis synovial fibroblast cells. *Rheumatol Int* 26(2):142-151, 2005.

52. Onik G et al: Percutaneous lumbar discectomy using a new aspiration probe: porcine and cadaver. *Radiology* 155(1):251-252, 1985.

53. Boswell MV et al: Interventional techniques: Evidence based practice guidelines in the management of chronic spinal pain. *Pain Physician* 10:107-111, 2007.

54. Hirsch JA et al: Automated percutaneous lumbar discectomy for the contained herniated lumbar disc: a systematic assessment of evidence. *Pain Physician* 12(3):601-620, 2009.

55. Gibson JNA, Waddell G. Surgical interventions for lumbar disc prolapse, *Cochrane Database Syst Rev* 1:CD001350, 2009.

56. *Percutaneous discectomy:* Washington State Department of Labor and Industries, Office of Medical Director, February 24, 2004.

57. Teng GJ et al: Automated percutaneous lumbar discectomy: a prospective multi-institutional study. *J Vasc Interv Radiol* 8(3):457-463, 1997.

58. Maroon JC, Allen AC: A retrospective study of 1,054 APLD cases: a twenty-month clinical follow-up at 35 US centers. *J Neurol Orthop Med Surg* 10:335-337, 1989.

59. Carragee EJ et al: 2009 ISSLS Prize Winner: Does discography cause accelerated progression of degeneration changes in the lumbar disc: a ten-year matched cohort study. *Spine* 34(21):2338-2345, 2009.

60. Lee SH, Kang HS: Percutaneous endoscopic laser annuloplasty for discogenic low back pain. *Surg Neurol* Epub ahead of print, March 2009.

61. Quigley MR et al: Laser discectomy: comparison of systems. *Spine* 19(3):319-322, 1994.

62. Schenk B et al: Percutaneous laser disk decompression: a review of the literature. *AJNR Am J Neuroradiol* 27:232-235, 2006.

63. Boswell MV et al: Interventional techniques: evidence-based practice guidelines in the management of chronic spinal pain. American Society of Interventional Pain Physicians. *Pain Physician* 10(1):7-111, 2007.

64. Singh V et al: Percutaneous lumbar laser disc decompression: a systematic review of current evidence. *Pain Physician* 12(3):573-588, 2009.

65. Choy DS et al: 23rd Anniversary of Percutaneous Laser Disc Decompression (PLDD. *Photomed Laser Surg* 27(4):535-538, 2009.

66. Mayer HM, Brock M, Stern E: Percutaneous endoscopic laser discectomy: experimental results. In Mayer HM, Mrock M, editors: *Percutaneous Lumbar Discectomy*, Heidelberg, 1989, Springer-Verlag.

67. Lierz P, Alò KM, Felleiter P: Percutaneous lumbar discectomy using the Dekompressor system under CT-control. *Pain Pract* 9(3):216-220, 2009. Epub March 3, 2009.

68. Amoretti N et al: Clinical follow-up of 50 patients treated by percutaneous lumbar discectomy. *Clin Imaging* 30(4):242-244, 2006.

69. Domsky R et al: Critical failure of a percutaneous discectomy probe requiring surgical removal during disc decompression. *Reg Anesth Pain Med* 31(2):177-179, 2006.

70. Singh V et al: Percutaneous disc decompression using coblation (nucleoplasty) in the treatment of chronic discogenic pain. *Pain Physician* 5(3):250-259, 2002. Erratum in *Pain Physician* 5(4):445, 2002.

71. Manchikanti L et al: A systematic review of mechanical lumbar disc decompression with nucleoplasty. *Pain Physician* 12(3):561-572, 2009.

72. Gerges FJ, Lipsitz SR, Nedeljkovic SS: A systematic review on the effectiveness of the nucleoplasty procedure for discogenic pain. *Pain Physician* 13(2):117-132, 2010.

73. Chou R et al: Nonsurgical interventional therapies for low back pain: a review of the evidence for an American Pain Society clinical practice guideline. *Spine* 34(10):1078-1093, 2009. Review.

74. Bhagia SM et al: Side effects and complications after percutaneous disc decompression using coblation technology. *Am J Phys Med* 85:6-13, 2006.

75. Smuck M et al: Epidural fibrosis following percutaneous disc decompression with coblation technology. *Pain Physician* 10(5):691-696, 2007.

76. Smith L: Enzyme dissolution of the nucleus pulposus in humans. *JAMA* 187:137-140, 1964.

77. Simmons JW, Fraser RD: The rise and fall of chemonucleolysis. In Kambin P, editor: *Arthroscopic and endoscopic spinal surgery: text and atlas*, ed 2, Totowa, NJ, 2002, Humana Press, pp 351-357.

78. McCulloch JA: Chemonucleolysis. *J Bone Joint Surg* 59:45-52, 1977.

79. McCulloch JA: Chemonucleolysis: experience with 2000 cases. *Clin Orthop* 146:128-135, 1980.

80. Benoist M: A randomized, double-blind study to compare low-dose with standard-dose chymopapain in the treatment of herniated lumbar intervertebral discs. *Spine* 18(1):28-34, 1993.

81. Sutton CJ, Jr: Repeat chemonucleolysis. *Clin Orthop* 206:45-49, 1986.

82. Nordby EJ, Fraser RD, Javid MJ: Chemonucleolysis. *Spine* 21:1102-1105, 1996.

83. Tsay YG et al: A preoperative chymopapain sensitivity test for chemonucleolysis candidates. *Spine* 9(7):764-768, 1984.

84. McKinnon RP: Allergic reactions during anaesthesia. *Curr Opin Anaesthesiol* 9:267-270, 1996.

85. Chymodiactin package insert (Knoll, Rockville, MD), Rev 2/9/98, Rec 2/4/99.

86. Smith L: Chemonucleolysis: personal history, trials, and tribulations. *Clin Orthop Relat Res* 287:117-124, 1993.

87. Bouillet R: Treatment of sciatica: a comparative survey of complications of surgical treatment and nucleolysis with chymopapain. *Clin Orthop* 251:145-152, 1990.

88. Couto JM, Castilho EA, Menezes PR: Chemonucleolysis in lumbar disc herniation: a meta-analysis. *Clinics (Sao Paulo)* 62(2):175-180, 2007. Review *Clinics* 2007.

89. Martins AN et al: Double-blind evaluation of chemonucleolysis for herniated lumbar discs: late results. *J Neurosurg* 49(6):816-827, 1978.

90. Simmons JW, Stavinoha WB, Knodel LC: Update and review of chemonucleolysis. *Clin Orthop Relat Res* 183:51-60, 1984.

91. Postacchini F, Lami R, Massobrio M: Chemonucleolysis versus surgery in lumbar disc herniations: correlation of the results to preoperative clinical pattern and size of the herniation. *Spine* 12(2):87-96, 1987.

92. Ramirez LF, Javid MJ: Cost effectiveness of chemonucleolysis versus laminectomy in the treatment of herniated nucleus pulposus. *Spine* 10(4):363-367, 1985.

93. Alden TD et al: Intraoperative chymopapain in lumbar laminotomy for disc disease: a less invasive technique. *Neurosurg Focus* 15:4(2):e10, 1998.

94. Moss J et al: Decreased incidence and mortality of anaphylaxis to chymopapain. *Anesth Analg* 64:1197-1201, 1985.

95. Andreula CF et al: Minimally invasive oxygen-ozone therapy for lumbar disk herniation. *AJNR Am J Neuroradiol* 24:996-1000, 2003.

96. Bocci V: Is it true that ozone is always toxic? The end of a dogma. *Toxicol Appl Pharmacol* 216(3):493-504, 2006. Epub Jun 27, 2006. Review.

97. Bocci V et al: Studies on the biological effects of ozone. Part 3. An attempt to define conditions for optimal induction of cytokines. *Lymphokine Cytokine Res* 12(2):121-126, 1993.

98. Oder B et al: CT-guided ozone/steroid therapy for the treatment of degenerative spinal disease—effect of age, gender, disc pathology and multi-segmental changes. *Neuroradiology* 50(9):777-785, 2008 Epub May 16, 2008.

99. Gallucci M et al: Sciatica: treatment with intradiscal and intraforaminal injections of steroid and oxygen-ozone versus steroid only. *Radiology* 242(3):907-913, 2007.

100. Muto M et al: Low back pain and sciatica: treatment with intradiscal-intraforaminal O(2)-O(3) injection: our experience. *Radiol Med* 113(5):695-706, 2008.

101. Wu Z et al: Percutaneous treatment of non-contained lumbar disc herniation by injection of oxygen-ozone combined with collagenase. *Eur J Radiol* 72(3):499-504, 2009.

102. Paoloni M et al: Intramuscular oxygen-ozone therapy in the treatment of acute back pain with lumbar disc herniation: a multicenter, randomized, double-blind, clinical trial of active and simulated lumbar paravertebral injection. *Spine* 34(13):1337-1344, 2009.

103. Bo W et al: A pyogenic discitis at C3-C4 with associated ventral epidural abscess involving C1-C4 after intradiscal oxygen-ozone chemonucleolysis: a case report. *Spine* 34(8):E298-304, 2009.

104. Gazzeri R et al: Fulminating septicemia secondary to oxygen-ozone therapy for lumbar disc herniation: case report. *Spine* 32(3):E121-123, 2007.

105. Devetag CF et al: Thunderclap headache caused by minimally invasive medical procedures: description of two cases. *Headache* 47(2):293-295, 2007.

12 Current Surgical Options for Intervertebral Disc Herniation in the Cervical and Lumbar Spine

W. Porter McRoberts and Kevin D. Cairns

CHAPTER OVERVIEW

Chapter Synopsis: The approaches to surgical intervention for disc herniation are multiple, varied, and contentious. The surgical aims remain reduction or elimination of pain, disability, and danger. Approaches may vary among not only individual practitioners but also specialties involved in surgical spine care. This chapter elucidates for the spinal interventionalist the most common surgical options for treatment of disc herniation with or without neural compression in the cervical and lumbar spines. In addition, criteria that guide patient selection, descriptions of surgical techniques, and outcomes and nuances of the particular therapies that influence surgical planning are discussed.

Important Points: Despite a multi-decade history, spine surgery for disc disease remains in its infancy. There exists little compelling evidence to consider disc surgery as a first line of treatment, and surgery should only be considered in cases refractory to conservative care.

Clinical Pearls: The natural history of disc disease still favors the likely resolution of pain and disability. Surgery may be a tempting option in the early disease process, but no bridges are burned from careful conservative care and watchful waiting. Surgical options exist and remain equally effective later in the disease course if conservative care is ultimately unsatisfactory.

Clinical Pitfalls: The early symptoms and signs of central neural compression and neural cell death are important sentinels. Education of patients and practitioners alike on the methods of surveillance for these signs will help keep patients safe. Should signs of irreversible neural death occur, rapid action towards decompression is mandatory.

Introduction

In 1990 nearly 15 million office visits to physicians occurred for mechanical low back pain, the fifth most common reason for seeking medical care.[1] Axial spinal disorders and associated pain present an enormous economic burden on Western health care systems. In the United States from 2003 to 2007 the rate of complex fusion procedures increased 15-fold, and the odds ratio of life-threatening complications from complex fusion vs. simple decompression was 2.95.[2] Little consensus exists regarding the choice of sole decompression vs. decompression combined with fusion.[3,4] In addition, it appears that individual surgeon preference may impact surgical approach more than the surgical pathology.[5] Success is highly varied, and long-term outcome studies are few. Great debate still surrounds disc surgery.

This chapter presents the current surgical options for disc herniation in the cervical and lumbar spines, recognizing that the approaches to each are as vastly different as the functional and structural targets. Surgical treatment of thoracic disc herniation is rarely indicated unless there is concomitant neural danger or recidivist infection; thus it is not included in the text. Cervical and lumbar disc surgery serves two main functions: elimination or control of pain and associated dysfunction or the elimination of danger from neural compression. Many factors must be considered in forming a surgical plan and approach such as pathology, age, gender, and co-morbidities.

Cervical disc herniation is a common cause of pain that can frequently lead to disability. Cote, Cassidy, and Carroll[6] reported that, among 2184 Canadian individuals randomly surveyed between the ages of 20 and 69 years of age, 54% noted significant neck pain in the prior 6 months, with 10% of those individuals rating their pain as "disabling." In a 5-year series examining the natural history of cervical disc disease, 23% of patients remained partially or totally disabled with nonoperative care.[7] Cervical symptoms can result from either direct compression of nerve roots by disc herniation or pain arising from the disc itself.

Cervical Disc Herniation Causing Neural Compression

Patient Selection

Neural compression from cervical intervertebral disc herniation often presents with severe neck pain with distal paresthesias with or without radiating interscapular pain.[8] Ideal surgical patients present with radicular symptoms and magnetic resonance imaging (MRI) findings that match the anticipated dermatomal level.[9] The most commonly involved cervical disc herniations occur at the C5-C6 and C6-C7 levels, with the most common objective sensory deficits affecting C6 and C7 dermatomes and motor deficits most commonly affecting the biceps and triceps muscles.[10] In addition, concordant neurological deficits such as motor weakness in the anticipated myotome, loss of associated motor reflex, and presence of Spurling's sign give further support to disc herniation causing the patient's symptoms and support consideration of surgical treatment. Ideal surgical candidates are those who have failed conservative treatment, including medication management, physical therapy, and epidural steroid injections. Patients with significant neurological symptoms, including worsening motor weakness, bowel or bladder dysfunction, or MRI findings showing significant cord compression, should be referred for surgical evaluation promptly. Younger patients more likely present with soft disc herniations level and are better surgical candidates than older patients with severe multilevel spondylosis.[9]

Surgical Approaches

Surgical treatments for cervical disc herniation depend largely on the location of the disc herniation itself. They can be engaged from an anterior approach with hardware, posterior/posterolateral decompression, or posterior decompression with fusion. Patients with far-lateral disc herniations potentially can be candidates for posterolateral approaches such as keyhole foraminotomy and posterior laminotomy and discectomy. Keyhole foraminotomy describes a technique whereby lateral disc herniations are resected from the inferior aspect of the neural foramen while using a curette or similar instrument to retract the posterior-superior aspect of the foramen and visualize the neural and vascular elements (**Fig. 12-1**). To perform this technique, the lamina of the involved intervertebral level is resected with a rongeur and resected with either a

Kerrison punch or high-speed drill. The lateral third of the ligamentum flavum is resected, the nerve is retracted superiorly, a microsurgical nerve hook is swept below the nerve root, and the disc is resected.[9] The superior aspect of the neuroforamen is often visualized further by resecting part of the cervical facet joint. In a series of 172 patients with cervical lateral disc herniation, 97% of patients noted relief of radicular symptoms at a follow-up period of between 1 and 2 years. In this cohort of patients 35% underwent single-level cervical foraminotomy, 25% underwent single level laminotomy with discectomy, and 40% underwent two-level foraminotomy.[9] Older patients often underwent two-level surgery (mean age 55) compared to younger patients who underwent single-level surgery (mean age 45).[9] Other studies involving microsurgical foraminotomy revealed similar results.[10-12] These studies also stressed the importance of selecting patients with soft lateral disc herniations, minimal myelopathy, and single-level disease.[9-12] Central and paracentral disc herniations sometimes cannot be accessed with a posterior or lateral approach given the position of the spinal cord and the fact that the spinal cord cannot be retracted without severe neurological compromise. Generally younger patients presenting with soft disc herniations without significant spondylitic disease are better suited for posterior/posterolateral discectomy.

A Cochrane database review of the literature in 2009 assessing the efficacy of posterior laminoforaminotomy for the treatment of cervical radiculopathy primarily due to soft lateral disc herniations or cervical spondylosis recommended posterior laminoforaminotomy as a surgical option with class III evidence.[13] Older patients with severe spondylosis with broad-based central disc herniation with calcific stenosis can make posterior surgery more challenging.[9] In addition, significant cervical spondylosis introduces additional pain generators, including cervical facet joints, cervical discogenic pain, uncovertebral joint pain, and cervical instability with Modic changes that may be better served by cervical fusion,

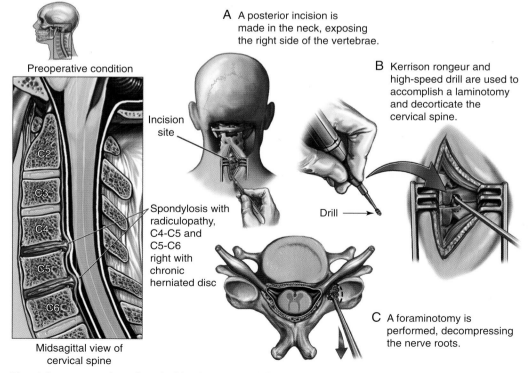

Preoperative condition

A A posterior incision is made in the neck, exposing the right side of the vertebrae.

B Kerrison rongeur and high-speed drill are used to accomplish a laminotomy and decorticate the cervical spine.

Incision site

Spondylosis with radiculopathy, C4-C5 and C5-C6 right with chronic herniated disc

Drill

C A foraminotomy is performed, decompressing the nerve roots.

Midsagittal view of cervical spine

Fig. 12-1 Pictorial representation of cervical laminotomy and foraminotomy. From Phototake Illustration/Stock Illustration Source.

which potentially addresses these additional pain generators. Multiple-level surgery increases the probability of instability since the posterior bony anatomy is weakened and may require the addition of posterior or anterior hardware to facilitate fusion, proper alignment, and stability.[14]

Potential advantages of posterior laminotomy/foraminotomy over anterior surgery/posterior fusion include maintaining segmental motion and proposed less common segmental disc degeneration in adjacent fused levels. The medical literature does not support one technique as being superior to the other either in the short or long term; the type of surgery performed is often a function of a surgeon's particular training and comfort level.[13]

Anterior surgical approach is a suitable approach for cervical radiculopathy and for patients with a large central or paracentral disc herniation. Most of the studies looking at an anterior approach and outcomes have looked at patients with significant myelopathy, which is the result of a variety of pathologies, including cervical disc herniation, uncovertebral joint hypertrophy, facet joint arthropathy, and hypertrophy of the ligamentum flavum, but who have generally shown neurological improvement in 80% to 90% of cases.[15,16] Advantages of anterior cervical discectomy and fusion (ACDF) include arthrodesis of the spine that better corrects cervical kyphosis, better ability to target central disc herniations, better ability to treat ossification of the posterior longitudinal ligament (OPLL), and positive postoperative pain relief.[16] Beginning in the 1950s there has been a shift from posterior to anterior surgery.[17] Anterior cervical surgery was first pioneered by Cloward in 1958[18] and involves retracting the trachea and vascular structures to visualize the involved intervertebral level, decorticating the vertebral endplates, resecting the disc preserving the posterior longitudinal ligament, and placing an anterior plate for stability (Fig. 12-2). The Robinson-Smith is similar to the Cloward procedure except that the vertebral endplates are preserved.[19] Comparisons for anterior and posterior surgical decompression for cervical disc herniation have yielded similar results.[20] Anterior fusion can better address the site of pathology with a central disc herniation. Nerve root trauma associated with a posterior approach can also be reduced with ACDF. In addition, the incidence of postoperative excessive neck flexion resulting from posterior surgical decompression and compromise of the ligamentous attachments to the C7 spinous process can be avoided with an anterior approach. Few studies specifically comparing anterior and posterior approaches for cervical herniated nucleus pulposus (HNP) exist, although studies evaluating cervical spinal myelopathy for anterior and posterior approaches have yielded similar results.[21,22]

Surgical Complications

Infection after cervical surgery overall occurs between 0% and 18% of the time.[23-28] Similar rates have been reported for anterior and posterior surgery, although some authors have reported lower rates for anterior surgery.[25,27] Higher infection rates have been reported in patients with systemic illness, patients on long-term steroids, and immunocompromised patients.[29] Other complications include nerve injury, pulmonary embolism, spinal cord injury, esophageal rupture, and death.[23-25] With anterior surgery plate nonunion or dislocation can occur, and with posterior decompressive surgery kyphotic deformity can develop.[14,30]

Cervical Disc Replacement

Cervical disc replacement is intended for one- or two-level disc disease, although other applications are emerging as well. Artificial disc replacement involves a polyurethane nucleus surrounded by two titanium alloy shells that contain a porous coating to help promote cortical anchoring. In a study of 103 patients with symptomatic radiculopathy and myelopathy, 90% of patients noted greater than 50% improvement of preoperative signs and symptoms with single-level disc replacement.[31] Data for 1 and 3 years have shown success for patients with one- and two-level disc disease, although longer-term studies evaluating device-related complications are needed.[31,32] This study did not show any significant device migration, although several incidences of anterolateral paravertebral ossification were noted on computed tomography (CT) scan. Longer-term data are needed to demonstrate long-term efficacy and the absence of complications, including device migration. A more recent application of placement of cervical arthroplasty after prior fusion and adjacent-level disc degeneration has also been reported that may be more beneficial than extending fusion levels for treating patients with adjacent-level stenosis.[33]

Conclusion

Current surgical solutions for cervical disc herniation involve decompressing the area of pathology and in instances of instability the addition of hardware to facilitate fusion. Several approaches are commonly performed. No clear data exist to show superiority of one technique over another, and decision making is based largely on the site of pathology and a surgeon's training.

Lumbar Disc Herniation and Surgical Approaches

Lumbar disc herniation commonly causes not only low back pain but also radicular pain. It is more common among males, and 70% of those affected are between ages 20 and 40 years; the gross majority of herniations occur at L4-L5 and/or L5-S1.[34] Surgery is indicated when conservative pain treatment measures have failed or there is significant risk of, or impending, neurological injury. This section discusses the various approaches, considerations for surgical planning and technique, and the reported outcomes for anterior decompression (discectomy) and fusion (anterior lumbar interbody fusion [ALIF]), extreme lateral interbody fusion (XLIF), transforaminal lumbar interbody fusion (TLIF), posterior lumbar interbody fusion (PLIF), and disc replacement.

Lumbar Discectomy

Oppenheim and Fedor Krause initially developed discectomy in 1906.[35] To obtain access to the anterior epidural space, fenestration, laminectomy, and hemilaminectomy were developed and are still

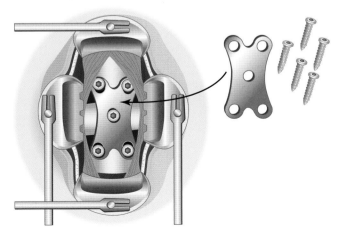

Fig. 12-2 Pictorial representation showing anterior plate typically used in anterior cervical discectomy and fusion procedure.

mainstream approaches to exposure to the large free-fragment disc pathology contributing to neural pressure. Today unilateral transflaval microdiscectomy is standard of care for treatment of patients with symptomatic disc herniation.[36] Historically percutaneous approaches, including chymopapain injection, automated percutaneous discectomy, and multiple other approaches were indicated as a whole for contained disc herniation. Nevertheless, the appeal of small incision and minimally invasive approaches led Casper,[37] Williams,[38] and Yasargil[39] to use microscopes to achieve less muscle and epidural scarring, resulting in diminished perioperative morbidity and higher satisfaction. In 1997 Foley and Smith pioneered the muscle-splitting technique of tubular discectomy, common with such surgical systems as the METRx (Medtronic, Minneapolis, Minn).[36] The gross majority of lumbar discectomies are performed by either open, microscope-assisted microdiscectomy or tubular approaches using either an endoscope or microscope.

The operative techniques are fairly similar, regardless of surgical approach. A posterior or posterolateral approach is taken ipsilateral to the disc bulge. With the open technique a small incision is made, and dissection is made to the lumbodorsal fascia and then deeper through the ipsilateral paravertebral musculature. Using a tubular system, fluoroscopic guidance is used to place a guidewire down to the posterior superior lamina, laterally toward the facet joint. Entry point is a 1.5- to 2-cm incision, about 1 to 1.5 cm lateral to the midline. A series of dilators are then introduced with subsequent dilation of the paraspinous muscles. The ultimate retractor is a 15- to 20-mm diameter tube through which direct observation of the posterior lamina is achieved. At this point either an endoscope is directed down to the operating depth, or a projection microscope allows the surgeon visualization of the field. Regardless of technique, flavectomy and/or laminotomy allow visualization of the dural margin, nerve root, and, with retraction, the offending disc. Free disc fragment is resected, and annulotomy can be performed. Disc forceps trim and resect annulus and nuclear material. After irrigation the field can be covered with Gelfoam (Pfizer, New York, NY), the retraction system of choice is removed, and the fascia and skin are sutured and closed.

Questions remain regarding superiority of technique, and the techniques are frequently compared by a variety of measures. In a randomized controlled trial, both techniques appear similar in terms of muscle injury, with nonsignificant differences in postoperative-to-preoperative creatine phosphokinase ratios and muscular atrophy at 1 year, however the tubular discectomy group had more back pain during the first year after surgery.[36] In an industry-supported study, the measures of cost and length of stay (LOS) tend to favor tubular systems: an 18% cost saving was seen, and LOS was 2 days for conventional approach vs. outpatient for most tubular approaches.[40] Lau and associates[41] compared a retrospective cohort of patients treated with either open microdiscectomy or minimally invasive approaches for lumbar disc herniation and found no statistically significant difference in operative time, length of stay, neurological outcome, complication rate, or pain improvement.

Until recently there was little high-level evidence comparing conservative care to surgery; and meta-analyses, including Cochrane reviews, concluded that little evidence existed to support decompressive lumbar surgery over conservative care.[42] However, the longest prospective cohort study, the Maine Lumbar Spine Study, found surgery superior to conservative care in the treatment of leg pain; but the predominant symptom and work and disability outcomes were similar, regardless of treatment.[43] Despite some methodological restrictions, in a prospective cohort of 100 patients Amundsen and colleagues[44] found surgical treatment to be considerably better than conservative care alone at 4 and 10 years but concluded an initial conservative approach to be superior to a surgical one because patients can later choose surgery.

The Spine Patient Outcomes Research Trial (SPORT) evaluated nonoperative treatment vs. open lumbar discectomy.[45,46] The SPORT trial presented three distinct components: randomized trial with 2-year data, observational study with data collected over 4 years, and combined randomized/observational data collected over 4 years. The initial SPORT trial 2-year data reported significant improvement in both operative and nonoperative groups with no significant statistical differences noted between the groups in primary outcome measures of SF-36 and Oswestry Disability Index. Near equivalence in outcomes at 2 years between both groups caused some concern in the surgical community, given the inherent risks of surgery compared to nonoperative care. However, a very large crossover rate was noted, with many patients in both groups switching their assigned randomized treatment, making it difficult to evaluate statistical benefit of one treatment over the other given the inherent bias created. Primary outcome measures, including SF-36 and Oswestry Disability Index, did not show any statistical differences between the two groups at 2 years; whereas secondary outcome measures of sciatica severity and patient satisfaction did show significance, with surgical patients showing improvement over nonsurgical care. When looking at the surgical (as treated) vs. nonsurgical (as treated) groups, surgical patients demonstrated superior outcomes compared to the nonoperative group at 4 years. The challenges in designing a randomized controlled trial that eliminates high crossover rates may be impossible given the dynamic nature of lumbar HNP and the fact that patients' symptoms change over time.

Increased time to surgery in the absence of neurological deficit does not increase likelihood of adverse outcomes and, in light of the high frequency of remittance of symptoms with conservative care, at least 3 to 6 months should elapse before surgical consideration.[44] Time on sick leave is also important as a clinical predictor of success for disc herniation surgery; sick leave less than 2 months yielded a satisfactory outcome (in both subjective and objective measures) 80% of the time, whereas sick leave longer than 3 months generated a satisfactory outcome in only 50%.[47] Heavy manual work, low vocational education, and jobs requiring significant physical strain harm outcomes over the ensuing decades following discectomy.[48] Gender may play a role in outcomes; before surgery females had more pronounced back pain and disability and, at 1-year follow-up after lumbar disc herniation surgery, reported a greater degree of back and leg pain, greater consumption of analgesics, and more disability than their male counterparts.[49]

The presence of concomitant degenerative disc disease or marrow or endplate changes may somewhat confound the decision to perform simple microdiscectomy vs. fusion or disc replacement. Chin and associates[51] in a prospective case-controlled study when performing microdiscectomy alone found a slight trend toward greater disability improvement in those without Modic changes, but otherwise found similarly compelling results in both groups: regarding lower back pain, visual analog scale at 6 months dropped from 6.9 to 2.3 in the Modic group and 6.3 to 1.6 in the non-Modic group.[50] Follow-up studies have corroborated these findings.[51] It appears the intensity of concomitant low back pain negatively affects outcome of decompressive surgery from a lumbar herniated disc.[52] In a retrospective case series comparing discectomy alone vs. decompression with interbody fusion for treatment of disc herniation with Modic changes, it was reported that both approaches improved leg pain but decompression with fusion was statistically superior over discectomy alone for the treatment of back pain over an average follow-up of 21 months.[53] The indications for discectomy alone vs. combination with fusion are neither clearly defined nor widely accepted and often depend on to whom the patient is referred, with neurosurgeons rarely fusing and orthopedists more often doing so.[54,55]

Lumbar Fusion

The data surrounding the surgical treatment of discogenic pain in the lumbar spine is at best miasmic, with few large prospective randomized controlled trials and much contest even within the spine community itself. Surveying the attendants at the 2009 American Orthopedic Association meeting, only 23% believed that degeneration of the intervertebral disc is the major source of low back pain. When asked if they themselves had single-level degeneration with low back pain, 61% responded they would choose nonoperative treatment and 38% would choose no treatment. Of 100 responders, one agreed to fusion, and one agreed to disc replacement.[56] Furthermore, the data surrounding instrumented fusion may bear the influential financial force of industry.[57]

Spinal fusion is designed to treat instability. Spinal stability is classically described as the ability of the spine under normal physiological loads to limit displacement to protect the neural structures it houses and prevent incapacitating pain or damage.[58] However, even by this strict definition, the decision to fuse is complicated because little consensus exists regarding the diagnosis of instability; it is also difficult to measure in the clinical realm. Finally little high-level evidence exists for lumbar fusion. Decisions are largely guided by the surgeon's knowledge of spinal biomechanics and indications and contraindications. Pedicle screw fixation is the most common approach to internal stabilization of the lumbar spine, after which fusion is performed.

Pedicle screws are inserted into the pedicles above and below the target motion segment. The inferior-lateral pedicle is exposed by subperiosteal dissection from a lateral approach using fluoroscopy as a guide. The entry to the pedicle is at the intersection of the superior articulating facet and the transverse process. Using fluoroscopy, a pedicle probe is used to establish the path of the screw, with attention to the exiting nerve root. The intended path should carry the screw through the pedicle and into the body laterally to medially, avoiding endplates and the anterior confines of the body. Screws are then linked with rods. The screws can be used to distract, reduce, or decompress the vertebral bodies and align and balance spondylolisthesis. Then the screws are tightened onto the contoured rods to maintain the desired architecture.

Posterior or posterolateral fusion can be performed with or without instrumentation. Noninstrumented fusion has a higher rate of pseudarthrosis and is contraindicated in settings of overt instability. The technique requires exposure of the posterior spine through a midline incision and is carried laterally to expose the facets and transverse processes. Posterior decompression may be performed through laminectomy or facetectomy. The facets and transverse processes are decorticated with a high-speed drill; then corticocancellous bone harvest material from a variety of donor sites (but usually iliac crest) can be used, packing the (decorticated) articular surfaces of the facets as well as the lateral aspects of the joints and transverse processes. If posterior elemental structure remains, as in the case of laminotomy only, similar efforts posteriorly can fuse the posterior elements as well.

Lumbar interbody fusion seeks to replace the diseased disc and space with bone. Interbody fusion not only presents a favorable environment since the bone is under natural compression, but it also restores intervertebral height often lost by the disease process.

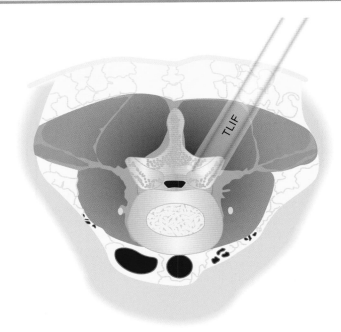

Fig. 12-3 Posterior oblique approach of the transforaminal interbody fusion. *TLIF,* Transforaminal lumbar interbody fusion.

It is often supplemented with pedicle screw fixation. Multiple approaches exist, all with various challenges and advantages.

TLIF (**Fig. 12-3**) presents a lateral oblique access to the intervertebral disc. Usually performed unilaterally, it can be performed in an open or a minimally invasive fashion. Partial facetectomy exposes the foramina to reveal nerve root, epidural space, and disc. Nerve root retraction is often required and may predispose to neuropraxia and fibrosis, but less nerve root tension is often required than in PLIF discussed in the next paragraph. The endplates are decorticated, and a crescent-shaped TLIF cage is inserted. However, this unilateral approach may only prepare 56% of the endplate surface area; thus the size of the bone cage is limited by both the size of the intervertebral foramen and the relatively small decortication possible.[59] In addition, there may be impaired muscular function secondary to dissection and distraction.[60] The TLIF approach yields many advantages; from one incision it achieves all the goals of surgery, including decompression, stabilization, and fusion, even circumferentially. Since the upper lumbar spinal segments are more sensitive to neuropraxia with distraction because they are closer to the conus medullaris, TLIF may be more advantageous than PLIF for these levels. In addition, TLIF can be performed in a minimally invasive manner using the tubular retractor systems discussed previously through two small paramedian incisions. If previous posterior surgery has been performed, avoiding scar tissue is possible, and it has proven to be an overall safe approach.[61]

First described by Briggs and Milligan[62] and then by Cloward[63] with a published series in 1953, the PLIF technique (**Fig. 12-4**) requires either laminectomy or a bilateral hemilaminectomy and medial hemifacetectomy to gain access to the posterior canal. Then the canal contents are retracted, allowing a bilateral approach to discectomy. Discectomy and decortication of the endplates are easily achieved. Neural elements are medially retracted as the bilateral interbody implants are introduced with fluoroscopic guidance. More traditional and older in technique, PLIF became synonymous with interbody fusion with numerous modifications through the

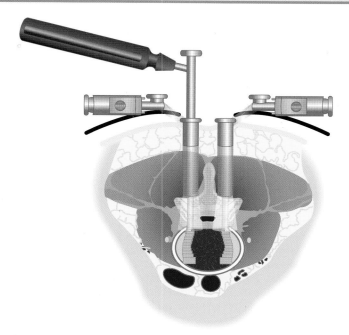

Fig. 12-4 Posterior lumbar interbody fusion. Note that bilateral access is required.

decades into the 1990s. PLIF does allow greater access for complete discectomy but may cause more neural tension than TLIF. Both PLIF and TLIF allow easy access to lamina and posterior instrumentation and permit a complete fusion and decompression with a single posterior incision. The PLIF is laborious and technically demanding and may lead to significant pain, resulting in increased LOS and possible chronic pain.[64]

Understanding the technical demands and potential weaknesses of both anterior and posterior approaches, the extreme lateral interbody fusion was developed by NuVasive (San Diego, Calif).[65] With the XLIF (**Fig. 12-5**) the spine is approached from the side of the body. The patient lies in the lateral decubitus position; two small incisions are made, the first through which most of the procedure is performed and the second slightly posterior to the first to allow finger dissection and guidance of the tubular dilators and instrumentation to the lateral access of the spine. Once the tissue retractor is secured to the table, lateral access to the disc is visible. An ipsilateral annulotomy allows discectomy. The lateral annuli and the nucleus are resected, leaving the anterior and posterior annuli in place. From the side a large intervertebral bone graft can be introduced. Fixation is done either by lateral plating of the vertebral bodies through the same retractor or via pedicle or posterior fixation. XLIF is challenging at the lower lumbar levels; the remaining levels are more easily approached. The XLIF requires blunt dissection through the psoas muscle and consequently the lumbar plexus. The system includes nerve root stimulation and monitoring hardware to diminish the likelihood of neuropraxic injury. However, traction injury to the lumbar plexus can still occur with the tubular cannula; as many as 30% of patients may complain of anterior thigh anesthesia.[66] XLIF avoids the surgical dissection anteriorly, which commonly requires a general or vascular surgeon for the retroperitoneal dissection and retraction of the great vessels. It avoids the often-concomitant nerve root retraction required to place interbody grafts from the posterior approach and may increase stabilization when fixation occurs laterally.[67]

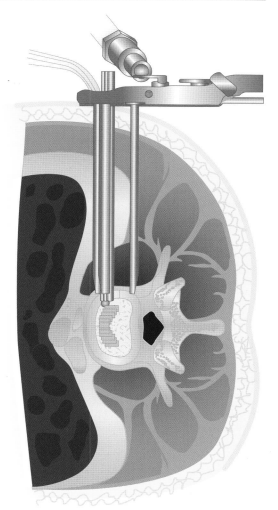

Fig. 12-5 Extreme lateral interbody fusion.

The anterior approach, or ALIF (**Fig. 12-6**), performed for the better part of the last century, usually requires the cooperation of a vascular or general surgeon for help with the dissection. Either a transperitoneal or an extraperitoneal approach can be used with either an open or a laparoscopic method. For the L5-S1 disc the approach takes the surgeon between the iliac vessels, but for the L4-L5 disc the level of the bifurcation of the abdominal aorta and the left iliac vein size determine the direction of retraction. The anterior longitudinal ligament and the anterior annulus are dissected, the nucleus is resected, and endplates are prepared. Implant is similar to the XLIF because excellent discal resection is possible with a large endplate surface area. When initially performed without fixation ALIF had a high incidence of pseudarthrosis.[68] Fixation can occur with pedicle screw fixation or anterior plating alone. Some studies found fusion rates with anterior plating equal to those with circumferential fusion[69]; in others plating was found to be inferior.[70] Although there are many advantages to ALIF, several weaknesses exist. Retrograde ejaculation in the male can result in up to 8% of retroperitoneal cases,[71] and transperitoneal approaches may increase that likelihood dramatically.[72] Approaches to lower disc levels are at greater risk of injury to the hypogastric plexus.

Overt instability readily ameliorates with fusion, as do the attendant symptoms. However, the data surrounding fusion for covert

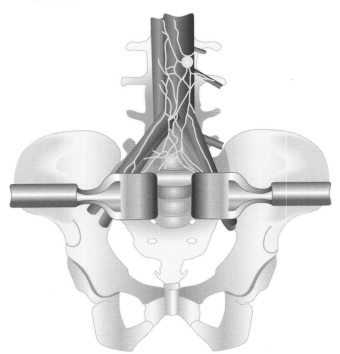

Fig. 12-6 Approach used for the anterior interior lumbar interbody fusion with retraction of the great vessels.

instability (when excessive motion is not readily indentified radiographically yet degeneration exists) do not provide clear direction. Although surgeons have put forth significant effort to elucidate fusion outcome data since 2005, at that time the Cochrane group concluded that very limited evidence was available to support fusion.[73] Several systematic reviews of trials have been published since. Mirza and Deyo[74] concluded that surgery may be more efficacious than unstructured nonsurgical care but may not be more efficacious than structured cognitive-behavior therapy.[74] A subsequent follow-up review agreed that fusion for discogenic low back pain was no more effective than intensive rehabilitation but may confer small-to-moderate benefit when compared to standard nonsurgical therapy.[75] Instrumentation is likely associated with higher fusion rates.[73]

In use in Europe before the United States, artificial disc replacement (ADR) sought to address the theoretical loss of range of motion and likely reduce the long-term degenerative changes at adjacent levels. ADR is approved for single-level disease in the lumbar spine caudal to L3 in otherwise healthy patients 60 years old or younger with absence of spondylolisthesis, neural deficit, or deformity.

With ADR an anterior approach must be used to fit the prosthesis. After dissection to the anterior spine, similar to that in ALIF, complete discectomy is performed. Then careful attention is paid to the preparation of the endplates extending to the posterior aspects of the vertebral bony body to fit the prosthetic disc and maximize surface area and contact with the metal implant.[76] Fluoroscopic confirmation of correct placement is paramount since the fulcrum must be midline in all planes. Patients are encouraged to mobilize as tolerated as early as the first day but instructed to avoid extension for 6 weeks.[77]

Two randomized trials exist comparing ADR and fusion. The first is a prospective, randomized controlled multicenter Food and Drug Administration (FDA)–regulated investigational device exemption (IDE) trial of 304 patients with the Charité disc.[78]

Patients were discographically positive for single-level concordance at either L5-S1 or L4-L5 but recalcitrant to 6 or more months of nonsurgical care and lacked radiographic evidence of neural compression. Randomized into ADR vs. fusion, the two groups failed to show a difference in either pain or functional status at 2 years, but the investigational group did reveal a significantly higher rate of satisfaction (73.7%) vs. the 53.1% satisfaction rate in the fusion group. However, 64% of ADR patients still required opioids. The ProDisc-L FDA-IDE trial generally reported more favorable outcomes.[79] Patients (286) were randomly assigned to either the ProDisc-L or circumferential fusion at one of the three disc levels: L3-L4, L4-L5, or L5-S1. Clinical success was higher in the ADR group (i.e., 53% vs. 41% in the control group). In addition, disability scores were superior in the ADR group early, with a decay of the difference, narrowing at 12 to 24 months. In both trials complication rates were similar. Of concern is the fact that high-quality, prospective, controlled, long-term follow-up studies are lacking. The longevity of the devices is yet to be determined; consequently safety must be held in question. The most recent systematic review yields the authors' conclusion that ADR be performed only within prospective scientific studies until further evidence for efficiency is provided.[80]

Conclusion

Surgical approaches to the cervical and lumbar spine for disc herniation are complex, and the surgical milieu is ripe for further technological development. The ultimate measures of surgical success in disc disease are similar to those used in pain treatments and thus are subject to the same confounding qualitative variables. The science surrounding technical improvement may lack the fidelity to reveal incremental advancement in outcomes since data sets are generally small and gains hard to quantify. Although this chapter seeks to investigate and present the available surgical options, the greater importance, already appreciated by many patients, may lie not in the selection of surgical method but rather in the selection of surgeon.

References

1. Hart LG, Deyo RA, Cherkin DC: Physician office visits for low back pain: frequency, clinical evaluation, and treatment patterns from a U.S. national survey. *Spine* 20(1):11-19, 1995.
2. Deyo R et al: Trends, major medical complications, and charges associated with surgery for lumbar spinal stenosis in older adults. *JAMA* 303(13):1259-1265, 2010.
3. Weinstein JN, Lurie JD, Olson PR et al: United States trends and regional variations in lumbar spine surgery, 1992-2003. *Spine* 31(23): 2707-2714, 2006.
4. Irwin ZN et al: Variation in surgical decision making for degenerative spinal disorders. I. Lumbar spine. *Spine* 30(19):2208-2213, 2005.
5. Katz JN et al: Lumbar laminectomy alone or with instrumented or noninstrumented arthrodesis in degenerative lumbar spinal stenosis: patient selection, costs, and surgical outcomes. *Spine* 22(10):1123-1131, 1997.
6. Cote P, Cassidy J, Carroll L: The factors associated with neck pain and its related disability in the Saskatchewan population. *Spine* 25(9):1109-1117, 2000.
7. Spurling R, Scoville WB: Lateral rupture of the cervical intervertebral discs: a common cause of shoulder and arm pain. *Surg Gynecol Obstet* 78:350-358, 1944.
8. Rothman R, Roshbaum R: Pathogenesis of signs and symptoms of cervical disc degeneration. In *American Academy of Orthopaedic Surgeons*. St. Louis, 1978, Mosby, pp 203-215.
9. Zeidman SM, Ducker TB: Posterior cervical laminoforaminotomy for radiculopathy: review of 172 case. *Neurosurgery* 33:356-362, 1993.

10. Henderson CM et al: Posterior-lateral foraminotomy as an exclusive operative technique for cervical radiculopathy: a review of 846 consecutively operated cases. *Neurosurgery* 13:504-512, 1983.

11. Aldrich F: Posterolateral microdiscectomy for cervical monoradiculopathy caused by posterolateral soft cervical disc sequestration. *J Neurosurg* 72:370-377, 1990.

12. Grieve JP et al: Results of posterior cervical foraminotomy for treatment of cervical spondylitic radiculopathy. *Br J Neurosurg* 14:40-43, 2000.

13. Heary R et al: Cervical laminoforaminotomy for the treatment of cervical degenerative radiculopathy. *J Neurosurg* 11:198-202, 2009.

14. Vaccaro AR et al: Early failure of long segment anterior cervical plate fixation. *J Spinal Disord* 11:410-415, 1998.

15. Bernard TN, Whitecloud TS: Cervical spondylotic myelopathy and myeloradiculopathy: anterior decompression and stabilization with autogenous fibula strut graft. *Clin Orthop* 221:149-160, 1987.

16. Hanai K, Fujiyoshi F, Kamei K: Subtotal vertebrectomy and spinal fusion for cervical spondylotic myelopathy. *Spine* 11:310-315, 1986.

17. Denaro V, Di Martino A: Cervical spine surgery: a historical perspective. *Clin Orthop Relat Res* 469(3):639-648, 2011.

18. Cloward RB: The anterior approach for removal of ruptured cervical discs. *J Neurosurg* 15:602-617, 1958.

19. Robinson RA, Smith GW: Anterolateral cervical disc removal and interbody fusion for cervical disc syndrome. *Bull John Hopkins Hosp* 96:223-224, 1955.

20. Herkowitz HN, Kurz LT, Overholt DP: Surgical management of cervical soft disc herniation: a comparison between the anterior and posterior approach. *Spine* 15:1026-1030, 1990.

21. Guidetti B, Fortuna A: Long-term results of surgical treatments of myelopathy due to cervical spondylosis. *J Neurosurg* 30(6):714-721, 1969.

22. Hukuda S et al: Operations for cervical spondylotic myelopathy: a comparison of the results of anterior and posterior procedures. *J Bone Joint Surgery [Br]* 67(4):609-615, 1985.

23. Kuriloff DB et al: Delayed neck infection following anterior spine surgery. *Laryngoscope* 97:1094-1098, 1987.

24. Cooper PR et al: Posterior stabilization of cervical spine fractures and subluxations using plates and screws. *Neurosurgery* 23:300-306, 1988.

25. Cuatico W: Anterior cervical discectomy without interbody fusion: an analysis of 81 cases. *Acta Neurochir* 57:269, 1981.

26. Martins AN: Anterior cervical discectomy with and without interbody bone graft. *J Neurosurg* 44:290, 1976.

27. Bohlman HH et al: Robinson anterior cervical discectomy and arthrodesis for cervical radiculopathy. *J Bone Joint Surg [Am]* 75:198-1307, 1993.

28. Segal LS et al: Complications of posterior arthrodesis of the cervical spine in patients who have Down's syndrome. *J Bone Joint Surgery [Am]* 73:1547-1554, 1991.

29. Wimmer C et al: Predisposing factors for infection in spine surgery: a survey of 850 spinal procedures. *J Spinal Disord* 11:124-128, 1998.

30. Bell DF et al: Spinal deformity after multiple level cervical laminectomy in children. *Spine* 4:406, 1994.

31. Goffin J et al: Intermediate follow-up after treatment of degenerative disc disease with the Bryan cervical disc prosthesis: single level and bi-level. *Spine* 28:2673-2678, 2003.

32. Goffin J, Casey A, Kehr P et al: Preliminary clinical experience with the Bryan cervical disc prosthesis. *Neurosurgery* 51: 840-847, 2002.

33. Sekhon L: Cervicothoracic junction arthroplasty after previous fusion surgery for adjacent segment degeneration: case report. *Operative Neurosurg* 56(suppl. 1):S-205, 2005.

34. Byrne TN, Benzel EC, Waxman SG: *Disease of the spine and spinal cord*, New York, 2000, Oxford University Press.

35. Mixter WJ, Barr JS: Rupture of the intervertebral disc with involvement of the spinal canal. *N Engl J Med* 211:210-215, 1934.

36. Arts M et al: Does minimally invasive lumbar disc surgery result in less muscle injury than conventional surgery? a randomized controlled trial. *Eur Spine J* 20:51-57, 2011.

37. Caspar W: A new surgical procedure for lumbar disc herniation causing less tissue damage through microsurgical approach. In

38. Williams RW: Microlumbar discectomy: a conservative surgical approach to the virgin herniated lumbar disc. *Spine* 3:175-182, 1978.

39. Yasargil MG: Microsurgical operation for herniated lumbar disc. In Wullenweber R et al, editors: *Advances in Neurosurgery*, Berlin, 1977, Springer-Verlag, p 81.

40. Palmer S: Tubular retractor system use in microscopic lumbar discectomy: clinical material and methods. *Neurosurg Focus* 13(2):E5, 2002.

41. Lau D et al: Minimally invasive compared to open microdiscectomy for lumbar disc herniation. *J Clin Neurosci* 18(1):81-84, 2011. E-publication Sept 20, 2010.

42. Gibson JN, Waddell G: Surgery for degenerative lumbar spondylosis: updated Cochrane review. *Spine* 30:2312-2320, 2005.

43. Atlas SJ et al: Long-term outcomes of surgical and nonsurgical management of sciatica secondary to a lumbar disc herniation: 10-year results from the Maine lumbar spine study. *Spine* 30(8):936-943, 2005.

44. Amundsen T et al: Lumbar spinal stenosis: conservative or surgical management? A prospective 10-year study. *Spine* 25:1424-1435, 2000.

45. Weinstein JN et al: Surgical vs nonoperative treatment for lumbar disc herniation: the Spine Patient Outcomes Research Trial (SPORT): a randomized trial. *JAMA* 296(20):2441-2450, 2006.

46. Weinstein JN et al: Surgical vs nonoperative treatment for lumbar disc herniation: the Spine Patient Outcomes Research Trial (SPORT) observational cohort. *JAMA* 296(20):2451-2459, 2006.

47. Silverplats K et al: Clinical factors of importance for outcome after lumbar disc herniation surgery: long-term follow-up. *Eur Spine J* 19(9):1459-1467, 2010. E-publication May 29, 2010.

48. Loupasis GA et al: Seven- to 20-year outcome of lumbar discectomy, *Spine* 24(22):2313-2317, 1999.

49. Strömqvist F et al: Gender differences in lumbar disc herniation surgery. *Acta Orthop* 79(5):643-649, 2008.

50. Chin KR et al: Success of lumbar microdiscectomy in patients with Modic changes and low-back pain: a prospective pilot study. *J Spinal Disord Tech* 21(2):139-144, 2008.

51. Ohtori S et al: Low back pain after lumbar discectomy in patients showing endplate Modic type 1 change. *Spine* 35(13):E596-600, 2010.

52. Kleinstueck FS et al: The outcome of decompression surgery for lumbar herniated disc is influenced by the level of concomitant preoperative low back pain. *Eur Spine J* E-publication ahead of print, Jan 12, 2011.

53. Yang YQ et al: Selection of surgical methods for lumbar disc herniation with degenerative endplates changes, *Zhonghua Yi, Xue Za, Zhi* 89(27):1902-1906, 2009.

54. Bärlocher C, Benini A: Long-term results of discectomy and primary spondylodesis in treatment of lumbar disc hernia. *Schweiz Arch Neurol Psychiatr* 145(5):14-24, 1994.

55. Benini A: Lumbar discectomy without or with spondylodesis? Revival of an old dilemma. *Z Orthop Ihre Grenzgeb* 127(3):276-285, 1989.

56. Hanley EN, Jr et al: Debating the value of spine surgery. *J Bone Joint Surg [Am]* 92(5):1293-1304, 2010.

57. Robaina-Padrón FJ: Controversies about instrumented surgery and pain relief in degenerative lumbar spine pain: results of scientific evidence. *Neurocirugia (Astur)* 18(5):406-413, 2007.

58. White AA, Panjabi MM: *Clinical biomechanics of the spine*, ed 2, Philadelphia, 1990, Lippincott, pp 300-342.

59. Javernick MA, Kuklo TR, Polly DW: Transforaminal lumbar interbody fusion: unilateral versus bilateral disc removal—an in vivo study. *Am J Orthop* 32:344-348, 2003.

60. Rantanen J et al: The lumbar multifidus muscle five years after surgery for a lumbar intervertebral disc herniation. *Spine* 18:568-574, 1993.

61. Hackenberg L et al: Transforaminal lumbar interbody fusion: a safe technique with satisfactory three- to five-year results. *Eur Spine J* 14(6):551-558, 2005. E-publication Jan 26, 2005.

62. Briggs H, Milligan P: Chip fusion of the low back following exploration of the spinal canal. *J Bone Joint Surg [Am]* 26:125-130, 1944.

63. Cloward RB: The treatment of ruptured lumbar intervertebral discs by vertebral body fusion. I. Indications, operative technique, after care. *J Neurosurg* 10:154-168, 1953.

Wullenweber R et al, editors: *Advances in neurosurgery*, Berlin, 1977, Springer-Verlag, pp 74-77.

64. Thomsen K et al: 1997 Volvo Award winner in clinical studies: the effect of pedicle screw instrumentation on functional outcome and fusion rates in posterolateral lumbar spinal fusion: a prospective, randomized clinical study. *Spine* 22:2813-2822, 1997.

65. Ozgur BM et al: Extreme lateral interbody fusion (XLIF): a novel surgical technique for anterior lumbar interbody fusion. *Spine J* 6(4):435-443, 2006.

66. Bergey DL et al: Endoscopic lateral transpsoas approach to the lumbar spine. *Spine* 29:1681-1688, 2004.

67. An HS et al: Biomechanical evaluation of anterior thoracolumbar spinal instrumentation. *Spine* 10:1979-1983, 1995.

68. Kumar A et al: Interspace distraction and graft subsidence after anterior lumbar fusion with femoral strut allograft. *Spine* 18(16):2393-2400, 1993.

69. Aryan HE et al: Stand-alone anterior lumbar discectomy and fusion with plate: initial experience. *Surg Neurol* 68(1):7-13; discussion 13, 2007.

70. Beaubien B et al: In vitro, biomechanical comparison of an anterior lumbar interbody fusion with an anteriorly placed, low-profile lumbar plate and posteriorly placed pedicle screws or translaminar screws. *Spine* 30:1846-1851, 2005.

71. Christensen FB, Bünger CE: Retrograde ejaculation after retroperitoneal lower lumbar interbody fusion. *Int Orthop* 21(3):176-180, 1997.

72. Sasso RC, Burkus J, LeHuec JC: Retrograde ejaculation after anterior lumbar interbody fusion: transperitoneal versus retroperitoneal exposure. *Spine* 28(10):1023-1026, 2003.

73. Gibson JA, Waddell G: Surgery for degenerative lumbar spondylosis, Cochrane Database of Systematic Reviews 2005, Issue 4, Art No CD001352. DOI 10.1002/14651858.CD001352.pub3.

74. Mirza SK, Deyo RA: Systematic review of randomized trials comparing lumbar fusion surgery to nonoperative care for treatment of chronic back pain. *Spine* 32(7):816-823, 2007.

75. Chou R et al: Surgery for low back pain: a review of the evidence for an American Pain Society Clinical Practice Guideline. *Spine* 34(10):1094-1099, 2009.

76. Geisler FH: Surgical technique of lumbar artificial disc replacement with the Charité artificial disc. *Neurosurgery* 56(suppl 1):S46-S57; discussion S46-S57, 2005.

77. Katsimihas M et al: Prospective clinical and radiographic results of Charité III artificial total disc arthroplasty at 2- to 7-year follow-up: a Canadian experience. *Can J Surg* 53(6):408-414, 2010.

78. Blumenthal S et al: A prospective, randomized, multicenter Food and Drug Administration investigational device exemptions study of lumbar total disc replacement with the Charité artificial disc versus lumbar fusion. Part I. Evaluation of clinical outcomes. *Spine* 30(14):1565-1575; discussion E387-391, 2005.

79. Zigler J et al: Results of the prospective, randomized, multicenter Food and Drug Administration investigational device exemption study of the ProDisc-L total disc replacement versus circumferential fusion for the treatment of 1-level degenerative disc disease. *Spine* 32(11):1155-1162; discussion 1163, 2007.

80. van den Eerenbeemt KD et al: Total disc replacement surgery for symptomatic degenerative lumbar disc disease: a systematic review of the literature. *Eur Spine J* 19(8):1262-1280, 2010. E-publication May 28, 2010.

13 Neuromodulation and Intrathecal Therapies for the Treatment of Chronic Radiculopathy Related to Intractable Discogenic Pain

José De Andrés and Stefano Palmisani

CHAPTER OVERVIEW

Chapter Synopsis: Although surgery for a herniated disc may be partly effective in relieving discogenic pain, the residual (and often severe) radiopathic leg pain often falls into a diagnosis of failed back surgery syndrome (FBSS). This chapter considers the nonsurgical therapies directed at discogenic radiculopathic pain, including spinal cord stimulation (SCS) and intrathecal drug delivery (IDD). SCS delivers electrical pulses to activate sensory nerves and has shown positive outcomes for chronic pain after herniated disc surgery. As with any procedure for chronic pain, good patient selection is a key factor in attaining successful outcomes. Although the paresthesias associated with SCS make a blinded placebo group virtually impossible, they do allow for a preimplantation trial, thereby increasing the odds of a successful treatment. IDD uses a pharmacological approach similar to conventional medication therapy, often with diminished side effects compared to systemic delivery. Opioids directly target receptors in spinal neurons (of the substantia gelatinosa) and supraspinal cells. The γ-aminobutyric acid receptor agonist baclofen and the calcium-channel blocker ziconotide have also been used in IDD for chronic pain. Although they are efficacious for cancer pain, evidence of long-term efficacy for chronic pain remains more questionable. The chapter reviews the technical aspects associated with the SCS and IDD implantation procedures. Risks and complications are also considered.

Important Points:

- FBSS is defined as persistent or recurrent low back and leg pain after technically and anatomically successful spine surgery; it affects approximately 10% to 40% of patients who had lumbar spinal surgery.
- Results of two randomized controlled trials (RCTs) suggest that SCS could be an appropriate therapy for FBSS patients who failed conventional medical management.
- No RCTs support the use of IDDs in treating chronic noncancer pain, despite FBSS still being considered one of the main indications for IDD implant in the United States.
- For both SCS and IDD, key points to success are patient selection and surgical techniques. All eligible patients should undergo a psychological screening and an evaluation trial period before being implanted by experienced operators.
- Long-term complication rates are high for both SCS and IDD, limiting the cost-effectiveness of the therapy. Incidence of complications, especially infection and mechanical failures of SCS leads in the system, could be reduced by a careful surgical technique performed in experienced, high-volume tertiary centers.

Clinical Pearls:

- Adequate patients selection
- Trial following protocol
- Responsible surgeons experienced in implant technique
- Duration of the implant operation as short as possible
- Perioperative antibiotic administration.
- Careful preparation of the surgical sites
- Placement of surgical incisions to avoid suture lines crossing over the implanted devices
- Intraoperative fluoroscopy
- Strategy in follow-up decisions

Introduction

Lumbosacral pain with leg radiculopathy following nerve injury from a prolapsed intervertebral disc is one of the most frequent causes of neuropathic pain.[1] Conventional patient management of neuropathic back and leg pain secondary to disc herniation includes surgery. However, when pain persists and no further surgical target exists, the patient is often described as suffering from failed back surgery syndrome (FBSS), defined as "persistent or recurrent pain, mainly in the region of the lower back and legs, even after technically, anatomically successful lumbosacral spine surgeries."[2] In these patients neuropathic pain is a main pain-generating mechanism characterized by predominant leg pain (radiculopathy). FBSS is common, affecting approximately 10% to 40% of patients who have undergone lumbar spinal surgery[3]; among the sources of the FBSS pain are recurrence of disc herniation, arachnoiditis, epidural fibrosis, and various radiculopathies.[4]

The most painful component in FBSS is the radiculopathy, as shown by the characteristics of an FBSS population compared to other chronic pain conditions.[5] The severity of pain in FBSS patients was on average moderate in the back (mean visual analog scale [VAS] 4.9) but severe in the legs (mean VAS 7.4); patients were severely disabled, as indicated by several validated scores (Oswestry Disability Index [ODI], SF-36, EQ-5D), and their health-related quality of life was very poor.[5] All patients had tried at least one class of drug or nondrug treatment before undergoing a trial of neuromodulation, and 87% had tried four or more types of drug and nondrug treatments.

Patients with FBSS typically have failed to respond to multiple therapies. Few options remain; these most prominently include a new surgical procedure, multidisciplinary rehabilitation, or neuromodulation. Neuromodulation, the reversible and adjustable blockade or manipulation of pain pathways to modify physiological function, may be applied to spinal cord, deep brain structures, motor cortex, and peripheral nerves.[6] Among all the available neuromodulation techniques, spinal cord stimulation (SCS) and intrathecal drug infusion are the most common and efficacious.

Spinal Cord Stimulation

SCS is an evidence-based therapy that has been used for many years in the treatment of several types of refractory neuropathic pain,[7] including chronic radiculopathy. As outlined in recent reviews,[7,8] the use of SCS in patients suffering from FBSS has been shown to provide (1) a sustained, long-term pain relief, with a reduction in concomitant pain medication; (2) an improvement in quality of life and functional status; (3) an increased ability to return to work; (4) an increased patient satisfaction; (5) minimal side effects; (6) a cost-effective alternative to conventional therapies; and (7) the opportunity for maximized combination therapy with oral and intrathecal methods.

Mechanism of Action

The introduction of SCS was inspired by Melzack and Wall's gate control theory in 1965.[9] This theory proposed that painful "nociceptive" information in the periphery is transmitted to the spinal cord in small-diameter, unmyelinated C-fibers and lightly myelinated A-delta fibers, which end in the superficial laminae of the dorsal horn (i.e., the gate) of the spinal cord. Other sensory information such as touch or vibration is carried in large, myelinated A-beta fibers that pass through this gate. As they do, they give off small branches that terminate in the dorsal horn, where they have an inhibitory effect on the nociceptive conduction. The basic premise of the gate control theory was that stimulation of large, low-threshold fibers would close the gate to the reception of small-fiber information. In the first volume of *Pain* more than 35 years ago, Lindblom and Meyerson[10] reported that SCS increased vibration thresholds and tactile thresholds but did not change the perception of cutaneous pain induced by pinching in five patients responding to SCS, suggesting that SCS affects A-beta fiber function but not C-fiber function.

The general mechanism of pain relief by SCS still is understood in these gating terms, even if there are several substantial problems with this understanding.[7] For example, both acute and chronic pain should be suppressed by SCS, but this is not the case. It became obvious that not all types of pain are modulated uniformly; whereas SCS primarily affects neuropathic pain and nonnociceptive pain, activation of large afferent fibers can still signal pain,[11] and only chronic pain appears to be affected. Thus the mechanism of action of SCS must involve more than a direct inhibition of pain transmission in the dorsal horn of the spinal cord.

Pain modulation by SCS may involve supraspinal activity via the posterior columns of the spinal cord (i.e., down-modulation involving loops or feedback mechanisms that influence rostral transmission of pain from higher centers to the spinal cord). In humans suffering from several types of neuropathic pain, electrical stimulation of the dorsal columns in the thoracic spinal cord generated antidromic action potentials, activating large myelinated fibers in pure sensory peripheral nerves[12]; and late cellular activation in the dorsal horn after SCS has been also hypothesized, as suggested by an increase in c-Fos immunoreactive cells in the dorsal horn after SCS.[13] Recent results in an animal model of neuropathic pain showed that the spinal serotonergic system plays a crucial role in the pain-relieving effect of SCS, suggesting an activation of serotonergic descending pathways that may inhibit spinal nociceptive transmission.[14] Moreover, evidences of SCS-induced activation of specific areas of the brain (primary and secondary sensorimotor cortex, cingulate cortex, insula, thalamus, and premotor cortex) have recently been published[15]; and regional cerebral blood flow measured by positron emission tomography in patients undergoing SCS therapy for intractable pain was increased in the right thalamus, superior parietal lobule, and left inferior parietal lobule after application of SCS. Thus SCS controls pain cognition by modulating the thalamus and parietal association area, and it also controls the emotional aspects of pain by modulating the prefrontal region.

However, spinal segmental inhibition still seems to be crucial. Animal studies show that second-order afferent nerves and inter-neurons can be activated by SCS,[16] and a proportion of these may manifest delayed inhibitory activity following brief stimulation.[17] SCS also selectively inhibits abnormal hypersensitivity in dorsal horn neurons[18] and significantly modulates neuronal activity in dorsal column nuclei.[19] It does not directly activate the neurons of the pars gelatinosa, but elicits inhibitory responses of these neurons via A-fibers by reducing excitatory neurotransmitters.[20] At the cellular level SCS was shown to stimulate the neurons of the dorsal horn of the spinal cord to release increased amounts of acetylcholine, substance P, serotonin, noradrenaline, glycine, and γ-aminobutyric acid (GABA).[21-23] In a series of acute experiments using microdialysis in the dorsal horn of nerve-lesioned rats, SCS reduces the release of excitatory amino acids (glutamate, aspartate) and at the same time increases the GABA release[24]; the reduction in excitatory amino acids is prevented by blockade of GABA recep-tors.[25] The state of central hyperexcitability manifested in the devel-opment of allodynia after peripheral nerve injury seems to be related to dysfunction of the spinal GABA systems, and it appears that SCS may act by restoring normal GABA levels in the dorsal horn.[25,26] Moreover, rats that were nonresponders to SCS (their mechanical allodynia was not attenuated by SCS) could be con-verted to responders with intrathecal administration of low doses of baclofen.[25] Similar results were obtained in a pilot clinical study in humans in which the SCS effect was enhanced by simultaneous intrathecal administration of low dose baclofen, and the obtained pain relief results appeared to be long lasting.[27,28] Thus experimen-tal and clinical evidences point toward a significant role played by the activation of the GABA system within the spinal cord in the analgesic mechanism of SCS.

SCS is effective on mechanical allodynia in animal models of neuropathic pain.[29] The antiallodynic effect was observed after 30 minutes of stimulation, with a complete return to preneuropathy levels, and it lasted up to 60 minutes after SCS cessation. However, a differential antiallodynic effect seems to be related to the degree of severity of the allodynia itself. SCS leads to faster and better pain relief in mildly allodynic rats compared to the more severely allo-dynic ones.[30]

Finally, SCS yields a marked sympatholytic effect. This effect is considered responsible for the effectiveness of SCS in peripheral ischemia, cardiac ischemia, and at least some cases of complex regional pain syndrome (CRPS) and FBSS.[7]

Spinal Cord Stimulation: An Evidence-Based Therapy?
Systematic Reviews   In the last 20 years several systematic reviews have been published on the efficacy and cost-effectiveness of SCS in FBSS patients; just two randomized controlled trials (RCTs) have been completed so far. Thus, despite all the efforts to perform a systematic review as accurately as possible, most of the reviews are redundant because of the paucity of the available data.[31,32]

According to one of the last published systematic reviews[32] and based on Guyatt criteria,[33] the recommendation for SCS in an FBSS patient should be rated as 1B/1C (strong recommendation with moderate-to-low quality of evidence), with a caveat that it may change when higher-quality evidence becomes available. The American Pain Society found fair evidence that SCS is moderately

effective for FBSS with persistent radiculopathy, although device-related complications are common[34]; and both the European Fed-eration of Neurological Society and the National Institute for Health and Clinical Excellence (UK) (NICE) guidelines support the effect of SCS in patients with FBSS.[35,36]

The last update (January 2009) of the Cochrane systematic review of SCS for chronic pain, the first that included only RCTs for the analysis, still found only two trials that assessed the effects of spinal cord stimulators for CRPS type I and FBSS. Despite the conclusions pointing toward the existence of limited evidence in favor of SCS, authors recognized the paucity of the existing trials and the need for debate about trial designs that will provide the best evidence for assessing this type of intervention.[37] So far SCS-induced paresthesia virtually abolishes the possibility of designing a placebo-controlled randomized trial.

SCS is an expensive technique. List prices for SCS systems are not publicly available, but the Association of British Healthcare Industries provided indicative SCS equipment costs: a midrange price based on the average cost of each manufacturer's best-selling product, a lower cost based on the average cost of each manufac-turer's least expensive product, and an upper cost based on the average cost of the most expensive product. The prices supplied were: SCS system, including neurostimulator, controller, and charger, if applicable, but excluding leads £9282 ($13,445.35), range £6858 to £13,289 ($9,934.09 to $19,249.66); and leads £1544 ($2,236.55), range £928 to £1804 ($1,344.25 to $2,613.17); or £1136 ($1,654.54), range £1065 to £1158 ($1,542.70 to $1,677.41) for surgical or percutaneous implantation, respectively. However, although initially expensive because of the upfront implant costs, SCS proffers improvements in generic health-related quality of life. Of the total mean additional cost of SCS, 15% is offset in 6-months' time by reducing the use of drugs for pain relief and other non-drug pain treatment.[38] At 6 months SCS increases health-related quality of life in patients with chronic back and leg pain with a neuropathic component after one or multiple surgeries at an addi-tional mean health care cost of £11,373 ($16,474.25) per patient.[38] Moreover, a cost-effectiveness analysis based on data from another trial indicates that, at a mean follow-up period of 3.1 years, SCS is more cost-effective than reoperation in selected FBSS patients and should be the initial therapy of choice.[39] A recent systematic review assessing the cost-effectiveness of SCS in FBSS patients pooled all the available data and confirmed the hypothesis that SCS is both more effective and less costly in the long term.[40]

Clinical Trials   Two RCTs investigated the effect of SCS on the treatment of FBSS. One trial (PROCESS) compared SCS in com-bination with conventional medical management (CMM) with CMM alone;[41] interestingly, most of the patients recruited had persistent radicular pain following anatomically successful surgery for herniated disc. The second trial compared SCS in combination with CMM with repeat operation in combination with CMM.[39] Follow-up in the PROCESS trial was at 6 and 12 months, with a further analysis published 24 months later[42]; in the second trial follow-up was at 6 months and after a mean of 2.9 years. The primary outcome in both studies was the proportion of people who had 50% or greater pain relief.

The PROCESS trial reported that SCS had a greater effect than CMM in terms of the proportion of people experiencing 50% pain relief at 6 months (48% and 9% in the SCS and CMM groups, respectively), 12 months (34% and 7% in the SCS and CMM groups, respectively) and 24 months (37% vs. 2%, respectively). The second trial also reported a statistically significant benefit in terms of those experiencing 50% pain relief, favoring SCS over repeat operation (39% and 12% in the SCS and repeat operation groups, respectively). In the PROCESS trial opioid use did not differ significantly between the two groups (56% and 70% using opioids in the SCS and CMM groups, respectively). However, the second trial reported that SCS resulted in a significantly greater number of people reducing or maintaining the same dose of opioids when compared with repeat operation (87% and 58% in the SCS and repeat operation groups, respectively). In the PROCESS trial the SCS group showed a significantly greater improvement in function compared with the CMM group for mean change in functional ability (ODI) and significant benefits in health-related quality of life (SF-36). The second trial reported no statistically significant differences between SCS and repeat operation for pain related to daily activities or neurological function.

However, not all of the evidence is pointing in the same direction. First, an SCS device manufacturer funded both trials, and in the large international trial this manufacturer managed all study logistics and collected and analyzed the data. We should remember that industry-sponsored studies of drugs and devices yield more favorable results than do nonindustry-funded studies.[43] Second, in the PROCESS trial the comparator was CMM, even though patients had already failed such treatment and would probably continue to do so.[44] Third, independent analysis showing little or no evidence that SCS is superior to alternative treatment.[45]

In summary, despite the fact that two quality RCTs have already been performed, a multicenter, independently funded definite trial should still be advocated.

Patient Selection

Patient selection is the key to having positive outcomes.[7] As with any procedure that has risk, choosing a patient who wants to get better and has an etiology that has been shown to benefit from SCS is a must. Although not all patients are suitable for treatment with SCS, careful patient selection and implantation after evaluation by a multidisciplinary pain management team can offer safe and effective treatment of refractory neuropathic pain.[46] The search for objective criteria that predict an optimal result using implantable systems must include psychological criteria in the decision algorithm.[36] However, at present there is insufficient empirical evidence that psychological screening before surgery or device implantation helps to improve treatment outcomes, even if the current literature suggests that psychological factors such as somatization, depression, anxiety, and poor coping are important predictors of poor outcome.[47]

One of the unique and inherent benefits of SCS is the ability to perform a trial before permanent implantation.[48] A 50% pain relief reported by the patient is the minimal yet usually the only efficacy measurement that needs to be met during the trial. Unfortunately, this 50% gold standard is purely subjective and is potentially biased by placebo effects. Therefore the need for valid objective test(s) that, along with the subjective report of pain relief, can help the implanter define a "successful" trial is obvious. In a small prospective pilot study of patients with FBSS or CRPS, Eisenberg and associates[49] showed that some quantitative sensory measures—vibration threshold and tolerance to electrical stimulation at 5 and 250 Hz—were changed with an SCS trial. These changes were also correlated with the decision regarding the permanent implantation, which was made independently of them.

The delay between the first back surgery and the trial of SCS seems to be a significant prognostic factor. In a study of 235 patients treated over 15 years, the success rate of SCS dropped from 93% in patients who had a 3-year delay between surgery and implantation to 9% for those who had a 12-year delay.[8] Thus SCS should be considered early in the management of FBSS, before a second operation and before the use of high-dose opioid analgesics.[50]

However, despite a proper patient selection some patients do not benefit adequately from SCS, in spite of the fact that stimulation-induced paresthesia covers the painful area.[24] In a recent retrospective analysis of a single-center experience with SCS over the past 22 years, Kumar, Hunter, and Demeria[51] reported an 84% early–SCS trial success in FBSS patients, the success rate dropped to 60% in the long-term follow-up (mean 98 months).[51] Interestingly, authors reported a lower failure rate (16%) in FBSS patients with a clear pain etiology and radicular distribution compared to a higher rate (33%) in FBSS patients who did not experience obvious neuropathic pain but had nonspecific pain in their arms or legs that was not in the distribution of any particular nerve root or roots and was not associated with radicular neurological deficits.

During the patient selection process some commonly accepted contraindications should be taken into consideration.[23] Absolute contraindications are (1) sepsis, coagulopathy, or other conditions associated with an unacceptable surgical risk; (2) previous surgery or trauma that obliterates the spinal canal; (3) localized infection at the implantation site; and (4) spinal bifida. Relative contraindications are (1) physical and/or cognitive/psychological disability, (2) unresolved major psychiatric disorder, (3) unmanaged substance abuse or cognitive disorders, (4) pregnancy, and (5) presence of a cardiac pacemaker or defibrillator.

Technical Issues

Briefly, SCS is applied through a subcutaneous electrical generator that delivers pulses by means of electrodes placed in the epidural space adjacent to a targeted spinal cord area presumed to be causing the pain. Definitive electrodes can be placed percutaneously or through a surgical procedure (most of the time, a laminectomy). Although electrodes placed via laminectomy in the thoracic region appear to be associated with significantly better long-term effectiveness,[52] no definitive evidence has been published so far. However, a percutaneous trial is always required before proceeding to the full implant of the system.[48,53,54]

Trial of Spinal Cord Stimulation

The patient is positioned in a comfortable prone position on a fluoroscopy table. A pillow underneath the abdomen may correct lordosis curve and open posterior interlaminar space, which can facilitate electrode insertion. The choice of level of electrode insertion is guided by several factors. A fundamental consideration is that several centimeters of the lead have to lie in the epidural space to ensure maximal stability of the electrode and minimize unwanted migration. To ensure this, insertion must take place at least two spine segments below the desired target.

The epidural space is accessed using median or paramedian approach and angling steeply up from below. It is recommended that the loss of resistance technique be used to access the epidural space since contrast may obscure lead placement and saline flush can decrease the consistency of paresthesias. Some physicians now believe that a single lead is sufficient, and the lead is manipulated up under fluoroscopic guidance to the target level. If dual leads are desired, most are placed parallel but can be staggered according the final electrical field elicited with the different configuration provided with the position of the electrodes. Manipulation of the leads up the epidural space can be a tricky and subtle technique. Several stylets are available with different tip configurations that aid in the placement of the lead to its desired location. Once satisfied with lead positioning (check for the position in the posterior epidural space), the next step is assessing paresthesia coverage.

Ultimately the patient must determine if the paresthesia that occurs in his or her back and/or legs is better than the back and/or leg pain that drove him or her to attempt the trial. During the trial period the patient should be encouraged to log activities, activity durations, and medications and possibly measure pain levels on a VAS equivalent. Pain treatment with SCS therapy is considered effective when a patient experiences a clinically significant (50% or greater) reduction in pain. When this occurs, the patient is then recommended for permanent SCS placement.

Full Implant of Spinal Cord Stimulation

If a two-electrode implant technique is chosen, usually two needles are inserted either on one side of the midline at two different levels or on both sides of midline. The first technique is preferred to perform leads anchoring through a single paramedian incision. The needles are inserted, and the leads are placed under fluoroscopy guidance using techniques similar to those described in the trial procedures.

The skin incision, starting at the stab wound around the needle shaft and extending 5 cm caudally, should be deep enough to expose either the supraspinous ligament or the fascia of the paravertebral muscles.

Several anchors to secure the lead to the ligament or fascia are marketed by different companies. A silicone anchor with percutaneous leads improved average time to mechanical failure compared to a rigid plastic anchor; moreover, supporting the lead with the tip of the anchor as it entered the lumbodorsal fascia improved average time to failure (fracture) by 60-fold compared to the non-supported condition.[55] Finally, bonding the lead to the silicone anchor with silicone adhesive was shown to be the only method that reliably prevented slippage of the lead through the anchor during cyclical loading.[55]

The positions of the leads are then documented again by fluoroscopy, and they are tunneled subcutaneously from the midline incision to the exit side where the pulse generator is going to be implanted. The skin incision is then irrigated (with or without antibiotic solution) and closed in layers using absorbable sutures for the subcutaneous tissue and nylon sutures for the skin (e.g., Vicryl sutures to close the subcutaneous tissue and 3.0 nylon sutures to close the skin).

No consensus exists regarding the best site for implanting the pulse generator (buttock, lower abdomen, subclavicular area) or the need of interposing an extension with safety loops between the lead and the implantable pulse generator (IPG) to release tension generated by patient's movements (especially bending). However, it seems that placement of the IPG in the buttock region may produce up to a fivefold increase in tensile loading compared with placement in the abdomen or midaxillary line, and that the configuration that places the least amount of mechanical strain on the anchor is a coil lead with strain relief loops.[55]

The totally IPG contains a lithium battery, and activation and control occurs through an external transcutaneous telemetry device (for the physician) or through a small portable controller (daily carried by the patient). Life span of the battery varies with usage and with the parameters used (i.e., voltage, rate, and pulse width). Most patients can expect the battery to last, under average usage, between 2.5 to 4.5 years.

Electrical Issues

Understanding the somatotopy of the spinal cord is paramount in understanding the technical aspects of implantation. It is generally agreed that SCS relieves pain only if it induces paresthesias in the area of the patient's pain, although scientific proof is lacking. To this end, correlation of the somatotopy and the level of the spinal cord is necessary. Barolat and associates[56] have published extensively about the mapping of the human spinal structures. A database was created to suggest areas of sensory response to dorsal SCS: the lead contact typically is several levels above the desired area for concordant paresthesia. Moreover, the low threshold of the dorsal root sensory fibers makes it imperative that the lead position is sufficiently midline to avoid recruitment of the root. However, despite an optimally placed electrode, differences in paresthesia coverage between subjects should be expected because of the large interpatient variability of the intraspinal geometry.[57]

It is clear that stimulation on the dorsal aspect of the epidural space creates complex electrical fields that affect a large number of structures.[54] Electrical stimulation depends on the conductivity of the intraspinal elements in relation to the lead position.[11] If a neuron is made more electrically positive or depolarized, it will produce an action potential. Thus the neuron is activated or caused to propagate an action potential. An external electrode that can produce this effect must be negatively charged or a cathode. These effects are called cathodal effects. When the neuron is hyperpolarized or its membrane made more negatively charged, its ability to propagate an action potential is reduced, or its threshold for propagation is raised. A positively charged external electrode or anode produces this anodal effect. Thus the active electrode for stimulation is the cathode, and the anode or positive electrode may shield neuronal structures from the effects of stimulation.

The relative positions of cathodes and anodes and their distance from the spinal cord were demonstrated to be major determinants of axonal activation and paresthesia.[11] As the distance between the cathode and anode increases, the influence of the anode diminishes. At larger distances the field about the cathode becomes a sphere, with little influence produced by the anode. Closer contact produces the greatest influence on the anode, significantly shaping the field by pulling it toward the positive contact.[58] Thus dorsal columns of the spinal cord are most efficiently stimulated with closely spaced longitudinal bipolar (+ −) or tripolar (+ − +) configurations placed on the physiological spinal cord midline because the main current component of the stimulation field corresponds with the orientation of these fibers.[59,60]

The deepest penetration of the cord without creation of a larger electrical field is produced by a technique termed *guarding*.[11] A tripole, in which there is an anode, is placed in close proximity to each side of the cathode. This prevents the cathodal field from expanding beyond the anode on either side. Thus the anode represents the ultimate boundary for the cathodal field. When a guarded cathode is placed in a longitudinal fashion, as in classic SCS, it produces a field with greater penetration of the spinal cord. On the other hand, a guarded cathode used to stimulate in a transverse fashion (using three parallel leads) has the effect of shielding the nerve root and allowing use of greater amplitude to produce better penetration of the cord, contributing to maximum dorsal column stimulation with minimal dorsal root stimulation and providing analgesia to the lower back.[60] Left and right anodes can be set at different voltages, and changes in their voltage ratio ("balance") can steer the electric field from one side of the dorsal columns to the other, thus changing the body area covered with paresthesia.[61] Results from a pilot clinical study showed that the best "steering" score was obtained when the central cathode was >3 mm dorsal to the spinal cord and centered <2 mm from the midline, whereas the electrical field "steering" was impossible when, because of the transverse geometry of the spinal canal, the electrode–spinal cord distance was small compared with the anode-cathode distance (≈3 mm).[61]

According to 22 years of experience of a single teaching center in treating patients with a predominance of axial pain combined with either unilateral or bilateral leg pain, staggered, parallel, multicontact electrodes seem to be more efficacious than parallel, nonstaggered configurations.[51] At present it is difficult to be clear about the electrophysiological explanation for the higher success rate achieved with staggered configuration. A possible explanation is that, by staggering the electrodes, the contact separation distance is reduced, providing more extensive paresthesia coverage.

However, when the paresthesia area can be covered with several configurations, it is beneficial for the patient to program a configuration with one cathode and either no or multiple anodes to decrease energy consumption and increase battery lifetime.[62]

Although how and where the SCS stimulus is applied determines what structures are activated or inactivated,[11] no evidence has been published about the best lead configuration for SCS, and little is known about the effects of frequency and pulse width on SCS efficacy. SCS at 4 and 60 Hz seems to be more effective in reducing hyperalgesia than higher frequencies (100 and 250 Hz).[63]

Failures

Most of the failures are hardware related. Electrode displacement in either the axial or transverse planes was the most frequently encountered complication in SCS,[51] occurring in 9.5% to 21.5% of the patients (according to the type of the implanted system), followed by lead fracture (5.9%) and infection (3.4%).

However, when trying to analyze the cause of failure of satisfactory pain relief at long-term follow-up, Kumar, Hunter, and Demeria[51] found that a certain number of patients begin to require increasing amplitude of current to maintain satisfactory pain control.[51] Over time these patients lose satisfactory pain control, even when the system is fully functional and stimulation continues to produce overlapping paresthesias in the territory of pain. For lack of any better terminology, the phenomenon has been labeled *tolerance* and, according to the authors' opinion, could be considered as the single most important causative factor in the 85 (26%) long-term failures observed in their 22-year retrospective analysis.

Intrathecal Drug Infusion

Pharmacological treatment is effective in most patients suffering from chronic pain, and it is the first step in a multidisciplinary pain program. However, a substantial proportion of patients fails to respond to medication or suffers intolerable side effects. One of the problems with oral or systemic administration of drugs is that the potency of many drugs and their therapeutic effects are limited or reduced because of the partial degradation (e.g., in the stomach or liver) that occurs before they reach the desired target in the body. Thus higher doses of the drug are needed to achieve a therapeutic effect; and it results in intolerable side effects, including tolerance, psychological dependency, and neurotoxicity.

Data from a recent Cochrane systematic review regarding the efficacy and safety of long-term opioid therapy for chronic noncancer pain indicated that many patients discontinued long-term opioid therapy because of adverse effects or incomplete pain relief. The review of 26 different studies, including 4893 patients, showed that as many as 23% of the patients receiving oral opioids interrupted the treatment because of adverse effects and almost 10% of them because of inefficacious analgesia.[64]

Methods to intrathecally deliver drugs as close to the spinal cord as possible have been developed (intrathecal pumps) as an alternative to oral and systemic drug administration in the effort of overcoming both drug-related side effects and treatment failures.[65]

Delivering equipotent analgesic doses of medications directly to the spinal receptors could minimize opioid-related adverse effects by markedly reducing systemic exposure.[66] As a result, it has been suggested that opioids given by the intrathecal route compared to oral administration are less likely to be the cause of patients abandoning treatment, either because of side effects (23% vs. 9%) or ineffective analgesia (10% vs. 8%).[64]

Although intrathecal therapy initially was used only in the treatment of cancer-related pain, today the majority of patients treated with spinally administered medication have non-cancer types of pain. In a recent survey of experienced neuromodulation centers (more than 10 implants a year), FBSS was identified as the top indication for both SCS and intrathecal drug infusion device implantation.[67]

Mechanism of Action

There is limited research into the precise mode of action of the various agents reported to provide analgesia following intrathecal delivery since most use has been empirical. Of the 18 agents for which clinical or preclinical data for intrathecal infusion were found, only one (ziconotide [Prialt, ziconotide intrathecal infusion, Azur Pharmaceuticals, Dublin, Ireland]) had extensive data as a result of a formal development program for intrathecal administration.[68]

The most frequent intrathecally administered drug class (i.e., opioids) seems to act at receptors in the substantia gelatinosa of the spinal cord dorsal horn to yield dose-dependent analgesia.[69] Opioids may act through multiple mechanisms, including inhibition of presynaptic neurotransmitter release from primary afferents via presynaptic inhibition of calcium channels. Furthermore, opening of G-protein gates, K+ channels in the central nervous system (G-protein–regulated inwardly-rectifying K+ channels [GIRKs]) may lead to postsynaptic neuronal hyperpolarization. However, recent evidence highlights that antinociception following intrathecal opioids involves both spinal and supraspinal opioid receptors.[70]

Several drugs have been injected intrathecally so far to treat chronic pain. A brief summary of their hypothesized mechanism of action could be found in **Table 13-1**.[65,71]

Drug Diffusion

Little is known about the spread of the intrathecally infused drugs along the neuraxis. However, recent evidence links both the high failure rate seen in some studies of chronic intrathecal drug delivery (IDD) and the very wide range of effective doses seen in others with different patterns of drug distribution within the cerebrospinal fluid (CSF) at different spinal cord levels. Walker and associates[72] reported a failure rate as high as 40% in treating patients implanted with intrathecal pumps for baclofen administration despite a successful intrathecal, single-shot baclofen bolus trial. The failure to improve despite much larger doses of the same drug administered by slow continuous infusion was explained as a pharmacokinetic failure (i.e., a failure of baclofen to distribute from the administration site to the target site in sufficient quantity to reproduce the previously demonstrated pharmacodynamic effect).

To study intrathecal drug distribution during chronic continuous slow infusion in an animal model (pig), continuous samples of CSF at multiple sites along the spinal cord were taken by means of microdialysis techniques while a solution of bupivacaine and baclofen was infused. The distribution of the drug resulted to be very limited compared with that which occurs with bolus administration, with most of the infused drug recovered in the CSF and spinal cord found within 1 cm of the administration site.[73]

Table 13-1: Drugs Frequently Infused Intrathecally

Drug	Class	Mechanism of Action
Morphine Hydromorphone fentanyl	Opioids	Inhibit C-fiber transmission by binding to presynaptic and postsynaptic opioid mu receptors in substantia gelatinosa and dorsal horn
Clonidine	α_2 Agonist	Binds to presynaptic and postsynaptic α_2 receptors in dorsal horn, inhibiting neurotransmission, and depresses release of C-fiber transmitters, including substance P
Ziconotide (Prialt)	Anticonvulsant (?)	Blocks N-type voltage-sensitive calcium channels (N-VSCCs)
Baclofen (Lioresal)	Anticonvulsant	Agonist of GABA$_B$ receptor
Bupivacaine	Local anesthetic	Binds to plasma membrane of nerve cells, causing distortion of the fast sodium channels, thus preventing the sodium influx that initiates the action potential

However, in an attempt to limit the frequency of pump refills, clinicians frequently use highly concentrated drug solutions for chronic intrathecal infusions, which seem to be mostly hyperbaric. The effect of baricity and posture on drug distribution in the CSF and spinal cord during the very slow infusion rates typically used for chronic intrathecal drug administration has been recently studied in an animal model.[74]

Significant differences were found in drug distribution in the CSF and spinal cord in both the rostrocaudal and anteroposterior axes as a function of animal position. Bupivacaine and baclofen distributions were biased caudally in animals placed in a vertical position and cephalad in those placed horizontally, whereas the vertical position favored the posterior location of the study drugs compared with the horizontal position (likely because of the posterior location of the infusion catheter combined with anatomical barriers to circumferential drug movement). Drug concentration decreased rapidly in the CSF and spinal cord as a function of distance from the site of administration in both groups, resulting in most drugs being located in very close proximity to the site of infusion. Therefore latest evidence supports the hypotheses that (1) drug distribution in the CSF and spinal cord during slow intrathecal infusions is much more limited than that which occurs after an intrathecal bolus; (2) drug baricity and patient position may be important factors in determining the drug spread; (3) the location of the intrathecal catheter tip relative to the targeted spinal cord segment is a potentially important determinant of efficacy; and (4) measurements of the density of custom-compounded drug solutions could be important in determining the distribution of chronic intrathecal infusions.

Intrathecal Drug Infusion: An Evidence-Based Therapy?

Despite the widespread use of intrathecal drug infusion to treat chronic noncancer pain, unremarkable evidence of its efficacy has not yet been published. The main controversy surrounding spinal analgesia is whether it is effective in the long term for nonmalignant pain.[75] Intrathecal opioids do provide short-term pain relief,[76] but their long-term ability to attenuate pain and improve function is less convincing because opioid-induced hyperalgesia seems to account for a significant component of narcotic tolerance.

As stated by the American Society of Interventional Pain Physicians, the evidence for implantable intrathecal infusion systems is strong for short-term improvement in pain of either malignant or neuropathic origin.[77] However, although reasonably strong evidence exists for the use of long-term intrathecal drug infusion in cancer pain,[69] the evidence supporting long-term efficacy in persistent noncancer pain is less convincing. Moreover, the high cost of both the implantable device and the patients' follow-up makes some physicians doubtful regarding cost-effectiveness of long-term intrathecal therapy in patients with chronic pain.

Contrary to the available SCS literature, a recently published systematic review on the effectiveness of intrathecal infusion devices in treating chronic noncancer pain found no RCTs and included just observational studies.[78] Pain relief (short-term ≤1 year, long-term >1 year) was considered as the primary outcome variable; measures of improvement in functional status, psychological status, return to work, and reduction in opioid intake were included as secondary outcomes. The authors concluded that, based on U.S. Preventive Services Task Force criteria, the level of evidence for intrathecal infusion systems should be graded as level II-3 or level III (limited evidence). However, the lack of properly designed RCTs and the heterogeneous designs of the included studies make useful comparisons of existing literature quite difficult. As a matter of fact, older systematic reviews reported a slightly superior level of evidence. Boswell and associates[77] concluded that there is moderate evidence for long-term management of chronic pain with intrathecal infusion systems at 1 year or longer follow-up. In a reassessment of an evidence synthesis by the American College of Occupational and Environmental Medicine guidelines, Manchikanti and colleagues[79] also found moderate evidence for long-term management of chronic noncancer pain with intrathecal infusion systems.

Moreover, several well-known research groups reported long-term (exceeding 3 years) excellent or good pain reduction in 50% to 75% of the treated patients originally suffering from noncancer chronic pain.[80-85]

Finally, a simple reduction in the VAS pain score may not be the only variable to be considered as the target primary outcome. Just as an example, in a prospective study evaluating the impact of intrathecal morphine infusions on pain perception and psychosocial functionality, Duse, Davia, and White[86] reported a significant improvement in both evaluative and affective components of the pain assessment over the 24-month study period. The evaluative component of the McGill Pain Questionnaire improved 66%, the affective component 59%, and the sensory component 32%. The reduced level of chronic pain leads to improved social, work, and family relationships and quality of life. Among 13 patients of working age, 12 returned to work full time; among 17 retired patients, 14 had a reduced need for assistance.

Intrathecal Drug Infusion in Failed Back Surgery Syndrome

Although SCS has been studied extensively in patients suffering from FBSS, no specific data regarding the use of intrathecal infusion in complex chronic pain of spinal origin have been published.

However, most of the noncancer pain studies included in the available systematic reviews recruited FBSS patients as a population suitable to represent mixed (neuropathic and nociceptive) pain, and the same general level of evidence (limited evidence) could be applied to this specific subset of patients. Nevertheless, few small studies suggest that intrathecal drug infusion could decrease pain scores and increase quality of life in patients with residual low back pain and radiculopathy.

A long-term evaluation (mean follow-up 27 months) of a treatment regimen consisting of intrathecal morphine mixed with bupivacaine, clonidine, or midazolam in 26 patients with chronic nonmalignant back and leg pain caused by FBSS showed excellent or good long-term results in 19 patients and sufficient results in 6; only 1 patient complained of poor therapeutic efficacy.[87] In a review of the efficacy of IDD in 136 patients with chronic low back pain identified from the U.S. National Outcomes Registry for Low Back Pain, numerical pain ratings had fallen by more than 47% for back pain and 31% for leg pain at the 12-month follow-up. A total of 65% of patients had reduced their ODI scores by at least one level after 12 months, 80% were satisfied with their therapy, and 87% said that they would undergo the procedure again.[88]

However, FBSS is a heterogeneous chronic pain condition, and patients could have different degrees of nociceptive and neuropathic pain at the same time. According to the authors' experience and to the results of a multicenter, retrospective study that surveyed pain physicians in the United States, patients with somatic pain seem to have greater analgesic benefit with intrathecal infusion than the ones suffering from pure neuropathic pain.[89] Numerous preclinical[90] and clinical[91] studies confirmed the hypothesis that neuropathic pain could be less responsive to opioids than nociceptive pain.

Despite being heavily criticized for its high initial costs, intrathecal drug therapy proved to be cost-effective in the long term in patients who respond to this treatment. Kumar, Hunter, and Demeria[92] looked at the cost of implanting a programmable drug delivery pump vs. conservative treatment of chronic pain from FBSS. The cumulative costs for IDD during a 5-year period were $29,410, as opposed to $38,000 for conservative treatments. High initial costs of equipment required for IDD were recovered by 28 months. After this time, managing patients with conservative treatments became more expensive for the remainder of the follow-up period. Kumar, Hunter, and Demeria's data are in agreement with an older cost-effectiveness evaluation, which showed that intrathecal morphine delivery results in low cumulative 60-month costs ($16,579 per year) vs. medical management ($17,037 per year).[93]

Patient Selection

Intrathecal drug infusion should be considered only when pain control with conventional oral and systemic administration is inadequate or associated with unmanageable side effects and when alternatives such as SCS have already failed[65] (**Box 13-1**). However the use of IDD systems in chronic nonmalignant pain is still controversial. Considering that chronic nonmalignant pain is complicated by physical, psychological, and behavioral factors, we should remember that to be successful a treatment must include a multidimensional approach that takes into account each of the elements of the biopsychosocial model.[94]

To optimize the chances for a successful treatment outcome, patients should be selected carefully and undergo a trial period. This may be carried out by inserting a temporary intrathecal catheter and running a continuous infusion of the drug, usually over 1 to several days or less invasively and more frequently by means of intrathecal injection or continuous epidural infusion. In a recent

> **Box 13-1: Criteria for Appropriate Use of Intraspinal Drug Delivery**
>
> 1. The oral route and other less invasive methods cause excessive side effects and/or inadequate relief.
> 2. Spinal analgesics provide better pain relief and quality of life than other methods of analgesia.
> 3. The effectiveness of analgesia is tested by a preimplantation trial.
> 4. The caregiver and the patient are trained, and there is good communication among the staff, the patient, and the patient's supporters.
> 5. The general and psychological status is stable and favorable.
> 6. The drug delivery system is cost-effective.

prospective, randomized trial of intrathecal injection vs. epidural infusion in the selection of patients for IDD, it was found that bolus intrathecal injection of morphine was equally as effective as epidural infusion and was less costly.[95]

A standard intrathecal bolus dose has not yet been established, most likely because of the large intersubject response variability. A recent prospective, randomized, double-blind investigation assessed the dose-effect characteristics of postoperative nausea and vomiting after intrathecal administration of small doses of morphine (from 0.015 to 0.25 mg) in nonsurgical patients suffering from noncancerous chronic back-pain.[96] In this study, the authors concluded that the onset and incidence of minor opioid-related side effects after intrathecal morphine administration do not depend on its dose (i.e., they occurred with even very small doses [0.015 mg]).[96]

Technical Issues

Drug Choice Opioids are the most commonly used agents for long-term spinal drug therapy for pain control.[65,75] Until recently only morphine had U.S. Food and Drug Administration (FDA) approval for long-term intrathecal infusion.[69] Patients with a neuropathic pain component should be considered initially for monotherapy with morphine or its derivative hydromorphone,[97] both of which are supported by extensive clinical experience and published preclinical and clinical data.[65] Selected patients with pure or predominant neuropathic pain should be considered for initial treatment with an opioid plus adjuvant medication such as the local anesthetic bupivacaine or the α_2-agonist clonidine. In case of failure of intrathecal morphine, combination with nonopioid drugs such as the anticonvulsant baclofen or the local anesthetic bupivacaine[98,99] also is possible and has been shown to be effective in patients with central pain and those with peripheral, nociceptive, or neuropathic pain mechanisms.

Ziconotide Results from this observational study suggest that combination intrathecal ziconotide and opioid therapy may be a safe and potentially effective treatment option for patients with refractory chronic pain.[100]

Ziconotide is a nonopioid analgesic; results from animal studies suggest that it inhibits neurotransmission from primary nociceptive afferents in the dorsal horn of the spinal cord by binding to and blocking N-type voltage-sensitive calcium channels (N-VSCCs).[101,102] Direct blockade of N-VSCCs inhibits the activity of a subset of neurons, including pain-sensing primary nociceptors. This mechanism of action distinguishes ziconotide from all other analgesics, including opioid analgesics. Moreover, in contrast to opiates, tolerance to ziconotide is not observed.

On the basis of relevant new literature and clinical experience, The Polyanalgesic Conference 2007, a panel of experts known for their expertise in intrathecal therapy, believed that ziconotide should be upgraded to a first-line intrathecal agent; currently ziconotide and morphine are the only drugs approved by the FDA for administration for intrathecal pain therapy.

Evidence from double-blinded controlled trials, open-label studies,[103] case series, and case studies suggests that ziconotide, as either monotherapy or in combination with other intrathecal drugs, is a potential therapeutic option for patients with refractory neuropathic pain.[104] In preclinical studies ziconotide demonstrated antiallodynic effects on neuropathic pain, and clinical data indicated that patients with neuropathic pain reported a mean percent improvement in pain score with ziconotide monotherapy that ranged from 15.7% to 31.6%. The main adverse effects of ziconotide in clinical trials were cerebellovestibular disorders such as ataxia, dizziness, and gait disorders; confusion; hallucinations (increased in cases of overdose); nausea; vomiting; postural hypotension; and urine retention. Approximately 40% of patients had an elevation in muscle creatine kinase activity through an unknown mechanism. A low starting dose and slow titration of ziconotide resulted in an improved safety profile and a better side-effects profile.[105]

However, the efficacy of ziconotide in relieving neurogenic pain is still questioned by some authors.[106] In particular:

- Clinical evaluation of ziconotide does not include any trials vs. morphine in patients with nociceptive pain or any trials vs. tricyclic or antiepileptic drugs in patients with neurogenic pain.
- In a trial of 220 patients in whom systemic morphine had failed, the mean pain score on a 100-mm VAS was 69.8 mm after 3 weeks on ziconotide compared to 75.8 mm with placebo. This difference, although statistically significant, is clinically irrelevant. The proportion of responders (reduction of at least 30% in the initial pain score) was respectively 16.1% and 12.0% (no statistically significant difference).
- The two other placebo-controlled trials included 112 patients with pain linked to cancer or human immunodeficiency virus infection and 257 patients with noncancer pain. After a titration phase lasting 5 to 6 days, a combined analysis of the two trials showed that the mean pain score was 48.8 mm with ziconotide and 68.4 mm with placebo (statistically significant difference). However, many patients did not complete the titration phase.
- Efficacy also appeared to differ according to the type of pain; ziconotide was more effective for cancer pain than for neurogenic pain, and some patients might experience a paradoxical increase in pain with ziconotide.

Patient-Controlled Analgesia

In a general sense patient-controlled analgesia (PCA) refers to a process in which patients can determine when and how much medication they receive, regardless of analgesic technique. However, the term is more commonly used to describe a method of pain relief that uses disposable or electronic infusion devices and allows patients to self-administer analgesic drugs, usually intravenous (IV) opioids, as required.

The PCA concept has been extended to implanted programmable pumps to control unpredictable pain fluctuations in patients whose constant pain is otherwise well controlled by a continuous spinal drug infusion. Medtronic (Minneapolis, Minn) developed an external device (personal therapy manager [PTM]), that the patient can use to trigger the pump to deliver a predetermined dose of drug. The number of boluses permitted and lock-out periods can also be programmed.[107] The system has been evaluated in a multicenter, open-label registry conducted in seven European countries enrolling chronic pain patients (92% noncancer pain, mainly FBSS) during a follow-up period of up to 12 months. Of the 168 patients enrolled, 79 had a preexisting pump, and 89 received a pump after their enrollment in the registry. Although more than half of the subjects experienced benign complications (essentially drug-related side effects) and despite the fact that not all patients experienced significantly greater pain relief as a result of PTM use, 75% of patients with a preexisting pump were more satisfied with the PTM system than with their pump alone.

Surgical Technique

An intrathecal pump consists of a small battery-powered, programmable pump that is implanted under the subcutaneous tissue of the abdomen and connected to a small catheter tunneled to the site of spinal entry.[94] The surgical technique consists of catheter placement under fluoroscopy followed by implantation of the pump.[94] The patient is placed in a lateral decubitus position, prepped, and draped in sterile fashion. Skin bacterial colonization can be decreased before the operation by having the patient wash with an antibacterial soap the night before and the morning of surgery. If a patient is a known carrier of methicillin-resistant *Staphylococcus aureus* (MRSA), it is wise to obtain a nasal swab before surgery and treat with vancomycin if found to be positive.[94] Repeat nasal swabs should be done until clear before proceeding with the procedure. Prophylactic antibiotic agents have been shown to decrease the risk of shunt-related infections and are recommended for operations involving the implantation of pumps, although data are not available to confirm their effectiveness. The double-gloving practice is advisable and has been shown to be associated with a lower infection rate in studies involving shunt surgery and in orthopedic studies.

A posterior midline incision approximately 5 to 7 cm long is made from the skin to the supraspinous fascia at approximately L2-L3 or L3-L4. A 16-g Tuohy spinal needle is advanced through the incision into the epidural space with a shallow angled paramedian approach. Some surgeons place a purse-string 2-0 silk suture around the Tuohy needle before removing the needle to prevent CSF from entering the subcutaneous tissue and creating a hygroma. After removing the needle, the catheter is anchored to the supraspinous fascia using a Silastic anchor provided by the manufacturer. Remember that it is possible to puncture or occlude the catheter when suturing it. Therefore, before proceeding, the end of the catheter should be checked for free-flowing CSF and clamped to prevent excessive leakage.

Surgical techniques that minimize CSF leakage are essential to successful intrathecal baclofen therapy. CSF leaks usually develop within 2 weeks of pump/catheter insertion and may present as subcutaneous swelling posteriorly beneath the lumbar incision, anteriorly over and around the pump, or both. These leaks impair wound healing; and, if CSF transgresses through the incision to the exterior, an infection usually develops.

A shallow-angle paramedian catheter insertion technique can reduce the incidence of CSF leakage because the catheter obliquely traverses several centimeters of paravertebral musculature before the dura is punctured and because the purse-string circumferential suture is inserted around the Tuohy needle before it is withdrawn.

After the pump is prepared, an incision for the pump pocket is made in the right or left lower quadrant of the abdomen at or about the umbilical level. The pump should be placed below the belt line but not too close to the anterior rib or iliac crest because it may lead to prolonged discomfort. Because of refilling requirements, it is important not to place the pump too deep.

After creating the pump pocket, a tunneling device is used to tunnel the catheter subcutaneously from the back wound to the pump pocket. The catheter should then be measured, trimmed if needed, and connected to the pump. Before connecting the catheter, it is important to once again verify the free flow of CSF. The pump is now placed into the pocket reservoir side up. Any excess catheter should be placed behind the pump to prevent damage to the catheter during refilling. The pump should be secured to the pocket by suturing to the abdominal fascia under the pump pocket. Before closing the wounds, it is important to establish adequate hemostasis to prevent the risk of postoperative infections and to irrigate the surgical site with a pulse irrigator and a diluted iodine solution. The wounds should be closed in a two-layer closure according to the preference of the surgeon.

Recently the ITB Therapy Best Practice Forum developed recommendations to help surgeons implant pumps effectively while minimizing surgical complications.[108] The following technical key points should be considered:

- Subfascial placement is particularly advisable in thin, small children (baclofen infusion); but the technique has some advantages even in obese patients, in whom it may reduce the risk of the pump becoming flipped if the retaining sutures break.
- Incisions under tension often heal poorly, and pumps often erode through thin tissues.
- The L2-L3 or L3-L4 levels are associated with less movement than the L4-L5 level and therefore less wear-and-tear on the catheter.
- Insertion of the Tuohy needle in an oblique, shallow-angle, paramedian trajectory allows easy rostral advancement of the catheter into the intrathecal space.
- Use of a suture ligature around the Tuohy needle at its exit site from the fascia minimizes the incidence of cerebrospinal fluid (CSF) leakage.
- Anchor the catheter to the fascia or muscle with a Silastic butterfly flap and a nonabsorbable suture to minimize the risk of outward migration.
- To prevent catheter kinks, it is important that the needle enter the supraspinous fascia at the rostral end of the incision to ensure that the catheter has room caudally to gently exit and connect to the pump catheter.

Complications

Although intrathecal infusion is considered to be a safe treatment, a recent paper underlined the fact that patients with noncancer pain treated with intrathecal opioid therapy experience increased mortality compared to similar patients treated with other therapies, including SCS and low back surgery.[109] Respiratory depression as a direct consequence of intrathecal drug overdose or mixed intrathecal and systemic drug interactions is one plausible, but hypothetical, cause. Despite the low mortality rate reported (mortality rate of 0.088% at 3 days after implantation, 0.39% at 1 month, and 3.89% at 1 year), the report should be considered to be a serious concern and needs further investigation.

Technical Complications

A significant proportion of side effects and complications related to long-term intrathecal analgesic infusion has been reported: in a retrospective analysis of 419 patients with at least 6 months of infusion time, a rate as high as 21.6% was reported.[89] In a 12-year retrospective review of a tertiary center with long-term experience in intrathecal infusion, the annual rate for complications requiring surgical measures was 10.5%; 35% were pump related and 65% were catheter related.[110] After 3 years of continuous treatment, catheter-related technical problems (catheter dislocation, obstruction, kinking, disconnection, or rupture) can be observed in as many as 11% of patients,[80] whereas pump malfunctions are quite rare (5%) and usually limited to older pump types.

Intrathecal Granuloma

Intrathecal granuloma formation is a serious complication that carries the potential to produce spinal cord compression and paralysis caused by the development of an inflammatory mass at the distal tip of spinal infusion catheters.[111] Over 100 cases have been reported, the first of which was in 1991, with an estimated incidence ranging between 0.1% and 5% and an increased rate associated with the long-term infusions.[112,113]

Based on published data from human and animal studies, the most plausible explanation for the formation of these lesions include the properties of opioids (especially morphine), the dynamics of CSF and the location of the distal tip of the catheter. Formation of a granuloma is associated specifically with high concentrations of opioids at a low administration rate and a low CSF flow rate.[114-116] However, 39% of cases occurred with morphine concentrations less than 25 mg/mL, and 30% received daily morphine doses less than 10 mg/day. Some were also noted within 1 month of the initiation of therapy.[69]

Studies published so far suggest the absence of a specific role for opioid receptors in the formation of a granuloma, whereas the etiology does appear to be related to the drug-induced release of histamine and other inflammatory mediators by the mast cells in the dura mater. Long-term intrathecal infusion of morphine significantly increases the spinal levels of inflammatory cytokines and induces a slight but significant phosphorylation of mitogen-activated protein kinase.[117] A significant expression of tumor necrosis factor–α was observed in catheter-tip granulomas and in macrophages in the perivascular cuffs.[118] Degranulation of dural mast cells occurs after exposure to morphine or hydromorphone in vivo and in vitro.[119] These mast cells have a phenotype similar to that of skin mast cells in terms of response to opioid drugs.[119] Based on these findings, it has been suggested that the inflammatory cells derive from dural microvascularization near the tip of the catheter[120]—its activation and the consequent release of inflammatory mediators (such as cytokines and histamine) being responsible, at least in part, for the formation of inflammatory masses around the tip of the catheter.

Opioid-Induced Side Effects

Almost all intrathecal opioid-related side effects are mediated by opioid receptors.[121] The majority of the commonly seen pharmacological side effects during intrathecal morphine therapy such as pruritus nausea/vomiting, urinary retention, constipation, mental status change, and respiratory depression can be easily antagonized by the mu antagonist, naloxone. However, the analgesic effect may or may not be maintained. Side effects of intrathecal morphine therapy are usually common at the initiation phase of the treatment and generally resolve with standard medical management during the first 3 months with few exceptions (e.g., sweating, peripheral edema, constipation).[75,122]

Finally, patients receiving intrathecal opioids exhibit changes in their neuroendocrine function. In a case series of 73 patients with noncancer pain, the majority of patients developed hypogonado-tropic hypogonadism, 15% developed central hypocortisolism, and 96% of men and 69% of women who received intrathecal opioids reported decreased libido.

Infections Related to Implanted Devices

Spinal Cord Stimulation Infection

Device-related infection is the most common, potentially reducible, serious adverse event associated with IDD or SCS devices.[123] Treatment of an established infection often involves temporary or permanent removal of the device, which causes cessation of drug or stimulation therapy, exposing the patient to additional risks (abrupt cessation of intrathecal drug therapy may precipitate drug withdrawal symptoms), discomfort, and inconvenience. The results of postmarket surveillance of 114 infections that involved Medtronic implantable SCS devices in the period between September 2000 and July 2002 showed that in 94% of the cases, physicians decided to completely or partially remove the infected SCS devices, and in 91% of all SCS cases, patients experienced resolution of their infections without major morbidity.[123] No episodes of meningitis or mortality were reported, and the IPG pocket proved to be the most vulnerable site (54%) followed by the tract connecting the IPG to the lead (17%).

Intrathecal Drug Delivery Infection

Infection does seem to be more frequent in intrathecal device implants compared with stimulators.[123] Acute (within 60 days of the surgery) infection rate after the implant of an IDD system ranges between 4% to 12%,[69] and the probability of developing a late infection was 1% per year of follow-up.[124] In experienced centers the incidence of infections can be as low as 0.7% per year, with all the infections reported occurring during the first 3 months after implantation of the pump.[110] System removal should no longer be considered the first treatment option in infections of intrathecally delivering pumps, especially those caused by non-adherent bacteria, with mild clinical symptomatology.[125] An initial attempt should always be made to treat conservatively; intrapocket administration of antibiotics helps to achieve high drug levels locally.

Infection Prevention

Pertinent information from the most recent version of surgical site infection prevention guidelines published by the Centers for Disease Control and Prevention is summarized in **Box 13-2**. Additional recommendations derived from a review of the CSF shunt literature and from postmarket surveillance data on IDD and SCS device infections are also included in the class II recommendations in **Box 13-2**.[123]

Box 13-2: Surgical Site Infection Prevention Guidelines Published by the Centers for Disease Control and Prevention

Patient Selection, Preparation, Surgical Planning, and Preoperative Hand and Forearm Antisepsis
CATEGORY IA
- Identify and treat all remote infections before elective operation; postpone surgery until cured.
- Do not remove hair unless removal is necessary to facilitate surgery.
- If hair is removed, do so immediately before surgery, preferably with electric clippers.

CATEGORY IB
- Control serum blood glucose perioperatively.
- Patients should discontinue tobacco use 30 days before surgery.
- Do not withhold necessary blood products to prevent surgical site infections (SSIs).
- Require patients to shower or bathe with an antiseptic agent at least the night before surgery.
- Perform surgical scrub for at least 2 to 5 minutes with an appropriate antiseptic.
- After scrub, keep hands up and away from body, and dry hands with sterile towel; don sterile gown and gloves.
- Wash incision site before performing antiseptic skin preparation with approved agent.

CATEGORY II
- Prepare skin in concentric circles from incision site.
- Keep preoperative stay in hospital as short as possible.
- Device implantation may proceed, albeit at increased risk, in patients (especially those with spasticity or cancer pain) in whom remote infections or other risk factors cannot be eradicated or resolved completely.
- Select device or model suitable for patient's size and body habitus.
- Consider surgical scars, ostomies, seat belt or wheelchair use, and clothing or belt line in selection of device pocket site.

- If practical, mark the device pocket site before surgery with the patient in the standing and/or sitting position.

Surgical and Operating Room Management
CATEGORY II
- Perform implant surgery in an operating room rather than a procedure room.
- Minimize operating room traffic during implant surgery.
- Use sterile draped fluoroscope to expedite case and avoid contamination by portable x-ray equipment.

Antimicrobial Prophylaxis
CATEGORY IA
- Administer antimicrobial agent only when indicated and if effective against most common pathogens.
- Use intravenous route to achieve adequate serum concentrations during surgery and for at most a few hours after incision is closed.

CATEGORY IB
- Do not routinely use vancomycin for antimicrobial prophylaxis.

Surgical Procedure
CATEGORY II
- Use double-glove and minimal-touch or no-touch surgical techniques.
- Avoid implanting devices directly under incision lines.
- Close the implant site incisions in anatomical layers, consider subfascial placement in small or underweight patients.

Postoperative Care
CATEGORY II
- Apply occlusive, antiseptic wound dressings; perform the initial dressing change using sterile technique.
- Treat threatened incisions and external cerebrospinal leaks promptly and aggressively.

Adapted from Mangram AJ et al: Guideline for prevention of surgical site infection, 1999: Hospital Infection Control Practices Advisory Committee, *Infect Control Hosp Epidemiol* 20:250-278, 1999.

Other practical advice could be suggested, despite not being supported by scientific evidence and not included in the guidelines[123]:

- Avoid the potentially contaminated temporary lead-extension tract when internalizing SCS leads after the trial period.
- Place the neurostimulator pocket on the side of the body opposite the location of the temporary lead or extension wire tract.
- If the permanent electrode or extension wire or both must be implanted at the same cutaneous/subcutaneous site used for the temporary trial, a delay between removal of the trial system and implantation of the permanent SCS system should be considered.
- Permanent internalization of percutaneously inserted SCS trial leads during a second-stage neurostimulator implant operation requires careful removal of the temporary extension wires (withdrawn by having a nonscrubbed assistant pull on the external extension from outside the sterile operative field after the implanter has disconnected it from the extraspinal end of the stimulation lead).

After a small series of infections associated with SCS and IDD devices, Burgher and associates[126] found the implementation of a series of prevention measures to be effective, albeit not statistically significant because of the general low rate of infections. These included: (1) a traditional air exchange operating room venue rather than a procedure suite for implantation of all devices, (2) perioperative IV antibiotic prophylaxis, (3) patient antiseptic bathing prior to surgery, (4) 10-minute scrub of the surgical site using chlorhexidine followed by povidone-iodine paint, (5) double gloving of operative personnel, (6) optimal scrub procedure classes and anatomy-based suturing instruction for all pain fellows involved in device implantation, and (7) intraoperative wound irrigation with an antibiotic-containing solution.

The role of povidone-iodine paint as both a skin antiseptic and wound sterilizing agent is still controversial, especially when compared to chlorhexidine-alcohol for preventing surgical site infection after clean-contaminated surgery.[127] Povidone-iodine has bactericidal activity against a wide spectrum of pathogens, including MRSA. In experimental studies povidone-iodine solution has been found to be maximally effective against MRSA in a dilution of 1:25 to 1:200 (0.5% to 4% Betadine). Cytotoxicity has been observed in the osteoblasts of cultured chicken tibias at a Betadine concentration of 5%, but few (if any) cytotoxic effects occur at a lower Betadine concentration of 0.5%. Moreover, the inhibitory effects on osteoblast and fibroblast have been reported in animal studies only.[128] After spinal surgery procedures, soaking surgical wounds with dilute povidone-iodine solution for 3 minutes followed by wound irrigation with normal saline resulted in no wound infections in an RCT enrolling 414 patients undergoing spinal surgery.[129] Conversely, one superficial infection and six deep infections (total infection rate 3.4%) were noted in the control group when wound irrigation with normal saline alone was performed. An identical protocol was applied in another study aimed to evaluate the effect of wound irrigation with povidone-iodine not only on infection rates, but also on wound healing, fusion status, and clinical outcome of spinal surgeries.[130] Authors obtained results similar to the ones of the previous RCT (0% vs. 4.8% infection rates) and concluded that diluted povidone-iodine solution can be used safely in spinal surgeries without influencing wound healing, bone union, and clinical outcomes.

References

1. Dworkin RH et al: Advances in neuropathic pain: diagnosis, mechanisms, and treatment recommendations. *Arch Neurol* 60:1524-1534, 2003.
2. Leveque J et al: Spinal cord stimulation for failed back surgery syndrome. *Neuromodulation* 4:1-9, 2001.
3. North RB et al: Failed back surgery syndrome: 5-year follow-up in 102 patients undergoing repeated operation. *Neurosurgery* 28:685-690; discussion 90-1, 1991.
4. Mekhail NA et al: Clinical applications of neurostimulation: forty years later. *Pain Pract* 10(2):103-112, 2010.
5. Thomson S, Jacques L: Demographic characteristics of patients with severe neuropathic pain secondary to failed back surgery syndrome. *Pain Pract* 9:206-215, 2009.
6. Bittar RG, Teddy PJ: Peripheral neuromodulation for pain. *J Clin Neurosci* 16:1259-1261, 2009.
7. De Andres J, Van Buyten JP: Neural modulation by stimulation. *Pain Pract* 6:39-45, 2005.
8. Van Buyten JP: Neurostimulation for chronic neuropathic back pain in failed back surgery syndrome. *J Pain Symptom Manage* 31:S25-S29, 2006.
9. Melzack R, Wall PD: Pain mechanisms: a new theory. *Science* 150:971-979, 1965.
10. Lindblom U, Meyerson BA: Influence on touch, vibration and cutaneous pain of dorsal column stimulation in man. *Pain* 1:257-270, 1975.
11. Oakley JC, Prager JP: Spinal cord stimulation: mechanisms of action. *Spine* 27:2574-2583, 2002.
12. Buonocore M, Bonezzi C, Barolat G: Neurophysiological evidence of antidromic activation of large myelinated fibres in lower limbs during spinal cord stimulation. *Spine* 33:E90-E93, 2008.
13. Smits H et al: Spinal cord stimulation induces c-Fos expression in the dorsal horn in rats with neuropathic pain after partial sciatic nerve injury. *Neurosci Lett* 450:70-73, 2009.
14. Song Z et al: Pain relief by spinal cord stimulation involves serotonergic mechanisms: an experimental study in a rat model of mononeuropathy. *Pain* 147:241-248, 2009.
15. Stancak A et al: Functional magnetic resonance imaging of cerebral activation during spinal cord stimulation in failed back surgery syndrome patients. *Eur J Pain* 12:137-148, 2008.
16. Dubuisson D: Effect of dorsal-column stimulation on gelatinosa and marginal neurons of cat spinal cord. *J Neurosurg* 70:257-265, 1989.
17. Lindblom U, Tapper DN, Wiesenfeld Z: The effect of dorsal column stimulation on the nociceptive response of dorsal horn cells and its relevance for pain suppression. *Pain* 4:133-144, 1977.
18. Yakhnitsa V, Linderoth B, Meyerson BA: Spinal cord stimulation attenuates dorsal horn neuronal hyperexcitability in a rat model of mononeuropathy. *Pain* 79:223-233, 1999.
19. Qin C et al: Modulation of neuronal activity in dorsal column nuclei by upper cervical spinal cord stimulation in rats. *Neuroscience* 164:770-776, 2009.
20. Baba H et al: Synaptic responses of substantia gelatinosa neurones to dorsal column stimulation in rat spinal cord in vitro. *J Physiol* 478 (Pt 1):87-99, 1994.
21. Schechtmann G et al: Cholinergic mechanisms involved in the pain relieving effect of spinal cord stimulation in a model of neuropathy. *Pain* 139:136-145, 2008.
22. Meyerson BA, Linderoth B: Mechanisms of spinal cord stimulation in neuropathic pain. *Neurol Res 2000* 22:285-292, 2000.
23. Jeon Y, Huh BK: Spinal cord stimulation for chronic pain. *Ann Acad Med Singapore* 38:998-1003, 2009.
24. Meyerson BA, Linderoth B: Mode of action of spinal cord stimulation in neuropathic pain. *J Pain Symptom Manage* 31:S6-S12, 2006.
25. Cui JG et al: Spinal cord stimulation attenuates augmented dorsal horn release of excitatory amino acids in mononeuropathy via a GABAergic mechanism. *Pain* 73:87-95, 1997.
26. Stiller CO et al: Release of gamma-aminobutyric acid in the dorsal horn and suppression of tactile allodynia by spinal cord stimulation

in mononeuropathic rats. *Neurosurgery* 39:367-374; discussion 74-75, 1996.

27. Lind G et al: Intrathecal baclofen as adjuvant therapy to enhance the effect of spinal cord stimulation in neuropathic pain: a pilot study. *Eur J Pain* 8:377-383, 2004.

28. Lind G et al: Baclofen-enhanced spinal cord stimulation and intrathecal baclofen alone for neuropathic pain: long-term outcome of a pilot study. *Eur J Pain* 12:132-136, 2008.

29. Truin M et al: The effect of spinal cord stimulation in mice with chronic neuropathic pain after partial ligation of the sciatic nerve. *Pain* 145:312-318, 2009.

30. Smits H et al: Effect of spinal cord stimulation in an animal model of neuropathic pain relates to degree of tactile "allodynia." *Neuroscience* 143:541-546, 2006.

31. Simpson EL et al: Spinal cord stimulation for chronic pain of neuropathic or ischaemic origin: systematic review and economic evaluation. *Health Technol Assess* 13:iii, ix-x, 1-154, 2009.

32. Frey ME et al: Spinal cord stimulation for patients with failed back surgery syndrome: a systematic review. *Pain Physician* 12:379-397, 2009.

33. Guyatt G et al.: Grading strength of recommendations and quality of evidence in clinical guidelines: report from an American college of chest physicians task force. *Chest* 129:174-181, 2006.

34. Chou R et al: Nonsurgical interventional therapies for low back pain: a review of the evidence for an American Pain Society clinical practice guideline. *Spine* 34:1078-1093, 2009.

35. Cruccu G et al: EFNS guidelines on neurostimulation therapy for neuropathic pain. *Eur J Neurol* 14:952-970, 2007.

36. (NICE) NIfHaCE: Spinal cord stimulation for chronic pain of neuropathic or ischaemic origin. *NICE technology appraisal guidance* 159: 1-31, 2008.

37. Mailis-Gagnon A, et al: Spinal cord stimulation for chronic pain. Cochrane Database Syst Rev 2, CD003783, 2004.

38. North RB et al: Spinal cord stimulation versus reoperation for failed back surgery syndrome: a cost effectiveness and cost utility analysis based on a randomized, controlled trial. *Neurosurgery* 61:361-368; discussion 8-9, 2007.

39. North RB et al: Spinal cord stimulation versus repeated lumbosacral spine surgery for chronic pain: a randomized, controlled trial. *Neurosurgery* 56:98-106; discussion 106-107, 2005.

40. Bala MM et al: Systematic review of the (cost-)effectiveness of spinal cord stimulation for people with failed back surgery syndrome. *Clin J Pain* 24:741-756, 2008.

41. Kumar K, Taylor RS, Jacques L et al: Spinal cord stimulation versus conventional medical management for neuropathic pain: a multicentre randomised controlled trial in patients with failed back surgery syndrome. *Pain* 132:179-188, 2007.

42. Kumar K et al: The effects of spinal cord stimulation in neuropathic pain are sustained: a 24-month follow-up of the prospective, randomized controlled multicenter trial of the effectiveness of spinal cord stimulation. *Neurosurgery* 63:762-770; discussion 70, 2008.

43. Bhandari M et al: Association between industry funding and statistically significant pro-industry findings in medical and surgical randomized trials. *CMAJ* 170:477-480, 2004.

44. Chou R: Generating evidence on spinal cord stimulation for failed back surgery syndrome: not yet fully charged. *Clin J Pain* 24:757-758, 2008.

45. Turner JA et al: Spinal cord stimulation for failed back surgery syndrome: outcomes in a workers' compensation setting. *Pain* 148: 14-25, 2010.

46. Monsalve V, De Andres J, Valia J: Application of a psychological decision algorithm for the selection of patients susceptible of implantation of neuromodulation systems for the treatment of chronic pain: A proposal. *Neuromodulation* 3:191-200, 2000.

47. Celestin J, Edwards RR, Jamison RN: Pretreatment psychosocial variables as predictors of outcomes following lumbar surgery and spinal cord stimulation: a systematic review and literature synthesis. *Pain Med* 10:639-653, 2009.

48. Brook AL, Georgy BA, Olan WJ: Spinal cord stimulation: a basic approach. *Tech Vasc Interv Radiol* 12:64-70, 2009.

49. Eisenberg E et al: Quantitative sensory testing for spinal cord stimulation in patients with chronic neuropathic pain. *Pain Pract* 6:161-165, 2006.

50. Kumar K et al: Epidural spinal cord stimulation for treatment of chronic pain—some predictors of success: a 15-year experience. *Surg Neurol* 50:110-120; discussion 120-121, 1998.

51. Kumar K, Hunter G, Demeria D: Spinal cord stimulation in treatment of chronic benign pain: challenges in treatment planning and present status, a 22-year experience. *Neurosurgery* 58:481-496; discussion 496, 2006.

52. Villavicencio AT et al: Laminectomy versus percutaneous electrode . placement for spinal cord stimulation. *Neurosurgery* 46:399-405; discussion 405-406, 2000.

53. de Leon-Casasola OA: Spinal cord and peripheral nerve stimulation techniques for neuropathic pain. *J Pain Symptom Manage* 38:S28-S38, 2009.

54. Falowski S, Celii A, Sharan A: Spinal cord stimulation: an update. *Neurotherapeutics* 5:86-99, 2008.

55. Henderson JM et al.: Prevention of mechanical failures in implanted spinal cord stimulation system. *Neuromodulation* 9:183-191, 2006.

56. Barolat G et al: Mapping of sensory responses to epidural stimulation of the intraspinal neural structures in man. *J Neurosurg* 78:233-239, 1993.

57. Holsheimer J, Wesselink WA: Effect of anode-cathode configuration on paresthesia coverage in spinal cord stimulation. *Neurosurgery* 41:654-659; discussion 59-60, 1997.

58. Holsheimer J, Wesselink WA: Optimum electrode geometry for spinal cord stimulation: the narrow bipole and tripole. *Med Biol Eng Comput* 35:493-497, 1997.

59. North RB et al: Spinal cord stimulation for chronic, intractable pain: superiority of "multi-channel" devices. *Pain* 44:119-130, 1991.

60. Buvanendran A, Lubenow TJ: Efficacy of transverse tripolar spinal cord stimulator for the relief of chronic low back pain from failed back surgery. *Pain Physician* 11:333-338, 2008.

61. Holsheimer J et al: Clinical evaluation of paresthesia steering with a new system for spinal cord stimulation. *Neurosurgery* 42:541-547; discussion 7-9, 1998.

62. de Vos CC et al: Electrode contact configuration and energy consumption in spinal cord stimulation. *Neurosurgery* 65:210-216; discussion 6-7, 2009.

63. Maeda Y, Wacnik PW, Sluka KA: Low frequencies, but not high frequencies of bi-polar spinal cord stimulation reduce cutaneous and muscle hyperalgesia induced by nerve injury. *Pain* 138:143-152, 2008.

64. Noble M, et al: Long-term opioid management for chronic noncancer pain, Cochrane Database Syst Rev, CD006605, 2010.

65. Erdine S, De Andres J: Drug delivery systems. *Pain Pract* 6:51-57, 2006.

66. Prager JP: Neuraxial medication delivery: the development and maturity of a concept for treating chronic pain of spinal origin. *Spine* 27:2593-2605; discussion 2606, 2002.

67. Peng PW et al: Survey of the practice of spinal cord stimulators and intrathecal analgesic delivery implants for management of pain in Canada. *Pain Res Manag* 12:281-285, 2007.

68. Hassenbusch SJ et al: Polyanalgesic Consensus Conference 2003: an update on the management of pain by intraspinal drug delivery—report of an expert panel. *J Pain Symptom Manage* 27:540-563, 2004.

69. Smith HS et al: Intrathecal drug delivery. *Pain Physician* 11:S89-S104, 2008.

70. Goodchild CS, Nadeson R, Cohen E: Supraspinal and spinal cord opioid receptors are responsible for antinociception following intrathecal morphine injections. *Eur J Anaesthesiol* 21:179-185, 2004.

71. Wallace M, Yaksh TL: Long-term spinal analgesic delivery: a review of the preclinical and clinical literature. *Reg Anesth Pain Med* 25:117-157, 2000.

72. Walker RH et al: Intrathecal baclofen for dystonia: benefits and complications during six years of experience. *Mov Disord* 15:1242-1247, 2000.

73. Bernards CM: Cerebrospinal fluid and spinal cord distribution of baclofen and bupivacaine during slow intrathecal infusion in pigs, *Anesthesiology* 105:169-178, 2006.

74. Flack SH, Bernards CM: Cerebrospinal fluid and spinal cord distribution of hyperbaric bupivacaine and baclofen during slow intrathecal infusion in pigs. *Anesthesiology* 112:165-173, 2010.

75. Cohen SP, Dragovich A: Intrathecal analgesia. *Med Clin North Am* 91:251-270, 2007.

76. Walker SM et al: Combination spinal analgesic chemotherapy: a systematic review. *Anesth Analg* 95:674-715, 2002.

77. Boswell MV et al: Interventional techniques: evidence-based practice guidelines in the management of chronic spinal pain. *Pain Physician* 10:7-111, 2007.

78. Patel VB et al: Systematic review of intrathecal infusion systems for long-term management of chronic non-cancer pain. *Pain Physician* 12:345-360, 2009.

79. Manchikanti L et al: Reassessment of evidence synthesis of occupational medicine practice guidelines for interventional pain management. *Pain Physician* 11:393-482, 2008.

80. Koulousakis A et al: Intrathecal opioids for intractable pain syndromes. *Acta Neurochir* 97(suppl):43-44, 2007.

81. Angel IF, Gould HJ, Jr, Carey ME: Intrathecal morphine pump as a treatment option in chronic pain of nonmalignant origin. *Surg Neurol* 49:92-98; discussion 8-9, 1998.

82. Anderson VC, Burchiel KJ: A prospective study of long-term intrathecal morphine in the management of chronic nonmalignant pain, *Neurosurgery* 44:289-300; discussion 301, 1999.

83. Hassenbusch SJ et al: Long-term intraspinal infusions of opioids in the treatment of neuropathic pain. *J Pain Symptom Manage* 10:527-543, 1995.

84. Kumar K, Kelly M, Pirlot T: Continuous intrathecal morphine treatment for chronic pain of nonmalignant etiology: long-term benefits and efficacy. *Surg Neurol* 55:79-86; discussion 86-88, 2001.

85. Thimineur MA, Kravitz E, Vodapally MS: Intrathecal opioid treatment for chronic non-malignant pain: a 3-year prospective study. *Pain* 109:242-249, 2004.

86. Duse G, Davia G, White PF: Improvement in psychosocial outcomes in chronic pain patients receiving intrathecal morphine infusions. *Anesth Analg* 109:1981-1986, 2009.

87. Rainov NG, Heidecke V, Burkert W: Long-term intrathecal infusion of drug combinations for chronic back and leg pain. *J Pain Symptom Manage* 22:862-871, 2001.

88. Deer T et al: Intrathecal drug delivery for treatment of chronic low back pain: report from the National Outcomes Registry for Low Back Pain. *Pain Med* 5:6-13, 2004.

89. Paice JA, Penn RD, Shott S: Intraspinal morphine for chronic pain: a retrospective, multicenter study. *J Pain Symptom Manage 1996* 11:71-80, 1996.

90. Idanpaan-Heikkila JJ, Guilbaud G: Pharmacological studies on a rat model of trigeminal neuropathic pain: baclofen, but not carbamazepine, morphine or tricyclic antidepressants, attenuates the allodynia-like behaviour. *Pain* 79:281-290, 1999.

91. Hanks GW, Forbes K: Opioid responsiveness. *Acta Anaesthesiol Scand* 41:154-158, 1997.

92. Kumar K, Hunter G, Demeria DD: Treatment of chronic pain by using intrathecal drug therapy compared with conventional pain therapies: a cost-effectiveness analysis. *J Neurosurg* 97:803-810, 2002.

93. Mueller-Schwefe G, Hassenbusch SJ, Reig E: Cost-effectiveness of intrathecal therapy for pain. *Neuromodulation* 2:77-84, 1999.

94. Knight KH et al: Implantable intrathecal pumps for chronic pain: highlights and updates. *Croat Med J* 48:22-34, 2007.

95. Anderson V, Burchiel K, Cooke B: A prospective, randomized trial of intrathecal injection vs. epidural infusion in the selection of patients for continuous intrathecal opioid therapy. *Neuromodulation* 142-152, 2003.

96. Raffaeli W et al: Opioid-related side-effects after intrathecal morphine: a prospective, randomized, double-blind dose-response study. *Eur J Anaesthesiol* 23:605-610, 2006.

97. Du Pen S, Du Pen A, Hillyer J: Intrathecal hydromorphone for intractable nonmalignant pain: a retrospective study. *Pain Med* 7:10-15, 2006.

98. Deer TR et al: Clinical experience with intrathecal bupivacaine in combination with opioid for the treatment of chronic pain related to failed back surgery syndrome and metastatic cancer pain of the spine. *Spine J* 2:274-278, 2002.

99. Kumar K et al: Use of intrathecal bupivacaine in refractory chronic nonmalignant pain. *Pain Med* 10:819-828, 2009.

100. Deer TR et al: Intrathecal ziconotide and opioid combination therapy for noncancer pain: an observational study. *Pain Physician* 12:E291-296, 2009.

101. Miljanich GP: Ziconotide: neuronal calcium channel blocker for treating severe chronic pain. *Curr Med Chem* 11:3029-3040, 2004.

102. Williams JA, Day M, Heavner JE: Ziconotide: an update and review, *Expert Opin Pharmacother* 9:1575-1583, 2008.

103. Wallace MS et al: Intrathecal ziconotide for severe chronic pain: safety and tolerability results of an open-label, long-term trial. *Anesth Analg* 106:628-637, 2008.

104. Rauck RL et al: Intrathecal ziconotide for neuropathic pain: a review. *Pain Pract* 9:327-337, 2009.

105. Rauck RL et al: A randomized, double-blind, placebo-controlled study of intrathecal ziconotide in adults with severe chronic pain. *J Pain Symptom Manage* 31:393-406, 2006.

106. Ziconotide: new drug: limited analgesic efficacy, too many adverse effects. *Prescrire Int* 17:179-182, 2008.

107. Ilias W et al: Patient-controlled analgesia in chronic pain patients: experience with a new device designed to be used with implanted programmable pumps. *Pain Pract* 8:164-170, 2008.

108. Albright AL, Turner M, Pattisapu JV: Best-practice surgical techniques for intrathecal baclofen therapy. *J Neurosurg* 104:233-239, 2006.

109. Coffey RJ et al: Mortality associated with implantation and management of intrathecal opioid drug infusion systems to treat noncancer pain. *Anesthesiology* 111:881-891, 2009.

110. Fluckiger B et al: Device-related complications of long-term intrathecal drug therapy via implanted pumps. *Spinal Cord* 46:639-643, 2008.

111. Miele VJ et al: A review of intrathecal morphine therapy related granulomas: two case reports. *Eur J Pain* 102(5):16-18, 2006.

112. Yaksh TL et al: Inflammatory masses associated with intrathecal drug infusion: a review of preclinical evidence and human data. *Pain Med* 3:300-312, 2002.

113. Deer TR: A prospective analysis of intrathecal granuloma in chronic pain patients: a review of the literature and report of a surveillance study. *Pain Physician* 7:225-228, 2004.

114. Gradert TL et al: Safety of chronic intrathecal morphine infusion in a sheep model. *Anesthesiology* 99:188-198, 2003.

115. Allen JW et al: Opiate pharmacology of intrathecal granulomas. *Anesthesiology* 105:590-598, 2006.

116. Allen JW et al: Time course and role of morphine dose and concentration in intrathecal granuloma formation in dogs: a combined magnetic resonance imaging and histopathology investigation. *Anesthesiology* 105:581-589, 2006.

117. Tai YH et al: Amitriptyline suppresses neuroinflammation-dependent interleukin-10-p38 mitogen-activated protein kinase-heme oxygenase-1 signaling pathway in chronic morphine-infused rats. *Anesthesiology* 110:1379-1389, 2009.

118. Yaksh TL et al: Chronically infused intrathecal morphine in dogs. *Anesthesiology* 99:174-187, 2003.

119. Allen JW et al: Degranulation of dural mast cells by in vivo and ex vivo opiate exposure. *Toxicol Sci* 78:88, 2004.

120. Kerber CW, Newton TH: The macro and microvasculature of the dura mater. *Neuroradiology* 6:175-179, 1973.

121. Ruan X: Drug-related side effects of long-term intrathecal morphine therapy. *Pain Physician* 10:357-366, 2007.

122. Kanoff RB: Intraspinal delivery of opiates by an implantable, programmable pump in patients with chronic, intractable pain of non-malignant origin. *J Am Osteopath Assoc* 94:487-493, 1994.

123. Follett KA et al: Prevention and management of intrathecal drug delivery and spinal cord stimulation system infections. *Anesthesiology* 100:1582-1594, 2004.

124. Borowski A et al: Complications of intrathecal baclofen pump therapy in pediatric patients. *J Pediatr Orthop* 30:76-81, 2010.

125. Boviatsis EJ et al: Infected CNS infusion pumps. Is there a chance for treatment without removal? *Acta Neurochir (Wien)* 146:463-467, 2004.

126. Burgher AH et al: Introduction of infection control measures to reduce infection associated with implantable pain therapy devices. *Pain Pract* 7:279-284, 2007.

127. Darouiche RO et al: Chlorhexidine-alcohol versus povidone-iodine for surgical-site antisepsis. *N Engl J Med* 362:18-26, 2010.

128. Kaysinger KK et al: Toxic effects of wound irrigation solutions on cultured tibiae and osteoblasts. *J Orthop Trauma* 9:303-311, 1995.

129. Cheng MT et al: Efficacy of dilute Betadine solution irrigation in the prevention of postoperative infection of spinal surgery. *Spine* 30:1689-1693, 2005.

130. Chang FY et al: Can povidone-iodine solution be used safely in a spinal surgery? *Eur Spine J* 15:1005-1014, 2006.

Index

Page numbers followed by *f*, *t*, and *b* indicate figures, tables, and boxes, respectively.